Current Topics in Microbiology

241 **and Immunology**

Springer
Berlin
Heidelberg
New York
Barcelona
Hong Kong
London
Milan
Paris
Singapore
Tokyo

Gastroduodenal Disease and *Helicobacter pylori*

Pathophysiology, Diagnosis and Treatment

Edited by T. U. Westblom, S. J. Czinn,
and J. G. Nedrud

With a Foreword by B. Marshall

With 35 Figures and 13 Tables

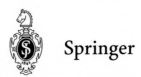 Springer

Professor T. Ulf Westblom, M.D.
Texas A&M University, College of Medicine
Chief, Medical Service (111)
Central Texas Veterans Health Care System
1901 S. First Street
Temple, TX 76504, USA

Professor Steven J. Czinn, M.D.
Case Western Reserve University
Department of Pediatrics
Division of Pediatric Gastroenterology
Rainbow Babies and Children Hospital
2074 Abington Road
Cleveland, OH 44106, USA

Associate Professor John G. Nedrud, Ph.D.
Institute of Pathology
Case Western Reserve University
Biomedical Research Building, Rm. 919
10900 Euclid Avenue
Cleveland, OH 44106-4943, USA

Cover Illustration: Genta G (1996) Helicobacter pylori in a Gastric Pit. N Engl J Med 335:250–250. Copyright© 1998 Massachusetts Medical Society. All rights reserved.

Cover Design: Design & Production GmbH, Heidelberg

ISSN 0070-217X

ISBN 3-540-65084-9 Springer-Verlag Berlin Heidelberg New York

© Springer-Verlag Berlin Heidelberg 1999
Library of Congress Catalog Card Number 15-12910
Printed in Germany

The use of general descriptive names, registered names, trademarks, etc. in this publication does not imply, even in the absence of a specific statement, that such names are exempt from the relevant protective laws and regulations and therefore free for general use.

Product liability: The publishers cannot guarantee the accuracy of any information about dosage and application contained in this book. In every individual case the user must check such information by consulting other relevant literature.

Typesetting: Scientific Publishing Services (P) Ltd, Madras

Production Editor: Angélique Gcouta

SPIN: 10633960   27/3020 – 5 4 3 2 1 0 – Printed on acid-free paper

Foreword

I am delighted to be able to write the foreword for this new book on *Helicobacter pylori* by three pioneers in the field, Ulf West-blom, Steven Czinn and John Nedrud. Because of their long experience in both basic and clinical aspects of *H. pylori*, the editors have been able to produce a volume which is authoritative and up to date in the science of *H. pylori*, while still being concise and interesting for the practicing physician or *H. pylori* novice. To achieve this, they have collected a very distinguished group of authors from within the United States and around the world.

The chapters are sequenced in approximately the same order as developments in *H. pylori* science over the past 15 years. The first chapter on the discovery of *H. pylori* is by Cliodna McNulty, who was the first person to culture the organism in Europe. The epidemiology is then described followed by the main clinical associations, which are gastritis and dyspepsia, peptic ulcers, cancers and lymphoma. This naturally leads to discussion of the laboratory aspects of *H. pylori*, especially the microbiology, including essential information on antibiotic resistance patterns. Next, virulence and pathogenicity of *H. pylori* are explained as defined in studies using animal models, then by discussion of the metabolism of the organism. Finally, the interaction of the bacterium with the host immune systems is dealt with, including the implications of these findings as they relate to the development of future vaccines.

Chapters by the editors themselves are particularly useful, especially that on the diagnosis of *H. pylori* infection, co-authored by Ulf Westblom and Bankim Bhatt, and the one on the host response and vaccine development, by Steven Czinn and John Nedrud together with Thomas Blanchard. The book also addresses very controversial areas of *H. pylori* with a chapter on economic aspects of *H. pylori* treatment, which ties in very well with the specific chapter on new *H. pylori* therapies by Peter Unge, the actual discoverer of the potentiation effect between proton pump inhibitors and antibiotics. Finally, Nirmal Mann and Ulf Westblom predict the future developments in *H. pylori* clinical and basic research. This is important reading for those planning new studies in the field.

With this concise new volume, Westblom, Czinn and Nedrud will simplify the learning process for *H. pylori* enthusiasts, ensuring that the mysterious spiral organism continues to be properly detected, studied and eradicated.

Barry Marshall

Preface

Summer was not yet over, but the morning air felt chilly and crisp. My eyes wandered down the mountainside, followed the narrow gravel road, and rested on a large complex of log cabins. This was Keystone, Colorado. The year was 1986. I had signed up for the trip just a few weeks earlier without really knowing what to expect. The program was still preliminary, and I hadn't even seen it when I arrived. Still, there was something magically attractive about the first American meeting on *Helicobacter pylori*. In my own humble way, I had entered the field just a year earlier, and up till now most of the researchers had been just names on photocopied articles. At Keystone the names took on faces. I was impressed, but also excited. Every presented paper created new questions and challenges in my mind. *Helicobacter pylori* turned out to be an even more enigmatic organism than I had imagined, and I felt blessed to be in the midst of all this bursting research.

At the end of the meeting, during an evening barbecue, I met Steven Czinn. He, like me, had published his first *H. pylori* paper just the year before. Inspired by the meeting, both of us were eager to continue our work. We had entered the field from two different angles, one from pediatric gastroenterology, the other from adult infectious diseases. These were fields that could complement each other, and over a couple of hot dogs we decided to collaborate on several future projects. Later I got to know John Nedrud, and his background in pathology and immunology provided us with yet another valuable point of view. We are now several years down the road. Though not yet gray like the sages, we feel that this book bridges a lot of the things we have worked with in the past. It also presents the exciting and insightful work of our many talented contributors. We have aimed at compiling a book that can appeal to both researchers and practicing physicians. You will find cutting-edge information as well as chapters with specific clinical recommendations. We are honored to have been asked by Springer-Verlag to put this book together, and it has been a very rewarding experience. We hope you will enjoy it too.

T. Ulf Westblom

List of Contents

List of Contributors

(Their addresses can be found at the beginning of their respective chapters.)

BHATT, B.D.   215

BLANCHARD, T.G.   181

CZINN, S.J.   181

EATON, K.A.   123

ESLICK, G.D.   31

GOLD, B.D.   71

INADOMI, J.M.   237

KALANTAR, J.   31

LEE, A.   47

MANN, N.S.   301

MARAIS, A.   103

MARSHALL, B.   V, VI

McGEE, D.J.   155

McNULTY, C.A.M.   1

MÉGRAUD, F.   103

MITCHELL, H.M.   11

MOBLEY, H.L.T.   155

MONTEIRO, L.   103

MUKHOPADHYAY, P.   57

NEDRUD, J.G.   181

SONNENBERG, A.   237

TALLEY, N.J.   31

UNGE, P.   261

VELDHUYZEN VAN
   ZANTEN, S.J.O.   47

WESTBLOM, T.U.   215, 301

List of Contributors

The Discovery of *Campylobacter*-like Organisms

C.A.M. McNulty

1 Introduction

Work in the primary care setting in 1980 showed that about 1% of a United
Kingdom population presented to their general practitioner with food-related upper abdominal pain (GEAR and BARNES (1980). On investigation one third of these
patients had a peptic ulcer, a third had no obvious abnormality (non-ulcer dyspepsia) and the remainder various other disorders such as gallstones, irritable
bowel etc. The two main aims of management of peptic ulcer disease were healing
of the acute lesion and prevention of recurrence. In the late 1970s and early 1980s
numerous studies confirmed that this could be attained by controlling gastric acid
secretion with the histamine H_2 antagonists; thus proving Karl Schwarz' maxim –
no acid no ulcer – (SCHWARZ 1910; BURLAND and SIMKINS 1977; GUT MULTI-
CENTRE TRIAL 1979; WATT et al. 1981). Soon the histamine H_2 antagonist became
the mainstay of treatment; accounting for a substantial proportion of drug costs
worldwide. The outcomes of large drug company sponsored multicentre studies,
involving gastroenterologists across the world, supported the lifelong use of
maintenance H_2 antagonists (GOUGH et al. (1984).

Public Health Laboratory, Gloucestershire Royal Hospital, Great Western Road, Gloucester, GL1 3NN,
UK

2 First Reports

It is small wonder then that the initial report by WARREN (1983) and MARSHALL (1983) of the strong association of a *Campylobacter*-like organism (CLO) with gastritis and peptic ulceration was greeted with such scepticism by the gastro-enterology fraternity. How could a bacterium found in the gastric antrum play a role in the aetiology of duodenal ulceration which was, after all, caused by an acid diathesis?

As the organism was *Campylobacter*-like, it seemed natural for MARSHALL to present his work at the Second International Workshop on *Campylobacter* Infections in Brussels in September 1983. Here his work was received with great interest and prompted worldwide research which was initially led by microbiologists. Since 1980, WARREN had noted *Campylobacter*-like bacteria on tissue sections of the gastric antrum in patients with the histopathological appearance of chronic active gastritis. They were not obvious in sections stained with haematoxylin and eosin, but showed up clearly with Warthin-Starry silver staining. They were found in all 13 patients with duodenal ulcers, 80% of patients with gastric ulcer and 96% of patients with chronic active gastritis. By contrast, they were found in only two of 31 control patients. MARSHALL and WARREN'S initial attempts to culture organisms from the biopsy specimens in a microaerobic atmosphere at 37°C were unsuccessful. Their first positive culture was noted after plates had been left in the incubator for 6 days during the Easter holidays. Thereafter, with extended incubation, isolation of *Campylobacter*-like organisms (CLOs) was easily attained.

At the 1983 *Campylobacter* workshop WARREN and MARSHALL described the first use of tripotassium dicitrato bismuthate (De-Nol) for the treatment of *Helicobacter pylori*. The CLOs and inflammatory response disappeared during treatment although they reappeared after cessation of the bismuth salt. MARSHALL, using 'in house' bismuth discs, had confirmed that CLOs were very sensitive to bismuth.

Just before the workshop a positive culture was obtained at the Worcester Royal Infirmary, UK, from a woman with gastric ulcer, demonstrating that the organisms were not exclusively Australian (McNULTY and WATSON 1984). It was in Worcester, during informal discussions between SKIRROW, DYER and MARSHALL, that the extremely appropriate name *Campylobacter pyloridis* was proposed. The word pyloridis derived from the Greek *pylorus*, "gatekeeper", one who looks both ways, forward to the duodenum and back to the stomach.

MARSHALL'S findings stimulated great discussion between the medical microbiologists who had a great interest in *Campylobacter* spp., and the veterinary microbiologists amongst whom there was a wealth of knowledge of animal spiral bacteria adaptations allowing survival in the intestinal tract. How could these CLOs survive in such enormous numbers in the gastric acid milieu and in the presence of such an intense immune response? Were the CLOs of primary or secondary importance in the aetiology of peptic ulceration; were they commensals or pathogens?

3 Dissemination of Work

Following Brussels the worldwide search for *Campylobacter* began. In May 1984 the first of many letters in the columns of the 1984 *Lancet* appeared, corroborating the earlier reports of Warren and Marshall on the presence of CLOs in gastric biopsy specimens and the association of these organisms with peptic ulcer and histological evidence of gastritis (McNULTY and WATSON 1984). The *Lancet* was a very important source of information in 1984 and 1985 and its correspondence columns regularly featured new work on *Campylobacter pyloridis*.

Early workers in the field were mainly junior physicians whose minds were not cluttered with preconceived ideas or prejudices of gastroduodenal pathology, so with each short report something new about the CLOs was revealed. It was very exciting to be involved in this pioneering work and to be challenging the established ideas on gastroduodenal disease. However, it was very difficult to convince others that *C. pyloridis* was such an exciting development. Initially the organisms effect on the gastric physiology was not understood and some of the data seemed conflicting. Langenberg et al. (1984) found that *C. pyloridis* was present in both patients at risk of peptic ulceration with a high gastric acidity and 24% of healthy non-dyspeptic volunteers. Although *C. pyloridis* was always associated with chronic active gastritis, was it so commonly present that it could be considered part of the normal flora? It was also recognised that many pathogens produce a wide spectra of disease. LANGENBERG also first described the striking urease production of *C. pyloridis*. A positive urease test was visible only a few minutes after a suspension of a loopful of growth was added to Christensen's urea broth-could the production of urease be a protective mechanism against gastric acid? The *Lancet* columns also reported the early serological study by ELDRIDGE et al. (1984). They showed that the presence of complement fixing antibody (using a sonicate of the organism as antigen) was also correlated with gastritis; this work seemed to produce more concerns-how could this organism persist in the presence of such a good immune response?

4 Earlier Descriptions

If detection of the gastric CLOs was seemingly so easy, why had its relationship with gastritis and peptic ulceration not previously been described? Gastric spiral organisms had been seen by Rappin over a century before in the dog (RAPPIN 1881; quoted in BREED et al. 1948), and his observations were confirmed and extended in the dog and other mammalian species by other authors, (BIZZOZERO 1893). In 1906 KRIENITZ described spiral organisms in the stomach contents, including vomit of a patient with carcinoma of the lesser curvature of the stomach. He identified three types of spiral bacteria; one, like the new gastric CLO, a spirochaete, and one larger

organism such as the more recently described *Helicobacter heilmanii*, McNulty
et al. (1989). This study, however, did not include microscopy of the gastric mucosa. Doenges in 1938 was the first to describe spiral organisms in the human
gastric mucosa; they were present in 43% of patients in post-mortem specimens.
Others confirmed that this organism was commonly found in the gastric mucosa,
but Steer and Colin-Jones were the first to attempt culture in 1975. They gave a
detailed description of gram-negative bacteria that were found over extensive areas
of the gastric mucosa deep to the mucus layer. They observed that the organisms
were absent from areas of intestinal metaplasia, later confirmed by Thomas (1984).
Unfortunately, microaerobic incubation was not routinely available at this time
and so there was little chance of growing the CLOs. *Pseudomonas aeruginosa* was
isolated, and Steer and Colin-Jones wrongly assumed that this organism was
responsible for the loss of mucus and polymorphonuclear infiltrate.

   In the 1970s and early 1980s there was much work performed on the histological classification of gastritis (Strickland and MacKay 1973; Correa 1980),
but despite this plethora of work few mentioned the CLOs that are now so obvious
to us all. We are often so blinkered in our approach that we see only what we are
taught should be there, and ignore everything else.

   As Langenberg described, the intense urease reaction by *C. pyloridis* was
striking. In 1984 I started dabbling in gastric urease myself. Was the urease production so great that *C. pyloridis* could be detected in the gastric mucosa indirectly
by this method? I was very excited to find that this was indeed so (McNulty and
Wise 1985). The biopsy urease test became the most rapid diagnostic test and is
now used worldwide. The presence of urease in the gastric mucosa was the basis of
an MD by Fitzgerald and Murphy published in the *Irish Journal of Medical
Science* in 1950. They found high concentrations in the pyloric region and presumed that the amount of urea present could be related to its possible neutralisa-
tion or protective power. They also found that urease could be demonstrated in the
stomachs of all animals they studied (dog, cat, pig, mouse, rat, rabbit and frog) – of
course *Helicobacter* spp. have now been confirmed in most of these animals. They
were not able to demonstrate an association with dyspepsia but suggested that urea
administration should be of help in the treatment of peptic ulceration.

5 Escalation of Work

By the summer of 1984 over 500 dyspeptic patients had been studied worldwide,
confirming the strong association of *C. pyloridis* with chronic active type B gastritis
and duodenal ulceration, but although workers in the field felt that *C. pyloridis* was
responsible, there was no proof of causation. Koch's (1882) first two postulates
(a) that the organism must be found in all cases of the disease, and that its distribution should be in accordance with the lesions observed, and (b) that the organism should be cultured outside the body of the host in pure culture for several

generations, had been proven. The aim was then to prove all of KOCH's four postulates with animal inoculation and treatment studies.

KOCH's third postulate states 'the organism must reproduce the same disease in a susceptible animal' and the fourth states 'the organism should be found in the diseased areas produced in the susceptible animal'. Initial pig inoculation studies were unsuccessful (MARSHALL 1989); therefore MARSHALL et al. (1985a) planned their famous self-inoculation study. Gastric biopsy specimens taken before the study confirmed that MARSHALL had a normal gastric mucosa and *C. pyloridis* was absent. MARSHALL drank a pure broth culture of *C. pyloridis* (from a man with chronic active gastritis) on an empty achlorhydric stomach. Ten days later gastric biopsy specimens showed that he had developed a chronic active gastritis and CLOs could be seen adhering to the gastric mucosa. Cultures of antral mucosa grew *C. pyloridis*. MARSHALL had mild dyspeptic symptoms and putrid breath. Symptoms resolved within 24h of starting tinidazole. There was evidence, from published papers, that human inoculation had occurred accidentally in some gastroenterology volunteer studies. An infectious aetiology was suspected in an epidemic of hypochlorhydric gastritis that occurred in 1979 after gastric pH studies in 39 Texan volunteers (RAMSEY et al. 1979). Acute onset of gastritis with symptoms that lasted 1–4 days occurred in 17 of the 39 volunteers whose gastric pH was repeatedly measured using a common pH electrode over an 18 month period. A severe fundal gastritis was found in all 12 volunteers in whom histopathology was available. After MARSHALL contacted the study group, retrospective analysis of the tissue sections showed that the gastritis was associated with the presence of *C. pyloridis* in the gastric mucosa. It was presumed that the bacteria were transferred from one case to another on a wet pH electrode, with the source of infection being one of the volunteers or a previously studied patient with gastritis. These volunteer studies certainly helped to convince the sceptics that the *C. pyloridis* was responsible for gastritis, but naturally clinicians were interested in the clinical relevance of infection. They had no interest in KOCH's postulates proposed more than a century before! If *C. pyloridis* was treated would ulcers heal and would there be symptomatic improvement?

5.1 Believers and Non-believers

There was conflict between those with an interest in *C. pyloridis* (the believers) and the non-believers. Believers felt that should these organisms prove important in the aetiology of gastritis and duodenal ulceration, the current approach to treating these conditions was incorrect. Although H_2 receptor antagonists produced symptomatic and endoscopic resolution of peptic ulceration, they had no effect on histologically confirmed gastritis (FULLMAN et al. 1985), and relapse was higher with these agents than with the bismuth salts that had in vitro activity against *C. pyloridis* (MARTIN et al. 1981). Believers felt that the clinical difference between these agents was indeed due to their differing activity against *C. pyloridis*. The H_2 antagonists had little in vitro activity (GOODWIN et al. 1986), and this was confirmed in vivo (LANGENBERG et al. 1985).

Treatment trials using bismuth salts or antimicrobials started in earnest; we, the believers, felt convinced that we would be able to cure chronic active gastritis rapidly and effectively by the eradication of *C. pyloridis*. In vitro studies showed that the organism was susceptible to a wide range of antimicrobial agents, including erythromycin, amoxycillin and bismuth salts (McNULTY et al. 1985b) and these were used in the initial studies. By the next *Campylobacter* workshop in July 1985 preliminary results were available from four centres in Europe and Australia. Amoxycillin and bismuth both produced a striking effect on the gastric mucosa. In 75% of patients the *C. pyloridis* was cleared and the histology of the gastric mucosa had dramatically improved with the disappearance of polymorphonuclear cells and decrease in mononuclear cells (JONES et al. 1985; LANGENBERG et al. 1985; MAR-SHALL et al. 1985b; McNULTY et al. 1985a). Unfortunately long-term clearance of *C. pyloridis* was not maintained and recrudescence of the organism was associated with the return of the cellular infiltration. Erythromycin and spiramycin, which had excellent in vitro activity, did not clear or even suppress *C. pyloridis* (LANGENBERG et al. 1985; McNULTY et al. 1985a). Although these treatment studies confirmed the close association of *C. pyloridis* with gastritis and its pathogenic role; they were also very disappointing. *C. pyloridis* was not going to be so easy to eradicate as we first envisaged!

The first treatment trials in patients with peptic ulceration were performed by MARSHALL's group; because of the disappointing results with single agents, they combined De Nol with tinidazole or amoxycillin. Results were much better and only 2 of 17 patients cleared of *C. pyloridis* relapsed (MARSHALL et al. 1985b).

In July 1985, at the 3rd *Campylobacter* Workshop, workers from Australasia, Europe, North America and Japan presented their findings on *C. pyloridis*. All showed an association with gastritis, although the prevalence in some countries was notably higher than others (84% in Japan, 35% in the UK) thus giving a hint at the differences in worldwide prevalences that would later be described (ISHII et al. 1985; PEARSON et al. 1985; LEE et al. 1985).

By this meeting optimum cultural methods had been established (GOODWIN et al. 1985), and only quite minor modifications to selective medium have been made since. Much was known about the ultrastructural and biochemical characteristics. In many ways *C. pyloridis* was similar to other *Campylobacter* species in size, morphology, Gram-negativity, oxidase and catalase positivity, motility, need for microaerobic conditions, respiratory type of metabolism and guanine-cytosine content (MORRIS 1985). However, there was a growing list of differences apart from the intense urease production which was so distinctive; suggesting that placement in the genus *Campylobacter* should be regarded at tentative (MORRIS 1985). *C. pyloridis* had up to five sheathed flagellae (with bulbous tips) that exited the cell with no cell end modification as in *Campylobacter* spp. (CURRY et al. 1985). The major protein bands on electrophoresis (PEARSON et al. 1984), and major fatty acid detected by gas liquid chromatography (HUDSON and WAIT 1985), distinguished *C. pyloridis* from other *Campylobacter* spp.

It was becoming evident that *C. pyloridis* was specifically adapted to survival on the gastric mucosa, and in gastric mucus. Careful examination of the gastric

mucosa by HAZELL and LEE (1985) showed that *C. pyloridis* localised at intercellular junctions where it could utilize urea and other growth substances, and its
corkscrew motility allowed movement through highly viscous concentrations of
methyl cellulose (simulating mucus) that severely impeded the movement of more
conventional rod shaped bacteria. The organism could also survive on the gastric
mucosa despite an intense immunological response. Circulating antibodies to
C. pyloridis in patients with gastritis were now sufficiently specific to allow serodiagnosis. A number of dominant antigens relating to the outer membrane and
flagella had been identified (NEWELL 1985), and these were now being used in
ELISA serodiagnosis. These tests were to pave the way for extensive worldwide
seroepidemiological studies.

6 1985

A leader in the *Lancet* following the Ottawa meeting stated – the accumulating
evidence is tending to support rather than refute the Australian hypothesis; the
odds are shortening. Yet more work needs to be done before we accept a concept
that could radically change the management of dyspepsia and ulcer diseases (ANON
1985). The believers were making progress but were not thus far winning the debate!

Acknowledgements. Thanks to Jill Whiting for her patience in typing this manuscript.

References

Anon (1985) *Campylobacters* in Ottawa. Lancet ii:135
Bader JP, Morin T, Bernier JJ, Bertrand J, Bétourné C, Gastard J, Lambert R, Ribet A, Sarles H, Toulet
    J (1977) Treatment of gastric ulcer by cimetidine; a multicentre trial. In: Burland WL, Simkins MA
    (eds) Cimetidine: proceedings of the 2nd international symposium of histamine H_2 receptor an-
    tagonists. Excerpta Medica, Amsterdam, pp 287–292
Bizzozero G (1893) Über die schlauchförmigen Drüsen des Magendarmkanals und die Beziehungen ihres
    Epithels zu dem Oberflächenepithel der Schleimhaut. Arch Mikrosk Anat Entw Mech 42:82
Breed RS, Murray EGD, Hitchens AP (1948) Bergey's manual of determinative bacteriology, 6th edn.
    Williams and Wilkins, Baltimore, p 217
Burland WL, Simkins MA (eds) Cimetidine: proceedings of the 2nd international symposium of hista-
    mine H_2 receptor antagonists. Excerpta Medica, Amsterdam
Correa P (1980) The epidemiology and pathogenesis of chronic gastritis: three aetiological entities. Front
    Gastrointest Res 6:98–108
Curry A, Jones DM, Eldridge J, Fox AJ (1985) Ultrastructure of *Campylobacter pyloridis* – not a
    Campylobacter? In: Pearson AD, Skirrow MB, Lior H, Rowe B (eds) *Campylobacter* III. PHLS,
    London, p 195
Doenges JL (1938) Spirochaetes in gastric glands of Macacus rhesus and humans without definite history
    of related disease. Proc Soc Exp Biol Med 38:536–538
Eldridge J, Lessells AM, Jones DM (1984) Antibody to spiral organisms on gastric mucosa. Lancet i:1237

Fitzgerald O, Murphy P (1950) Studies on the physiological chemistry and clinical significance of urease and urea with special reference to the stomach. Ir J Med Sci 292:97–159

Fullman H, Van Deventer G, Schneidman D, Walsh J, Elashoff J, Weinstein W (1985) 'Healed' duodenal ulcers are histologically ill. Gastroenterology 88:1390 (abstract)

Gear MWL, Barnes RJ (1980) Endoscopic studies of dyspepsia in a general practice. Br Med J 280:1136–1137

Goodwin CS, Blincow ED, Warren JR, Waters TE, Sanderson CR, Easton L (1985) Evaluation of cultural techniques for isolating Campylobacter pyloridis from endoscopic biopsies of gastric mucosa. J Clin Pathol 38:1127–1131

Goodwin CS, Blake P, Blincow E (1986) The minimum inhibitory and bactericidal concentrations of antibiotics and antiulcer agents against Campylobacter pyloridis. J Antimicrob Chemother 17:309–314

Gough KR, Bardham KD, Crowe JP, Korman MG, Lee FI, Reed PI (1984) Ranitidine and cimetidine in prevention of duodenal ulcer relapse. Lancet ii:659–662

Hazell SL, Lee A (1985) The adaptation of motile strains of Campylobacter pyloridis to gastric mucus and their association with gastric epithelial intercellular spaces. In: Pearson AD, Skirrow MB, Lior H, Rowe B (eds) Campylobacter III. PHLS, London, pp 189–191

Hudson MJ, Wait R (1985) Cellular fatty acids of Campylobacter species with particular reference to Campylobacter pyloridis. In: Pearson AD, Skirrow MB, Lior H, Rowe B (eds) Campylobacter III. PHLS, London, pp 198–199

Ishii E, Inoeu H, Tsuynguchi T, Shimoyama T, Tanaka T, Wada M, Kishi T. Masui M, Tamura T, Yanagase Y, Shoji K (1985) Campylobacter-like organisms in cases of stomach diseases in Japan. In: Pearson AD, Skirrow MB, Lior H, Rowe B (eds) Campylobacter III. PHLS, London, pp 179–180

Jones DM, Eldridge DM, Whorwell PJ, Miller JP (1985) The effects of various antiulcer regimens and antibiotics on the presence of Campylobacter pyloridis and its antibody. In: Pearson AD, Skirrow MB, Lior H, Rowe B (eds) Campylobacter III. PHLS, London, p 161

Koch R (1882) Die Aetiologie der Tuberkulose. Berl Klin Wochenschr 19:221–230

Krienitz W (1906) Über das Auftreten von Spirochaten verschiedener Form im Mageninhalt bei Carcinoma ventriculi. Dtsch Med Wochenschr 28:872

Langenberg ML, Tytgat GNJ, Schipper MEI, Rietra PJGM, Zenen HC (1984) Campylobacter-like organisms in the stomach of patients and healthy individuals. Lancet i:1348

Langenberg ML, Raws EAJ, Schipper MEI, Widjojoko S, Tytgat GNJ, Rietra PJGM, Zanen HC (1985) The pathogenic role of Campylobacter pyloridis studied by attempts to eliminate these organisms. In: Pearson AD, Skirrow MB, Lior H, Rowe B (eds) Campylobacter III. PHLS, London, pp 162–163

Lee WK, Gourley WK, Buck GE, Subramanyam K (1985) A study of gastric Campylobacter-like organisms in patients with gastritis. In: Pearson AD, Skirrow MB, Lior H, Rowe B (eds) Campylobacter III. PHLS, London, pp 178–179

Marshall BJ (1983) Unidentified curved bacilli on gastric epithelium in active chronic gastritis. Lancet i:1273–1275

Marshall BJ (1989) History of the discovery of C. pylori. In: Blaser M (ed) Campylobacter pylori in gastritis and peptic ulcer disease. Igakushein, New York, pp 7–23

Marshall BJ, Armstrong JA, McGechie DB, Glancy RJ (1985a) Attempt to fulfil Koch's postulates for pyloric Campylobacter. Med J Aust 142:436–439

Marshall BJ, Armstrong JA, McGechie DB, Francis GJ (1985b) The antibacterial action of bismuth: early results of antibacterial regimens in the treatment of duodenal ulcer. In: Pearson AD, Skirrow MB, Loir H, Rowe B (eds) Campylobacter III. PHLS, London, pp 165–16–6

Martin DF, May SJ, Tweedle DEF, Hollanders D, Ravenscroft MM, Miller JP (1981) Difference in relapse rates of duodenal ulcer after healing with cimetidine or tripotassium dicitrato bismuthate. Lancet i:7–10

McNulty CAM, Watson DM (1984) Spiral bacteria of the gastric antrum. Lancet i:1068–1069

McNulty CAM, Wise R (1985) Rapid diagnosis of Campylobacter-associated gastritis. Lancet i:1443–1444

McNulty CAM, Crump B, Gearty JC, Lister DM, David M, Donovan IA, Melikian V, Wise R (1985a) A trial to compare treatment with Pepto-Bismol (bismuth subsalicylate), placebo and erythromycin for the eradication of Campylobacter pyloridis in patients with gastritis. In: Pearson AD, Skirrow MB, Lior H, Rowe B (eds) Campylobacter III. PHLS, London, pp 163–164

McNulty CAM, Dent JC, Wise R (1985b) Susceptibility of clinical isolates of Campylobacter pyloridis to 11 antimicrobial agents. Antimicrob Agents Chemother 28:837–838

McNulty CAM, Dent JC, Curry A, Uff JS, Ford GA, Gear MWL, Wilkinson SP (1989) New spiral bacterium in gastric mucosa. J Clin Pathol 42:585 591

Morris A (1985) *Campylobacter pyloridis*: its history, characteristics and clinical relevance. NZ J Lab Technol 169 171

Multicentre trial (1979) Comparison of two doses of cimetidine and placebo in the treatment of duodenal ulcer: a multicentre trial. GUT 20:68 74

Newell DG (1985) The outer membrane proteins and surface antigens of *Campylobacter pyloridis*. In: Pearson AD, Skirrow MB, Lior H, Rowe B (eds) *Campylobacter* III. PHLS, London, pp 199 200

Pearson AD, Ireland A, Bamford J, Walker C, Booth L, Hawtin P, Holdstock G, Millward-Sadler H (1984) Polyacrylamide gel electrophoreises of spiral bacteria from the gastric antrum. Lancet ii:1349 1350

Pearson AD, Ireland A, Holdstock G, Bamford J, Booth L, Du Boulay C, Hawtin P (1985) Clinical pathological correlates of *Campylobacter pyloridis* isolates from gastric biopsy specimens. In: Pearson AD, Skirrow MB, Lior H, Rowe B (eds) Campylobacter III. PHLS, London, pp 181 182

Ramsey EJ, Carey KV, Peterson WL, Jackson JJ, Murphy FK, Read NW, Taylor KB, Trier JS, Fordtran JS (1979) Epidemic gastritis with hypochlorhydria. Gastroenterol 74:1449 1457

Schwarz K (1910) Über penetrierende Magen und Jejunalgeschwüre. Beitr Klin Chir 67:96 128

Steer HW, Colin-Jones DG (1975) Mucosal changes in gastric ulceration and their response to carbenoxolone sodium. GUT 16:590 597

Strickland RG, MacKay IR (1973) A reappraisal of the nature and significance of chronic atrophic gastritis. Dig Dis 18:426 440

Thomas JM (1984) *Campylobacter*-like organisms in gastritis. Lancet ii:1217

Warren JR (1983) Unidentified curved bacilli on gastric epithelium in active chronic gastritis. Lancet i:1273

Watt RP, Male PJ, Rawlings J, Hunt RH, Milton-Thompson GJ Misiewicz JJ (1981) Comparison of the effects of ranitidine, cimetidine and placebo on the 24 hour intragastric acidity and nocturnal acid secretions in patients with duodenal ulcer. GUT 22:49 54

The Epidemiology of *Helicobacter pylori*

H.M. MITCHELL

1 Introduction

In the world of modern medicine it is rare that the understanding of a previously described clinical disease is so completely revolutionized that clinical textbooks must be rewritten. This, however, has been the outcome of the isolation of *Helicobacter pylori* from the human stomach. Only 15 years after its initial isolation, this bacterium has been proven to be the etiological agent of acute on chronic gastritis, and a predisposing factor in peptic ulcer disease, gastric carcinoma and B cell mucosa-associated lymphoid tissue (MALT) lymphoma (GRAHAM et al. 1992; IARC 1994; MARSHALL et al. 1985; PARSONNET et al. 1994).

School of Microbiology and Immunology, University of New South Wales, Sydney 2052, Australia

Although today many questions relating to the epidemiology of *H. pylori* have been delineated, a number of controversial issues still remain. In this chapter I hope to provide the reader with a clear picture of the established facts in relation to the epidemiology of *H. pylori*, to outline current areas of epidemiological research and to discuss the clinical implications of epidemiological studies.

1.1 Prevalence of Infection

Epidemiological studies have shown that *H. pylori* infection is ubiquitous, with approximately 50% of the world's population being estimated to be infected with this organism. The prevalence of *H. pylori* infection is similar in males and females and it is believed that once a subject is infected, the bacterium persists for life (POUNDER and NG 1995). Although infection with *H. pylori* may occur worldwide, significant differences in the prevalence of infection have been reported both between and within countries (MEGRAUD et al. 1989; MITCHELL et al. 1992a). In general, the prevalence of infection in developing countries has been shown to be higher than that in developed countries. For example, in developed countries such as the United States, the United Kingdom and Australia, the overall prevalence of infection has been found to range from 19% to 57% whereas in developing countries such as China, Thailand and India overall prevalence rates of between 44% and 79% have been reported (GRAHAM et al. 1991a,b; MITCHELL et al. 1992a; PEREZ PEREZ et al. 1990; SITAS et al. 1991; WHITAKER et al. 1993). Comparison of the age stratified prevalence rates from such countries indicates that the difference in prevalence between developed and developing countries relates to the rate of acquisition of *H. pylori* in childhood. For example, in a comparison of the prevalence of *H. pylori* infection in asymptomatic subjects living in Australia with that in a southern province of China we found 4% of Australian children under 10 years of age to be infected with *H. pylori* compared with 27% of Chinese children. Over this age, however, the increase in prevalence of infection was similar in both countries, being in the order of 1% per year (MITCHELL et al. 1992a).

Examination of epidemiological data from other developed and developing countries has supported this finding with the prevalence of *H. pylori* infection in children under 10 years resident in developed countries being approximately 0%–5%, compared with 13%–60% in children resident in developing countries. Over this age an increase in prevalence in the order of 0.5%–2% per annum is commonly observed (MOAGEL et al. 1990; GRAHAM et al. 1991b; JONES et al. 1986; MEGRAUD et al. 1989; MITCHELL et al. 1992a; PEREZ PEREZ et al. 1990). Initially this increase in prevalence with age was interpreted as acquisition of *H. pylori* over time; however, in recent years it has been proposed that this may relate to a cohort moving through the population. In this latter scenario, the increasing prevalence of *H. pylori* occurring from younger to older subjects would reflect the passage through the population of distinct cohorts. That is, all persons are infected in childhood and the decreased levels of *H. pylori* infection associated with younger age groups, particularly in developed countries are due to gradual improvements in medical care, sanitation and or living conditions.

Evidence to support this latter view has been provided by a number of studies (BANATVALA et al. 1993; CULLEN et al. 1993; REPLOGLE et al. 1996). For example, CULLEN et al. (1993) showed the prevalence of *H. pylori* in serum samples collected from 141 adults in 1969, 1978, and 1990 to be 39%, 40.9% and 34.8% respectively. Of 86 subjects who were seronegative in 1969, only six (7%) were found to be seropositive in 1990. As a result of this study CULLEN and associates (1993) concluded that the increasing prevalence of *H. pylori* with age was due to a cohort effect and that acquisition of infection in adults was rare. In contrast, Veldhuyzen van Zanten et al. (1994) have argued that the increase in *H. pylori* prevalence in adulthood is due to acquisition. In a prospective 3-year cohort study examining the seroprevalence, conversion, and reversion rate of *H. pylori* infection in 316 randomly selected Canadian non-patient subjects aged 18–72 years, they showed the crude annual *H. pylori* seroconversion rate to be 1% and the "spontaneous" seroreversion rate to be 1.6%. These authors considered that a continuous risk of acquisition of 1%/year best explained the pattern of *H. pylori* infection in this Canadian population. Although the sample size of this study is small it does show that seroconversion can occur after childhood.

Hence at the present time, the ability to clearly differentiate between the gradual acquisition of infection and a cohort effect remains unresolved. In order to obtain a true evaluation of the situation, large cohort studies using in the order of 1000 individuals followed for a period of at least 5 years will be required. At the end of this time, given an acquisition rate of 0.5%–2% per annum, one would expect to find that 25–100 subjects would have seroconverted (MITCHELL 1995).

1.2 Source of Infection

Humans appear to be the natural host for *H. pylori*, and it has been postulated that *H. pylori* has adapted itself to the ecological niche of the human stomach (LEE and HAZELL 1988).

Over the years a number of studies have suggested that animals may act as reservoirs for *H. pylori*; however, evidence to support this view is on the whole unconvincing. Two early epidemiological studies by MORRIS and associates (1986) and VAIRA et al. (1988) showed the prevalence of *H. pylori* infection to be significantly higher in meat workers and abattoir workers than that in subjects not involved in handling animals or animal products; this finding led these authors to suggest that *H. pylori* infection was a zoonosis. Although studies have shown that both germ-free and specific pathogen free pigs can be experimentally colonized with *H. pylori*, attempts to identify *H. pylori* in abattoir pigs using both cultural and serological techniques have failed (EATON et al. 1990; ENGSTRAND et al. 1990; GRASSO et al. 1996; ROCHA et al. 1992). It is now believed that the increased prevalence of *H. pylori* infection observed in abattoir and meat workers may have resulted from cross reactivity between *H. pylori* and antibodies to other gastrointestinal organisms such as *Campylobacter jejuni* present in the sera of these workers (Fox 1995; MITCHELL 1993).

Several groups have reported the isolation of *H. pylori* from rhesus monkeys; however, given the rare association between man and monkeys, it is doubtful whether this represents an important reservoir of infection (DUBOIS et al. 1994; Fox 1995; HANDT et al. 1997).

Domestic pets have also been suggested as a possible reservoir of *H. pylori*. Prior to the isolation of *H. pylori* researchers had observed that cats harboured gastric spiral organisms (LEE et al. 1988). Subsequent investigation of these spiral organisms using 16 S rRNA sequence analysis showed them to differ from *H. pylori* but to be sufficiently homologous to be included in the genus *Helicobacter*; they have since been named *H. felis* and *H. heilmanni* (Fox 1994; LEE et al. 1988). Interestingly, these organisms have been reported to be associated with chronic gastritis in a small percentage (0.08%–1%) of humans (HEILMANN and BORCHARD 1991; LEE et al. 1995; STOLTE et al. 1994). Recently, HANDT et al. (1994, 1995) reported an *H. pylori*-like organism to be present in the stomachs of an entire colony of pathogen free cats. This organism was shown by biochemical, phenotypic and 16 S rRNA sequencing techniques to be *H. pylori*. Although HANDT et al. have suggested that cats may represent an important reservoir of *H. pylori* it is important to remember that these cats were commercially reared and had been maintained in isolation. Seroepidemiological studies examining the relationship between pet ownership and the prevalence of *H. pylori* have in general failed to support such a relationship (ANSORG et al. 1995; WEBB et al. 1994).

1.3 Transmission of *H. pylori*

Failure to reproducibly isolate *H. pylori* from reservoirs other than man suggest that direct person to person contact is the most likely mode of transmission of this organism. In general, infectious diseases spread from person to person by close contact are found to have a higher prevalence in institutions due to close personal contact and lack of personal hygiene. This observation has been shown to be true for *H. pylori*, an early study by BERKOWICZ and LEE (1987) reporting the prevalence of *H. pylori* infection in residents of an institution for the mentally handicapped to be significantly higher than that in normal blood donors (61% vs 19.7%). Similar studies have corroborated this initial finding and have led to the view that close personal contact is important for the spread of *H. pylori* (LAMBERT et al. 1995; VINCENT et al. 1994). The finding that the prevalence of *H. pylori* infection is significantly higher in the family members of children infected with *H. pylori* than in family members of children not infected with *H. pylori* has led to the view that transmission of *H. pylori* occurs mainly within the family setting (DRUMM et al. 1990; MITCHELL et al. 1993). Indeed in a study by our group we have reported evidence of transmission of *H. pylori* within the family setting. In this study a 21-

month-old boy who presented with a bleeding gastric ulcer was shown to be acutely infected with *H. pylori*. Serological investigation of the child's family showed the mother to have an established asymptomatic infection and his twin brother, who had suffered an episode of vomiting at a similar time to his brother, to also be acutely infected with *H. pylori*. Follow-up studies of the family showed that the twins' father became infected with *H. pylori* 7 months after the first twin's episode (MITCHELL et al. 1992b). In a subsequent study we were able to show using random amplification of polymorphic DNA (RAPD) polymerase chain reaction (PCR), that the strains of *H. pylori* infecting these twin boys were identical and based on serological studies, that a third child born some years after the initial episode had become infected with *H. pylori* (MITCHELL et al. 1996a).

Although early studies examining the prevalence of *H. pylori* infection in spouses suggested that transmission between spouses was uncommon (PEREZ PEREZ et al. 1991; POLISH et al. 1991), recent studies have shown that a significant number of couples may be infected with the same strain of *H. pylori* (GEORGOPOULOS et al. 1996; SCHUTZE et al. 1995). In a study of the spouses of *H. pylori*-positive duodenal ulcer patients, GEORGOPOULOS et al. (1996) found 42/54 (78%) partners to be *H. pylori* positive compared with only 2/10 (20%) partners of *H. pylori*-negative patients. Examination of the ribopatterns of the *H. pylori* strains derived from 18 of these patients and their spouses showed that in each of eight couples a single strain had colonized both partners, while in the remaining ten couples, each partner was colonized by a distinct *H. pylori* strain. Although this study may suggest person-to-person transmission within couples, it is also possible that transmission occurred by exposure to a common source of infection, or from contact with a child already infected by one parent with *H. pylori*. Several studies have reported an association between the number of children in a family and the prevalence of *H. pylori* infection, suggesting that children may facilitate the spread of *H. pylori* (BREUER et al. 1996; TEH et al. 1994; WEBB et al. 1994).

1.4 Factors Influencing the Transmission of *H. pylori*

1.4.1 Socioeconomic Status

Studies conducted throughout the world have indicated that low socioeconomic status may be associated with an increased prevalence of *H. pylori* infection. In particular, the socioeconomic status of a subject during childhood is considered to be an important determinant of the development of *H. pylori* infection. Socioeconomic status, however, is a broad criterion and encompasses factors such as level of hygiene, sanitation, density of living and educational opportunities, some or all of which have been reported to influence the level of infection within a population. The role of socioeconomic status *per se* is particularly clear if one examines the prevalence of *H. pylori* infection in poorer racial groups living in developed countries. For example, in a study in the United States where the socioeconomic status in childhood was estimated in a black and Hispanic population, MALATY and GRAHAM (1994) showed the prevalence of *H. pylori* infection to be inversely related to the social class during childhood, with the prevalence of *H. pylori* infection in the lowest social class being significantly higher than that in the highest social class (85% vs 11%).

1.4.2 Density of Living

A factor that has been consistently related to an increased prevalence of *H. pylori* is density of living (McCALLION et al. 1996; MENDALL et al. 1992; MITCHELL et al. 1992a). For example, in a large cross-sectional seroepidemiological study in China, we have shown high density of living to be the major factor relating to the higher prevalence of *H. pylori* infection in a large city area as compared with a rural area of Guangdong province (MITCHELL et al. 1992a). The importance of overcrowding in the acquisition of *H. pylori* is further supported by the finding that bed sharing in childhood is associated with a higher prevalence of *H. pylori* infection (McCALLION et al. 1996; WEBB et al. 1994).

1.4.3 Educational Level

Several studies have identified educational level as an important determinant of *H. pylori* prevalence (FORMAN et al. 1993; GRAHAM et al. 1991a; ROSENSTOCK et al. 1996). For example, in a large seroepidemiological study in which the prevalence of *H. pylori* infection in 3194 asymptomatic subjects living in 17 different populations was determined, FORMAN et al. (1993) found the prevalence of *H. pylori* infection to be inversely related to educational level, 34% of subjects with a tertiary education being infected compared with 47% of those with a secondary education and 63% of those with only a primary school education.

1.4.4 Sanitation

Low levels of sanitation have also been associated with an increased prevalence of *H. pylori* infection al (MOAGEL et al. 1990; MENDALL et al. 1992; PEREZ PEREZ et al. 1990). For example, it has been reported that the absence of running water in the childhood home is a significant risk factor for *H. pylori* infection (MENDALL et al. 1992). In adults, however, Basso et al. (1994) found no significant change in the prevalence of *H. pylori* infection in 130 asymptomatic Irish soldiers following 6 months peace duty in Lebanon, despite the fact that these soldiers had been exposed to poor living conditions and sanitation (BASSO et al. 1994).

The importance of improved living conditions on the prevalence of *H. pylori* infection has been supported by the finding that in countries where socioeconomic conditions have improved over the last few decades, a decline in the prevalence of *H. pylori* infection has occurred. For example, in Japan ASAKA et al. (1992) found the prevalence of *H. pylori* infection to be significantly higher in subjects over 40 years (75%) compared with that in subjects 30 to 39 years (42%) and those 20 to

29 years (26%). ASAKA et al. (1992) suggested that this fall in prevalence is related to the significant improvement of the Japanese economy and hence living conditions, following the Second World War (ASAKA et al. 1992). Similarly, in Korea, a country that has recently undergone substantial improvements in standard of living, the prevalence of *H. pylori* infection has been reported to be changing, with a markedly lower prevalence of infection in children of families of higher socioeconomic status (MALATY et al. 1996).

1.4.5 Genetic Predisposition

In a study examining the importance of genetic factors on the acquisition of *H. pylori* MALATY et al. (1994) compared the seroprevalence of *H. pylori* infection in 100 monozygotic and 169 dizygotic twins reared together and reared apart. This study showed the correlation coefficient for the relative importance of genetic predisposition on acquisition of *H. pylori* infection to be approximately 0.66, the remaining variance being accounted for by shared rearing environmental factors (20%) and non-shared environmental factors (23%). MALATY et al. (1994) concluded that genetic effects influenced the acquisition of *H. pylori* infection due to greater similarities within monozygotic twin pairs and that sharing the same rearing environment also contributed to the familial tendency to acquire *H. pylori*.

2 Current Research

Although many areas in relation to the epidemiology of *H. pylori* continue to be investigated, it is probably true to say that the most studied and certainly the most controversial area of research today is the determination of the route of transmission of *H. pylori*. Clearly, if intervention strategies are to be introduced, such knowledge is essential.

Given the location of *H. pylori* infection and the basic need of this bacterium for gastric type mucosa for in vivo proliferation, it is probable that ingestion is the most common means of acquiring *H. pylori*. Whether *H. pylori* reaches the oral cavity via the faecal-oral or oral-oral route is, however, still open for conjecture. Numerous articles from proponents of both routes of transmission continue to appear in the literature, however, whether one or both of these routes of transmission is important in the spread of *H. pylori* remains unclear.

2.1 Faecal-Oral Transmission of *H. pylori*

In 1992 the first report of the isolation of *H. pylori* from human faeces appeared in the literature. In this study THOMAS et al. (1992) reported the isolation of *H. pylori* from the faeces of one infected adult and 9 of 23 randomly selected children living in a Gambian village. In 1994 KELLY and colleagues (1994), using the same isolation technique as THOMAS's group, also claimed to have isolated *H. pylori* from the faeces of 12 of 25 *H. pylori*-positive subjects with dyspepsia. Although based on various phenotypic and genotypic characteristics KELLY et al. claimed that the organisms isolated from the faeces of these patients were *H. pylori*, this study must be interpreted with some caution as proof that the organisms cultured were *H. pylori* was unconvincing. Attempts by other groups to isolate *H. pylori* from patient populations using these methods have failed, and it has been suggested that the ability of THOMAS et al. to culture *H. pylori* from Gambian children may be related to the fact that these children were malnourished and had a extremely short faecal transit time (MEGRAUD 1995).

Although there is some supportive evidence for the passage of *H. pylori* through the intestine (DYE et al. 1990), this bacterium is not well adapted for such passage. Several groups have shown that *H. pylori* is sensitive to the lethal effects of bile (MITCHELL et al. 1992c; RAEDSCH et al. 1989) hence survival of *H. pylori* after transit through the intestinal tract is unlikely.

Attempts to detect *H. pylori* DNA in faeces via PCR has produced variable results. In such studies, specific primers directed against *H. pylori* have been used to probe faecal samples from patients infected with *H. pylori*. While MAPSTONE et al. (1993a) and NOTARNICOLA et al. (1996) reported *H. pylori* DNA to be present in a high percentage (89.6% and 95.6%, respectively) of faecal samples obtained from patients known to be infected with *H. pylori*, NAMAVAR et al. (1995) found *H. pylori* DNA in the faeces of only 1 of 15 (7%) patients whose stomach biopsies were positive for *H. pylori* DNA. Although detection of *H. pylori* DNA in faeces may add to the evidence supporting the faecal-oral route of transmission, it is important to remember that the finding of *H. pylori* DNA does not necessarily mean that viable *H. pylori* are present in the faeces.

If *H. pylori* is transmitted by the faecal-oral route, one might predict that, as with other pathogens spread by the faecal-oral route, both food and water (via faecal contamination) represent a reservoir of infection. In a study of the prevalence of *H. pylori* infection in Peruvian children, KLEIN et al. (1991) have reported an association to exist between the prevalence of *H. pylori* infection and their source of drinking water. In this study, children whose homes had an external water supply were found to be three times more likely to be infected with *H. pylori* than those children whose home had an internal water source. Attempts to culture *H. pylori* from water samples at this time were unsuccessful; however, this group has sub-sequently reported the detection of *H. pylori* DNA using PCR in drinking water samples collected from the same areas (HULTEN et al. 1996). HOPKINS et al. (1993) have suggested that contamination of vegetables with water containing raw sewage and subsequent consumption of uncooked vegetables may be an important mode of transmission of *H. pylori*. In a study in Chile these authors found a correlation to exist between *H. pylori* seropositivity in children and the consumption of uncooked vegetables; however, this correlation was associated more with older children (> 5 years) and hence unknown confounding factors may be involved.

Epidemiological studies in China have failed to support the view that water is a significant factor in the dissemination of *H. pylori*. In a large seroepidemiological study in southern China, we found the prevalence of *H. pylori* infection to be high (45%) despite the fact that the majority of subjects in this study boiled their water prior to consumption (MITCHELL et al. 1992a). In a second study by our group examining the role of water in the transmission of *H. pylori*, we compared in the same Chinese population, the prevalence pattern of hepatitis A (an organism transmitted by the faecal-oral route) to that of *H. pylori*, for if *H. pylori* is indeed transmitted by the faecal-oral route, one would expect the prevalence pattern of hepatitis A to be similar to that of *H. pylori*. Although initial examination of the seroprevalence data from rural areas supported a correlation between *H. pylori* and hepatitis A, when the prevalence data from the urban area was examined it became evident that no such correlation existed. Although in this urban area the prevalence of *H. pylori* infection in subjects less than 10 years was high (approx. 32%), not one of these subjects was shown to be infected with hepatitis A. As a result of this study, we concluded that community-wide faecal-oral spread *of H. pylori* may be of limited importance (HAZELL et al. 1994). In a similar cross-sectional comparison of the patterns of hepatitis A and *H. pylori* seroprevalence in Stoke-on-Trent in the UK, WEBB et al. (1996) also found no correlation to exist between the prevalence of *H. pylori* and hepatitis A, a finding that led these authors to conclude that other modes of transmission, for instance, oral-oral contact, may be a more likely route of transmission.

2.2 Oral–Oral Transmission of *H. pylori*

Reports supporting the concept of oral-oral transmission of *H. pylori* have come from studies examining gastric secretions, oral secretions and dental plaque. *H. pylori* has been shown to be present in the gastric juice of up to 58% of patients (VAROLI et al. 1991) infected with *H. pylori*, and hence it is possible that refluxed gastric juice may represent a vehicle of transmission for this organism. Indeed a gastro-oral route of transmission has been suggested by a number of studies. For example, our group (1992b) and AXON et al. (1995) have postulated that in children, where regurgitation of gastric material into the mouth is fairly common, that gastric secretions may represent a possible vehicle of transmission. Direct contact with gastric secretions has also been implicated in the higher prevalence of *H. pylori* infection reported in gastroenterologists (LIN et al. 1994; MITCHELL et al. 1989) and in the reported epidemics of *Helicobacter* gastritis following gastric intubation experiments (GRAHAM et al. 1988; RAMSEY et al. 1979).

Although attempts to culture *H. pylori* from the oral cavity have in many cases proved to be fruitless, a number of studies have been successful. In a study investigating the route of transmission of *H. pylori*, KRAJDEN et al. (1989) isolated *H. pylori* from the dental plaque of 1 of 29 patients whose stomach biopsies were shown to be positive for *H. pylori*. Comparison using restriction endonuclease analysis of the *H. pylori* strains isolated from the stomach and dental plaque of this patient subsequently showed one of three strains of *H. pylori* isolated from dental plaque to be indistinguishable from that isolated from the stomach (SHAMES et al. 1989). Similar results have been reported by CELLINI et al. (1995), who isolated *H. pylori* from the dental plaque of 1 of 20 endoscopy patients whose gastric biopsy specimen were positive for *H. pylori*. Comparison of the protein patterns of whole cells obtained from the stomach biopsy and from the dental plaque of this patient showed these to be identical as was the restriction endonuclease pattern obtained from DNA extracted from both of these strains (CELLINI et al. 1995). In contrast to these studies, DESAI et al. (1991) in a study of Indian dyspeptic patients found *H. pylori* to be present in the dental plaque of 98% of patients. In this study, however, identification of *H. pylori* was based solely on the urease test, which due to the presence of other urease positive organisms in the mouth is likely to have resulted in false positive results. The possibility of falsely identifying normal flora from the oral cavity as *H. pylori* has recently been underlined by NAMAVAR et al. (1995) who showed that organisms isolated from the tongue and palate of one patient which were considered to be phenotypically identical to *H. pylori* (micro-aerophilic, urease, catalase and oxidase positive) were in fact negative by an *H. pylori* specific PCR. These authors concluded that use of routine enzyme reactions may lead to the false identification of *H. pylori*.

In 1993 FERGUSON et al. reported the isolation of low numbers of *H. pylori* from the saliva of one of nine patients in whom gastric biopsies were shown to be positive for *H. pylori*. Comparison of the strains obtained from the stomach and saliva of this patient using restriction fragment length polymorphism subsequently showed the strains isolated from dental plaque and gastric tissue to be identical (FERGUSON et al. 1993).

The results of studies examining samples collected from the oral cavity for the presence of *H. pylori* specific DNA have varied significantly (BANATVALA et al. 1994; BICKLEY et al. 1993; CAMMAROTA et al. 1996; MAPSTONE et al. 1993b; NGUYEN et al. 1993). For example, BANATVALA et al. (1994) using an *H. pylori*-species specific *ureA* (urease) gene internal sequence showed 39 of 54 (72%) dental plaque samples taken from patients attending for endoscopy to be positive for *H. pylori* DNA (BANATVALA et al. 1994). In contrast, MAPSTONE et al. (1993b) using a 16S rRNA probe found *H. pylori* DNA to be present in only 38% of dental plaque samples obtained from 13 patients with histologically confirmed *H. pylori*, while CAMMAROTA et al. (1996) and BICKLEY et al. (1993) failed to detect *H. pylori* DNA in the dental plaque of any *H. pylori*-positive patients (MAPSTONE et al. 1993b; BICKLEY et al. 1993; CAMMAROTA et al. 1996). It has been suggested that the differences in detection rate of *H. pylori* in these studies is related to the specificity of the primers used (MEGRAUD 1995). Again, it is important to remember that detection of *H. pylori* DNA does not mean that viable *H. pylori* are present in oral secretions.

A number of seroepidemiological studies have also suggested that oral secre-tions may be important in the transmission of *H. pylori*. For example, ALBENQUE et al. (1990) showed premastication of food by African mothers prior to feeding their children to be a risk factor for *H. pylori* infection (ALBENQUE et al. 1990) while CHOW et al. (1995) reported the use of chopsticks and communal eating habits to be associated with transmission of *H. pylori* within Chinese communities outside of China (CHOW et al. 1995).

The finding that the prevalence of *H. pylori* infection in dentists or dental workers is not increased has been used to argue against the oral-oral transmission of *H. pylori* (BANATVALA et al. 1995; MALATY et al. 1992; NGUYEN et al. 1995).

3 Clinical Implications

3.1 Role of *H. pylori* in Gastroduodenal Disease

It is now well established that *H. pylori* plays an important role in peptic ulcer disease, gastric cancer and B cell mucosa-associated lymphoid tissue (MALT) lymphoma (GRAHAM et al. 1992; IARC 1994; MARSHALL et al. 1985; PARSONNET et al. 1994). Although almost half the world's population is infected with *H. pylori* only a small proportion go on to develop more serious sequalae. Why such subjects are more susceptible to disease development is unknown; however, there is some evidence to suggest that this may relate to infection with strains of *H. pylori* showing enhanced virulence potential.

Over recent years a number of putative virulence determinants of *H. pylori* have been proposed including, urease, the heat shock protein, vacuolating cyto-toxin (*vacA*), the cytotoxin associated gene A (*cagA*) and the cytotoxin associated gene II (*cagII*) (CENSINI et al. 1996). Although each of these determinants has been investigated to some degree, it is *cagA* that has received most attention in relation to its role in disease development. *cagA* has been found to be present in approxi-mately 60% of *H. pylori* strains and has been shown to encode a protein with a molecular size of approximately 120–128 kDa. Serological studies have shown that patients infected with *cagA* positive strains of *H. pylori* produce both local and systemic antibodies to the *cagA* gene product, the CagA protein (COVER et al. 1995). Seroepidemiological studies in patient groups resident in developed countries have shown a higher prevalence of antibodies to the CagA protein in patients with peptic ulcer disease than in those with gastritis alone (COVACCI et al. 1993; COVER et al. 1990; TUMMURU et al. 1993). For example, COVER et al. (1990) showed 100% of patients with peptic ulcer disease to have antibodies to the CagA protein as compared with only 61.6% of those with gastritis alone (COVER et al. 1990). An association between the presence of *cagA* and the development of gastric cancer has also been reported (BLASER et al. 1995; CRABTREE et al. 1993; PARSONNET et al. 1997). In a recent study PARSONNET et al. (1997) found persons infected with CagA-positive strains of *H. pylori* to be three times more likely to develop intestinal gastric cancer than persons infected with CagA-negative strains. When subjects were evaluated by tumour type, this study showed that both phenotypes of *H. pylori* appeared to increase the risk for diffuse type cancer while only the CagA phenotype was associated with intestinal malignancy (PARSONNET et al. 1997).

While for some years evidence to support a role for *cagA* in the development of more serious gastroduodenal disease was quite compelling, recent studies in developing countries have questioned this view (MITCHELL et al. 1996b; LAGE et al. 1995; MIEHLKE et al. 1995; GRAHAM et al. 1996). In a study, examining the prevalence of antibodies to CagA in both asymptomatic and symptomatic subjects living in Australia and The People's Republic of China, our group has shown no significant difference to exist between the prevalence of antibody to CagA in asymptomatic Chinese subjects and in Chinese gastric cancer patients (85.7% vs 83.3%). In contrast, in the Australian population, as has been shown in other developed countries, peptic ulcer disease patients were shown to have a higher prevalence of antibody to CagA than patients with gastritis alone or an asymptomatic blood donor population (MITCHELL et al. 1996b). In a recent study to confirm the association between carriage of *cagA*-positive strains of *H. pylori* and more serious gastroduodenal disease, GRAHAM et al. (1996) in a North American population compared the prevalence of antibody to CagA in 100 patients with peptic ulcer disease with that in 77 asymptomatic subjects with *H. pylori* infection without ulcer disease. The results of this study showed no significant difference to exist between the prevalence of serum IgG antibodies to CagA in *H. pylori* infected patients with ulcers (59%) and that in healthy *H. pylori* infected volunteers (44%) (GRAHAM et al. 1996). Such findings have led to the view that there may be major geographic differences in the prevalence of *cagA*-positive strains.

Although more recent studies would suggest that *cagA* may not associated with the development of more serious disease, one cannot rule out the possibility that this gene is a necessary but not sufficient factor in the development of peptic ulcer disease and gastric cancer.

3.2 Infection with Multiple Strains

Recently it has been reported that patients may be infected with more than one strain of *H. pylori* (HIRSCHL et al. 1994; JORGENSEN et al. 1996). In a recent study by our group we have shown using RAPD-PCR fingerprinting techniques that 14 of 17 symptomatic Australian adult patients were infected with more than 1 strain of *H. pylori*. In this study patients infected with more than one strain of *H. pylori* were found to be predominantly Vietnamese and Greek, both ethnic groups known to have a high prevalence of infection (JORGENSEN et al. 1996).

Based on these findings, we have suggested that in developing countries due to increased exposure to *H. pylori*, colonisation with multiple strains may be more common. The finding that patients can harbour multiple strains of *H. pylori* may also explain differences in the correlation between *cagA* and disease outcome in different geographic locations.

3.3 Reinfection After Treatment

An important factor with regard to patient management in *H. pylori* infection is the
issue of whether, following successful treatment of *H. pylori* infection, reinfection
with *H. pylori* can occur. Several studies have examined the reinfection rate of
H. pylori in patients treated for peptic ulcer disease. In general, in developed
countries, where adequate antibiotic therapy and *H. pylori* detection methods have
been used, reinfection rates have been shown to be low (0% and 1.2%; BORODY
et al. 1994; GRAHAM et al. 1992). In a 9-year follow-up study of 1182 patients in
whom *H. pylori* appeared to have been successfully eradicated as indicated by a
well-validated [^{14}C]urea breath test, BELL and POWELL (1996) reported 45 of 57
reinfections to occur within 6 months of treatment. Based on the reinfection rate in
the first 6 months of this study an annual reinfection rate of 9.5% per year would
be predicted; however, after the first year of the study the 'reinfection' rate was in
fact less than 0.6% per year. When the treatment regimens used in this study were
arbitrarily divided into five groups based on the following eradication rates, less
than 20%, 20%–39%, 40%–59%, 60%–79% and over 80%, the 6-month reinfection rates were shown to be 28.8%, 15.8%, 16.4%, 4.6% and 1.7%, respectively.
As a result of this study BELL and POWELL (1996) suggested that in "Westernized"
countries, most so-called reinfections in adults are due to late recrudescence of a
suppressed infection rather than a true reinfection and that if an eradication
therapy has an efficacy of greater than 85% the true reinfection rate is very low.

To date there have been a limited number of studies examining reinfection
rates in developing countries. In Southeast Asia, GOH et al. (1996) examined the
reinfection rate over a 2-year period in 38 duodenal ulcer patients in whom *H. pylori*
had been successfully eradicated. The results of this study showed the reinfection
rate to be zero in this patient group over this time period (GOH et al. 1996). In
contrast, in a 1-year follow-up study in Chile, FIGUEROA et al. (1996) reported 2/47
H. pylori-eradicated patients to become reinfected after 1 year, giving a reinfection
rate of 4.2%/year. A similar reinfection rate (3.7%/year) has been reported in
Africa, where 2/27 patients in whom *H. pylori* had been eradicated were shown to
be reinfected over a 2-year period (LOUW et al. 1995). Further studies, examining
large numbers of subjects are required to determine the true rate of reinfection in
developing countries.

3.4 Association of *H. pylori* with Extra-gastric Conditions

3.4.1 Diminished Growth

H. pylori infection has been associated with diminished growth in children (PATEL
et al. 1994; RAYMOND et al. 1994). In a study by PATEL et al. (1994) the growth in
height of *H. pylori*-infected children between aged 7 and 11 years was shown to be
diminished by a mean of 1.1 cm (0.3–2.0 cm) over 4 years. This growth reduction,
however, was found to be largely confined to girls. As a result of this study the

authors suggested that *H. pylori* infection delays or diminishes the pubertal growth spurt. Further studies in this area are required to determine the relevance of *H. pylori* in short-stature syndrome.

3.4.2 Coronary Heart Disease

Although initial studies in patients with coronary heart disease suggested a significant correlation between *H. pylori* infection and coronary heart disease (MURRAY et al. 1995; PATEL et al. 1995), more recent studies have failed to support this association (DELANEY et al. 1996; RATHBONE et al. 1996; SANDIFER et al. 1996). It has been suggested that the association between coronary heart disease and *H. pylori* may be accounted for by confounding effects or factors related to relative poverty in childhood.

4 Conclusion

Given the association between *H. pylori* and peptic ulcer disease, gastric cancer and B cell mucosa-associated lymphoid tissue (MALT) lymphoma, there is an urgent need for the development of intervention strategies to prevent the spread of this bacterium. Although it would appear that the development of a vaccine against *H. pylori* is proceeding satisfactorily, it may well be 5–10 years before this becomes available. Antibiotic treatment of all subjects infected with *H. pylori* is clearly out of the question, hence public health measures based on epidemiological data have the potential to play an important role. Current epidemiological studies have shown that the major reservoir of *H. pylori* is man, and that the principal mode of transmission is person to person, probably within the family setting. The higher prevalence of *H. pylori* infection in developing countries as compared with developed countries has been shown to relate to acquisition of *H. pylori* in childhood, this period being the major period for acquisition for this bacterium. Increased acquisition of *H. pylori* has been related to social status, high density of living, low levels of sanitation and genetic factors. To date, the route of transmission of *H. pylori* remains unresolved with evidence for both oral-oral and faecal oral transmission being reported. Clarification of this issue is essential if public health measures are to be implemented to prevent the spread of *H. pylori*.

References

al Moagel MA, Evans DG, Abdulghani ME, Adam E, Evans DJJ, Malaty HM, Graham DY (1990) Prevalence of *Helicobacter* (formerly Campylobacter) *pylori* infection in Saudi Arabia, and comparison of those with and without upper gastrointestinal symptoms. Am J Gastroenterol 85:944–948

Albenque M, Tall F, Dabis F, Mégraud F (1990) Epidemiological study of *Helicobacter pylori* transmission from mother to child in Africa. Enferm Digest 78:48

Ansorg R, Vonheinegg EH, Vonrecklinghausen G (1995) Cat owners risk of acquiring a *Helicobacter pylori* infection. Zentralb Bakteriol (Int J Med Microbiol Vir Parasitol Infect Dis 283:122–126

Asaka M, Kimura T, Kudo M (1992) Relationship of *Helicobacter pylori* to serum pepsinogens in an asymptomatic Japanese population. Gastroenterology 102:760–766

Axon ATR (1995) Review article – is *Helicobacter pylori* transmitted by the gastro-oral route. Aliment Pharmacol Therapeut 9:585–588

Banatvala N, Mayo K, Megraud F, Jennings R, Deeks JJ, Feldman RA (1993) The cohort effect and *Helicobacter pylori*. J Infect Dis 168:219–221

Banatvala N, Lopez CR, Owen RJ, Hurtado A, Abdi Y, Davies GR, Hardie JM, Feldman RA (1994) Use of the polymerase chain reaction to detect *Helicobacter pylori* in the dental plaque of healthy and symptomatic individuals. Microb Ecol Health Dis 7:1–8

Banatvala N, Abdi Y, Clements L, Herbert A, Davies J, Bragg J, Shepherd JP, Feldman RA, Hardie JM (1995) *Helicobacter pylori* infection in dentists: a case-control study. Scand J Infect Dis 7:

Basso L, Beattie S, Lawlor S, Clune J, O'Morain C (1994) A descriptive follow-up study on *Helicobacter pylori* infection before and after exposition to a war area. Eur J Epidemiol 10:109–111

Bell GD, Powell KU (1996) *Helicobacter pylori* reinfection after apparent eradication – the Ipswich experience. Scand J Gastroenterol 31 [Suppl 215]:96–104

Berkowicz J, Lee A (1987) Person-to-person transmission of *Campylobacter pylori*. Lancet 2:680–681

Bickley J, Owen RJ, Fraser AG, Pounder RE (1993) Evaluation of the polymerase chain reaction for detecting the urease c gene of *Helicobacter pylori* in gastric biopsy samples and dental plaque. J Med Microbiol 39:338–344

Blaser MJ, Perez Perez GI, Kleanthous H, Cover TL, Peek RM, Chyou PH, Stemmermann GN, Nomura A (1995) Infection with *Helicobacter pylori* strains possessing cagA is associated with an increased risk of developing adenocarcinoma of the stomach. Cancer Res 55:2111–2115

Borody TJ, Andrews P, Mancuso N, Mccauley D, Jankiewicz E, Ferch N, Shortis NP, Brandl S (1994) *Helicobacter pylori* reinfection rate, in patients with cured duodenal ulcer. Am J Gastroenterol 89:529–532

Breuer T, Sudhop T, Hoch J, Sauerbruch T, Malfertheiner P (1996) Prevalence of and risk factors for *Helicobacter pylori* infection in the western part of Germany. Eur J Gastroenterol Hepatol 8:47–52

Cammarota G, Tursi A, Montalto M, Papa A, Veneto G, Bernardi S, Boari A, Colizzi V, Fedeli G, Gasbarrini, G (1996) Role of dental plaque in the transmission of *Helicobacter pylori* infection. J Clin Gastroenterol 22:174–177

Cellini L, Allocati N, Piattelli A, Petrelli I, Fanci P, Dainelli B (1995) Microbiological evidence of *Helicobacter pylori* from dental plaque in dyspeptic patients. Microbiologica 18:187–192

Censini S, Lange C, Xiang ZY, Crabtree JE, Ghiara P, Borodovsky M, Rappuoli R, Covacci A (1996) Cag, a pathogenicity island of *Helicobacter pylori*, encodes type I-specific and disease-associated virulence factors. Proc Natl Acad Sci USA 93:14648–14653

Chow T, Lambert JR, Wahlqvist ML, Hsuhage B (1995) *Helicobacter pylori* in Melbourne Chinese immigrants – evidence for oral-oral transmission via chopsticks. J Gastroenterol Hepatol 10:562–569

Covacci A, Censini S, Bugnoli M, Petracca R, Burroni D, Macchia G, Massone A, Papini E, Xiang ZY, Figura N, Rappuoli R (1993) Molecular characterization of the 128-kDa immunodominant antigen of *Helicobacter pylori* associated with cytotoxicity and duodenal ulcer. Proc Natl Acad Sci USA 90:5791–5795

Cover TL, Dooley CP, Blaser MJ (1990) Characterization of and human serologic response to proteins in *Helicobacter pylori* broth culture supernatants with vacuolizing cytotoxin activity. Infect Immun 58:603–610

Cover TL, Glupczynski Y, Lage AP, Burette A, Tummuru MKR, Perez Perez GI, Blaser MJ (1995) Serologic detection of infection with cagA(+) *Helicobacter pylori* strains. J Clin Microbiol 33:1496–1500

Crabtree JE, Wyatt JI, Sobala GM, Miller G, Tompkins DS, Primrose JN, Morgan AG (1993) Systemic and mucosal humoral responses to *Helicobacter pylori* in gastric cancer. Gut 34:1339–1343

Cullen DJE, Collins BJ, Christiansen KJ, Epis J, Warren JR, Surveyor I, Cullen KJ (1993) When is *Helicobacter pylori* infection acquired? Gut 34:1681–1682

Delaney BC, Hobbs F, Holder R (1996) Association of *Helicobacter pylori* infection with coronary heart disease – eradication of the infection on grounds of cardiovascular risk is not supported by current evidence. Br Med J 312:251–252

Desai HG, Gill HH, Shankaran K, Mehta PR, Prabhu SR (1991) Dental plaque: a permanent reservoir of *Helicobacter pylori*. Scand J Gastroenterol 26:1205–1208

Drumm B, Perez PGI, Blaser MJ, Sherman PM (1990) Intrafamilial clustering of *Helicobacter pylori* infection. N Engl J Med 322:359–363

Dubois A, Fiala N, Hemanackah LM, Drazek ES, Tarnawski A, Fishbein WN, Perez Perez GI, Blaser MJ (1994) Natural gastric infection with *Helicobacter pylori* in monkeys: a model for spiral bacteria infection in humans. Gastroenterology 106:1405–1417

Dye KR, Marshall BJ, Frierson Jr HF, Pambianco DJ, McCallum RW (1990) *Campylobacter pylori* colonizing heterotopic gastric tissue in the rectum. Am J Clin Pathol 93:144–147

Eaton KA, Morgan DR, Krakowka S (1990) Persistence of *Helicobacter pylori* in conventionalized piglets. J Infect Dis 161:1299–1301

Engstrand L, Gustavsson S, Jorgensen A, Schwan A, Scheynius A (1990) Inoculation of barrier-born pigs with *Helicobacter pylori*: a useful animal model for gastritis type B. Infect Immun 58:1763–1768

Eurogast Study (1993) Epidemiology of, and risk factors for, *Helicobacter pylori* infection among 3194 asymptomatic subjects in 17 populations. Gut 34:1672–1676

Ferguson DA, Chuanfu L, Patel NR, Mayberry WR, Chi DS, Thomas E (1993) Isolation of *Helicobacter pylori* from saliva. J Clin Microbiol 31:2802–2804

Figueroa G, Acuna R, Troncoso M, Portell DP, Toledo MS, Albornoz V, Vigneaux J (1996) Low H. pylori reinfection rate after triple therapy in Chilean duodenal ulcer patients. Am J Gastroenterol 91:1395–1399

Fox JG (1994) In vivo models of gastric *Helicobacter* infection. In: Hunt RH, Tytgat GNJ (eds) *Helicobacter pylori*: Basic mechanisms to clinical cure. Kluwer Academic, Dordrecht, pp 3–27

Fox JG (1995) Non-human reservoirs of *Helicobacter pylori*. Aliment Pharmacol Ther 9 [Suppl 2]:93–103

Georgopoulos SD, Mentis AF, Spiliadis CA, Tzouvelekis LS, Tzelepi E, Moshopoulos A, Skandalis N (1996) *Helicobacter pylori* infection in spouses of patients with duodenal ulcers and comparison of ribosomal RNA gene patterns. Gut 39:634–638

Goh KL, Navaratnam P, Peh SC (1996) Reinfection and duodenal ulcer relapse in south-east Asian patients following successful *Helicobacter pylori* eradication – results of a 2-year follow-up. J Gastroenterol Hepatol 8:1157–1160

Graham DY, Alpert LC, Smith JL, Yoshimura HH (1988) Iatrogenic *Campylobacter pylori* infection is a cause of epidemic achlorhydria. Am J Gastroenterol 83:974–980

Graham DY, Malaty HM, Evans DG, Evans DJJ, Klein PD, Adam E (1991a) Epidemiology of *Helicobacter pylori* in an asymptomatic population in the United States. Effect of age, race, and socioeconomic status. Gastroenterology 100:1495–1501

Graham DY, Adam E, Reddy GT, Agarwal JP, Agarwal R, Evans DJ, Malaty HM, Evans DG (1991b) Seroepidemiology of *Helicobacter pylori* infection in India. Comparison of developing and developed countries. Dig Dis Sci 36:1084–1088

Graham DY, Lew GM, Klein PD, Evans DG, Evans DJ, Saeed ZA, Malaty HM (1992) Effect of treatment of *Helicobacter pylori* infection on the long-term recurrence of gastric or duodenal ulcer, a randomized, controlled study. Ann Intern Med 116:705–708

Graham DY, Genta RM, Graham DP, Crabtree JE (1996) Serum cagA antibodies in asymptomatic subjects and patients with peptic ulcer – lack of correlation of IgG antibody in patients with peptic ulcer or asymptomatic *Helicobacter pylori* gastritis. J Clin Pathol 49:829–832

Grasso GM, Ripabelli G, Sammarco ML, Ruberto A, Iannitto G (1996) Prevalence of *Helicobacter*-like organisms in porcine gastric mucosa – a study of swine slaughtered in Italy. Comp Immunol Microbiol Infect Dis 19:213–217

Handt LK, Fox JG, Dewhirst FE, Fraser GJ, Paster BJ, Yan LL, Rozmiarek H, Rufo R, Stalis IH (1994) *Helicobacter pylori* isolated from the domestic cat: public health implications. Infect Immun 62:2367–2374

Handt LK, Fox JG, Stalis IH, Rufo R, Lee G, Linn J, Li XT, Kleanthous H (1995) Characterization of feline *Helicobacter pylori* strains and associated gastritis in a colony of domestic cats. J Clin Microbiol 33:2280–2289

Handt LK, Fox JG, Yan LL, Shen Z, Pouch WJ, Ngai D, Motzel SL, Nolan TE, Klein HJ (1997) Diagnosis of *Helicobacter pylori* infection in a colony of rhesus monkeys (Macaca mulatta). J Clin Microbiol 35:165–168

Hazell SL, Mitchell HM, Hedges M, Shi X, Hu PJ, Li YY, Lee A, Reisslevy E (1994) Hepatitis A and evidence against the community dissemination of *Helicobacter pylori* via feces. J Infect Dis 170:686–689

Heilmann KL, Borchard F (1991) Gastritis due to spiral shaped bacteria other than *Helicobacter pylori*: clinical, histological, and ultrastructural findings. Gut 32:137–140

Hirschl AM, Richter M, Makristathis A, Pruckl PM, Willinger B, Schutze K, Rotter ML (1994) Single and multiple strain colonization in patients with *Helicobacter pylori*-associated gastritis: detection by macrorestriction DNA analysis. J Infect Dis 170:473–475

Hopkins RJ, Vial PA, Ferreccio C, Ovalle J, Prado P, Sotomayor V, Russell RG, Wasserman SS, Morris J (1993) Seroprevalence of *Helicobacter pylori* in Chile – vegetables may serve as one route of transmission. J Infect Dis 168:222–226

Hulten K, Han SW, Enroth H, Klein PD, Opekun AR, Gilman RH, Evans DG, Engstrand L, Graham DY, Elzaatari F (1996) *Helicobacter pylori* in the drinking water in Peru. Gastroenterology 110:1031–1035

IARC (1994) IARC monographs on the evaluation of carcinogenic risks to humans. World Health Organisation, Lyon, pp 177–240

Jones DM, Eldridge J, Fox AJ, Sethi P, Whorwell PJ (1986) Antibody to the gastric *Campylobacter*-like organism ("*Campylobacter pyloridis*") – clinical correlations and distribution in the normal population. J Med Microbiol 22:57–62

Jorgensen M, Daskalopoulos G, Warburton V, Mitchell HM, Hazell, SL (1996) Multiple strain colonization and metronidazole resistance in *Helicobacter pylori*-infected patients – identification from sequential and multiple biopsy specimens. J Infect Dis 174:631–635

Kelly SM, Pitcher MCL, Farmery SM, Gibson GR (1994) Isolation of *Helicobacter pylori* from feces of patients with dyspepsia in the United Kingdom. Gastroenterology 107:1671–1674

Klein PD, Graham DY, Gaillour A, Opekun AR, Smith EO (1991) Water source as risk factor for *Helicobacter pylori* infection in Peruvian children. Gastrointestinal Physiology Working Group. Lancet 337:1503–1506

Krajden S, Fuksa M, Anderson J, Kempston J, Boccia A, Petrea C, Babida C, Karmali M, Penner JL (1989) Examination of human stomach biopsies, saliva, and dental plaque for Campylobacter pylori. J Clin Microbiol 27:1397–1398

Lage AP, Godfroid E, Fauconnier A, Burette A, Goutier S, Butzler JPAB, Glupzynski Y (1995) Frequency of cagA in *Helicobacter pylori* strains isolated from Belgian and Moroccan patients. Gut 37:A69

Lambert JR, Lin SK, Sievert W, Nicholson L, Schembri M, Guest C (1995) High prevalence of *Helicobacter pylori* antibodies in an institutionalized population – evidence for person-to-person transmission. Am J Gastroenterol 90:2167–2171

Lee A, Hazell SL (1988) *Campylobacter pylori* in health and disease: An ecological perspective. Microb Ecol Health Dis 1:1–16

Lee A, Hazell SL, O'Rourke J Kouprach S (1988) Isolation of a spiral-shaped bacterium from the cat stomach. Infect Immun 56:2843–2850

Lee A, O'Rourke JL, Kellow JE (1995) Gastrospirillum hominis ("Helicobacter heilmannii") and other gastric infections in humans. In: Blaser MJ, Smith PD, Ravdin JI, Greenberg HB, Guerrant RL (eds) Infections of the gastrointestinal tract. Raven, New York, pp 589–601

Lin SK, Lambert JR, Schembri MA, Nicholson L, Korman MG (1994) *Helicobacter pylori* prevalence in endoscopy and medical staff. J Gastroenterol Hepatol 9:319–324

Louw JA, Lucke W, Jaskiewicz K, Lastovica AJ, Winter TA, Marks IN (1995) *Helicobacter pylori* eradication in the African setting, with special reference to reinfection and duodenal ulcer recurrence. Gut 36:544–547

Malaty HM, Evans DJ, Abramovitch K, Evans DG, Graham DY (1992) *Helicobacter pylori* infection in dental workers: a seroepidemiology study. Am J Gastroenterol 87:1728–1731

Malaty HM, Engstrand L, Pedersen NL, Graham DY (1994) *Helicobacter pylori* infection: genetic and environmental influences. Ann Intern Med 120:982–986

Malaty HM, Graham DY (1994) Importance of childhood socioeconomic status on the current prevalence of *Helicobacter pylori* infection. Gut 35:742–745

Malaty HM, Kim JG, Kim SD, Graham DY (1996) Prevalence of *Helicobacter pylori* infection in Korean children – inverse relation to socioeconomic status despite a uniformly high prevalence in adults. Am J Epidemiol 143:257–262

Mapstone NP, Lewis FA, Tompkins DS, Lynch DAF, Axon ATR, Dixon MF, Quirke P (1993a) PCR identification of *Helicobacter pylori* in faeces from gastritis patients. Lancet 341:447

Mapstone NP, Lynch DAF, Lewis FA, Axon ATR, Tompkins DS, Dixon MF, Quirke P (1993b) Identification of *Helicobacter pylori* DNA in the mouths and stomachs of patients with gastritis using PCR. J Clin Pathol 46:540–543

Marshall BJ, Armstrong JA, McGechie DB, Glancy RJ (1985) Attempt to fulfill Koch's postulates for pyloric Campylobacter. Med J Aust 142:436-439

McCallion WA, Murray LJ, Bailie AG, Dalzell AM, Oreilly D, Bamford KB (1996) *Helicobacter pylori* infection in children – relation with current household living conditions. Gut 39:18-21

Megraud F (1995) Transmission of *Helicobacter pylori* – faecal-oral versus oral-oral route. Aliment Pharmacol Ther 9 [Suppl 2]:85-91

Megraud F, Brassens Rabbe MP, Denis F, Belbouri A, Hoa DQ (1989) Seroepidemiology of Campylobacter pylori infection in various populations. J Clin Microbiol 27:1870-1873

Mendall MA, Goggin PM, Molineaux N, Levy J, Toosy T, Strachan D, Northfield TC (1992) Childhood living conditions and *Helicobacter pylori* seropositivity in adult life. Lancet 339:896-897

Miehlke S, Kim JG, Small SM, Graham DY, Go MF (1995) Lack of association between the presence of the cagA gene in *Helicobacter pylori* and gastric adenocarcinoma. Gut 37:A77

Mitchell HM (1993) The epidemiology of *Helicobacter pylori* infection and its relation to gastric cancer. In: Goodwin CS, Wormsley BW (eds) *Helicobacter pylori*: biology and clinical practice. CRC Press, Boca Raton, pp 95-114

Mitchell H (1995) *Helicobacter pylori* infection: a clinical viewpoint. In: Gilbert G (eds) Recent advances in microbiology. Australian Society for Microbiology, Melbourne

Mitchell HM, Lee A, Carrick J (1989) Increased incidence of Campylobacter pylori infection in gastroenterologists: further evidence to support person-to-person transmission of C. pylori, Scand J Gastroenterol 24:396-400

Mitchell HM, Li YY, Hu PJ, Liu Q, Chen M, Du GG, Wang ZJ, Lee A, Hazell SL (1992a) Epidemiology of *Helicobacter pylori* in Southern China – identification of early childhood as the critical period for acquisition. J Infect Dis 166:149-153

Mitchell JD, Mitchell HM, Tobias V (1992b) Acute *Helicobacter pylori* infection in an infant, associated with gastric ulceration and serological evidence of intra-familial transmission. Am J Gastroenterol 87:382-386

Mitchell HM, Li Y, Hu P, Hazell SL, Du G, Byrne DJ, Lee A (1992c) The susceptibility of *Helicobacter pylori* to bile may be an obstacle to faecal transmission. Eur J Gastro Hepatol 4 [Suppl 1]:S79-S83

Mitchell HM, Bohane T, Hawkes RA, Lee A (1993) *Helicobacter pylori* infection within families. Zentralbl Bakteriol Int J Med Microbiol 280:128-136

Mitchell HM, Hazell SL, Kolesnikow T, Mitchell J, Frommer D (1996a) Antigen recognition during progression from acute to chronic infection with a cagA-positive strain of *Helicobacter pylori*. Infect Immun 64:1166-1172

Mitchell HM, Hazell SL, Li YY, Hu PJ (1996b) Serological response to specific *Helicobacter pylori* antigens – antibody against cagA antigen is not predictive of gastric cancer in a developing country. Am J Gastroenterol 91:1785-1788

Morris A, Nicholson G, Lloyd A, Haines D, Rogers A, Taylor D (1986) Seroepidemiology of Campylobacter pyloridis. NZ Med J 99:657-659

Murray LJ, Bamford KB, Oreilly D, McCrum EE, Evans AE (1995) *Helicobacter pylori* infection – relation with cardiovascular risk factors, ischaemic heart disease, and social class. Br Heart J 74:497-501

Namavar F, Roosendaal R, Kuipers EJ, Degroot P, Vanderbijl MW, Pena AS, Degraaff J (1995) Presence of *Helicobacter pylori* in the oral cavity, oesophagus, stomach and faeces of patients with gastritis. Eur J Clin Microbiol Infect Dis 14:234-237

Nguyen AMH, Engstrand L, Genta RM, Graham DY, Elzaatari FAK (1993) Detection of *Helicobacter pylori* in dental plaque by reverse transcription polymerase chain reaction. J Clin Microbiol 31:783-787

Nguyen A, Elzaatari F, Graham DY (1995) *Helicobacter pylori* in the oral cavity. Oral Surg Oral Med Oral Pathol Oral Radiol Endodontics 79:705-709

Notarnicola M, Russo F, Cavallini A, Bianco M, Jirillo E, Pece S, Leoci, C, Dimatteo G, Dileo A (1996) PCR identification of *Helicobacter pylori* DNA in faeces from patients with gastroduodenal pathology. Med Sci Res 24:785-787

Parsonnet J, Hansen S, Rodriguez L, Gelb AB, Warnke RA, Jellum E, Orentreich N, Vogelman JH, Friedman GD (1994) *Helicobacter pylori* infection and gastric lymphoma. N Engl J Med 330:1267-1271

Parsonnet J, Friedman GD, Orentreich N, Vogelman H (1997) Risk for gastric cancer in people with CagA positive or CagA negative *Helicobacter pylori* infection. Gut 40:297-301

Patel P, Mendall MA, Khulusi S, Northfield TC, Strachan DP (1994) *Helicobacter pylori* infection in childhood: Risk factors and effect on growth. Br Med J 309:1119-1123

Patel P, Mendall MA, Carrington D, Strachan DP, Leatham E, Molineaux N, Levy J, Blakeston C, Seymour CA, Camm AJ, Northfield TC (1995) Association of *Helicobacter pylori* and Chlamydia pneumoniae infections with coronary heart disease and cardiovascular risk factors. Br Med J 311:711–714

Perez Perez GI, Taylor DN, Bodhidatta L, Wongsrichanalai J, Baze W B, Dunn BE, Echeverria PD, Blaser, MJ (1990) Seroprevalence of *Helicobacter pylori* infections in Thailand. J Infect Dis 161:1237–1241

Perez Perez GI, Witkin SS, Decker MD, Blaser MJ (1991) Seroprevalence of *Helicobacter pylori* infection in couples. J Clin Microbiol 29:642–644

Polish LB, Douglas JMJ, Davidson AJ, Perez Perez, GI, Blaser MJ (1991) Characterisation of risk actors for *Helicobacter pylori* infection among men attending a sexually transmitted disease clinic: lack of evidence for sexual transmission. J Clin Microbiol 29:2139–2143

Pounder RE, Ng D (1995) The prevalence of *Helicobacter pylori* infection in different countries. Aliment Pharmacol Ther 9 [Suppl 2]:33–39

Raedsch R, Pohl S, Plachky J, Stiehl A, Kommerell B (1989) The growth of Campylobacter pylori is inhibited by intragastric bile acids. In: Megraud F, Lamouliatte H (eds) Gastroduodenal pathology and campylobacter pylori. Elsevier, Amsterdam, pp 409–412

Ramsey EJ, Carey KV, Peterson W, Jackson JJ, Murphy FK, Read NWT (1979) Epidemic gastritis with hypochlorhydria. Gastroenterology 76:1449–1457

Rathbone B, Martin D, Stephens J, Thompson JR, Samani NJ (1996) *Helicobacter pylori* seropositivity in subjects with acute myocardial infarction. Heart 76:308–311

Raymond J, Bergeret M, Benhamou PH, Mensah K, Dupont C (1994) A 2-year study of *Helicobacter pylori* in children. J Clin Microbiol 32:461–463

Replogle ML, Kasumi W, Ishikawa KB, Yang SF, Juji T, Miki K, Kabat GC, Parsonnet J (1996) Increased risk of *Helicobacter pylori* associated with birth in wartime and post-war Japan. Int J Epidemiol 25:210–214

Rocha GA, Queiroz DMM, Mendes EN, Oliveira AMR, Moura SB, Silva RJA (1992) Source of *Helicobacter pylori* infection: studies in abattoir workers and pigs. Am J Gastroenterol 87:1525

Rosenstock SJ, Andersen LP, Rosenstock CV, Bonnevie O, Jorgensen T (1996) Socioeconomic factors in *Helicobacter pylori* infection among Danish adults. Am J Public Health 86:1539–1544

Sandifer QD, Lo SV, Crompton G (1996) Association of *Helicobacter pylori* infection with coronary heart disease – association may not be causal. Br Med J 312:

Schutze K, Hentschel E, Dragosics B, Hirschl AM (1995) *Helicobacter pylori* reinfection with identical organisms – transmission by the patients spouses. Gut 36:831–833

Shames B, Krajden S, Fuksa M, Babida C, Penner JL (1989) Evidence for the occurrence of the same strain of Campylobacter pylori in the stomach and dental plaque. J Clin Microbiol 27:2849–2850

Sitas F, Forman D, Yarnell JW, Burr ML, Elwood PC, Pedley S, Marks KJ (1991) *Helicobacter pylori* infection rates in relation to age and social class in a population of Welsh men. Gut 32:25–28

Stolte M, Wellens E, Bethke B, Ritter M, Eidt H (1994) Helicobacter heilmannii (formerly Gastro-spirillum hominis) gastritis: an infection transmitted by animals? Scand J Gastroenterol 29:1061–1064

Teh BH, Lin JT, Pan WH, Lin SH, Wang LY, Lee TK, Chen CJ (1994) Seroprevalence and associated risk factors of *Helicobacter pylori* infection in Taiwan. Anticancer Res 14:1389–1392

Thomas JE, Gibson GR, Darboe MK, Dale A, Weaver LT (1992) Isolation of *Helicobacter pylori* from human faeces. Lancet 340:1194–1195

Tummuru MKR, Cover TL, Blaser MJ (1993) Cloning and expression of a high-molecular-mass major antigen of *Helicobacter pylori* – evidence of linkage to cytotoxin production. Infect Immun 61:1799–1809

Vaira D, D'Anastasio C, Holton J, Dowsett J, Londei M, Salmon P, Gandolfi L (1988) Is *Campylobacter pylori* a zoonosis? Lancet 2:725

Vanzanten SJOV, Pollak PT, Best LM, Bezanson GS, Marrie T (1994) Increasing prevalence of *Helicobacter pylori* infection with age – continuous risk of infection in adults rather than cohort effect. J Infect Dis 169:434–437

Varoli O, Landini MP, LaPlaca M, Tucci A, Corinaldesi R, Paparo GF, Stanghellini V, Barbara L (1991) Presence of *Helicobacter pylori* in gastric juice. Am J Gastroenterol 86:249

Vincent P, Gottrand F, Pernes P, Husson MO, Lecomtehoucke M, Turck D, Leclerc H (1994) High prevalence of *Helicobacter pylori* infection in cohabiting children – epidemiology of a cluster, with special emphasis on molecular typing. Gut 35:313–316

Webb PM, Knight T, Greaves S, Wilson A, Newell DG, Elder J, Forman D (1994) Relation between infection with *Helicobacter pylori* and living conditions in childhood – evidence for person to person transmission in early life. Br Med J 308:750–753

Webb PM, Knight T, Newell DG, Elder JB, Forman D (1996) *Helicobacter pylori* transmission – evidence from a comparison with hepatitis a virus. Eur J Gastroenterol Hepatol 8:439–441

Whitaker CJ, Dubiel AJ, Galpin OP (1993) Social and geographical risk factors in *Helicobacter pylori* infection. Epidemiol Infect 111:63–70

Chronic Gastritis and Nonulcer Dyspepsia

J. Kalantar, G.D. Eslick and N.J. Talley

1 Introduction

The relationship between *Helicobacter pylori* gastritis and non-ulcer dyspepsia (NUD; operationally defined as chronic or recurrent pain or discomfort centred in the upper abdomen in the absence of peptic ulceration) has remained in contention for many years. Recently, increasing data have accumulated that support the null hypothesis that there is no true relationship between *H. pylori* infection and NUD, although there remains healthy scepticism in the scientific community. In this chapter, the epidemiological and pathophysiological data linking gastritis and dyspepsia are reviewed, and the clinical trial evidence is then summarized.

Department of Medicine, University of Sydney, Nepean Hospital, PO Box 63, Penrith NSW 2751 Australia

2 Review of Current Research

2.1 Epidemiology

Dyspepsia is very common in the community, as is *H. pylori* infection (TALLEY et al. 1991). Approximately 25% of the population report recurrent pain or discomfort in the upper abdomen annually; this is reasonably consistent from country to country in the developed world, although comparable data are largely absent from the developing world (TALLEY et al. 1991; KNILL-JONES 1991). Similarly, the prevalence of *H. pylori*, while dependant on age, ethnicity and socioeconomic status, has a prevalence of 20%–50% in developed countries (MEGRAUD et al. 1989). A key question is whether the overlap of *H. pylori* and dyspepsia is causal or coincidental as both conditions are common and could overlap by chance. *H. pylori* gastritis is found in 30%–70% of patients with NUD (LOFFELD et al. 1988; GREENBERG et al. 1990). In a meta-analysis of clinical studies by ARMSTRONG (1996), the relative risk of *H. pylori* infection was 2.3 times higher in patients with NUD than in controls (95%, CI 1.9–2.7). However, there were methodological problems with many of the referral-based studies included; in some studies inappropriate control groups were used. To avoid or minimise referral and selection bias, population-based studies have been conducted to try and determine the 'true' magnitude of the association between *H. pylori* infection and NUD.

One of these studies was conducted on a Swedish population using a postal questionnaire which assessed 1260 adults aged between 20 and 79 years for abdominal and gastrointestinal symptoms; 1097 (87%) responded and a sub-sample of this population (50 symptom free and 100 with dyspepsia or irritable bowel syndrome) was randomly selected to determine whether their *H. pylori* status was associated with any of the 24 abdominal symptoms. The sub-sample was tested for *H. pylori* antibodies (IgG); 55 (38%) were positive for *H. pylori*. The prevalence increased with age but no gender difference was found. In the dyspepsia group (*n* = 49), the prevalence of *H. pylori* infection was 33% which was less than the symptom-free group (*n* = 48), where 48% were positive for *H. pylori*. The major limitation of this study was that it did not apply endoscopy and hence any *H. pylori*-related pathology (particularly peptic ulcer disease) could not be excluded (AGREUS et al. 1995). NANDURKAR et al. (1998) similarly evaluated dyspeptic symptoms using a validated questionnaire in consecutive healthy blood donors. *H. pylori* status was determined by serology. They found that smoking and aspirin use but not *H. pylori* were significant risk factors for dyspepsia but again endoscopy was not employed.

In a Dutch study, healthy employees undergoing periodic medical examination were tested by *H. pylori* serology and filled in a questionnaire regarding dyspeptic symptoms in the preceding 3 months. They found that there was an association between dyspepsia and *H. pylori*, but that this disappeared when subjects with a past history of peptic ulcer disease were excluded. They concluded that the presence of peptic ulcer disease completely accounted for the association of *H. pylori* with dyspepsia in this population (SCHLEMPER et al. 1995).

In an excellent population-based endoscopic study from Norway, all 2027 persons in Sorreisa between 20 and 69 years of age received a questionnaire inquiring about abdominal complaints. Of those sent a questionnaire, 1802 (89%) responded, and 782 subjects were invited to undergo an endoscopy with 619 accepting. A total of 309 subjects were classified as dyspeptic and 310 as nondyspeptic controls. *H. pylori* infection was determined by histology and microbiological culture; 48% of dyspeptic subjects had *H. pylori* infection, compared with 36% of the controls, which was statistically significant ($p = 0.004$). However, after age and gender adjustment, the prevalence of *H. pylori* in dyspeptic subjects and controls with normal endoscopic findings was 53% and 35%, which was reported to be not significant (BERNERSEN et al. 1992) although an unadjusted analysis suggests that this difference is significant (OR 2.07; 95%, CI 1.16–3.71). Overall, if age, socioeconomic status, race and country of origin are taken into account and other diseases such as peptic ulcers excluded, the prevalence of infection with *H. pylori* in NUD may be increased over that of asymptomatic controls but the difference is very small.

2.2 Symptoms and *H. pylori* Status

The specific anatomical location of *H. pylori* makes it conceivable that characteristic symptoms exist for *H. pylori* related pathologies (ARMSTRONG 1996). However, a direct link between symptoms and *H. pylori* has been difficult to demonstrate. Upper gastrointestinal symptoms are likely to be due to many different interactive pathogenic mechanisms, and therefore investigating a single specific factor to try and explain these symptoms may be inadequate.

2.2.1 Symptoms in Peptic Ulcer Disease and *H. pylori*

Peptic ulcer disease (PUD) is unequivocally linked to *H. pylori*, but even in this setting the association with symptoms is not clear cut. Asymptomatic ulceration is a well-described condition. In the population-based study of BERNESEN et al. (1990), 1% had silent ulcers. In clinical trials conducted prior to the *H. pylori* era, ulcer recurrence and symptom recurrence were not always linked (JORDE et al. 1986). Moreover, cure of *H. pylori* in patients with ulcer disease does not always lead to symptom abolition (LABENZ et al. 1997).

2.2.2 Individual Symptoms in Non-ulcer Dyspepsia and *H. pylori*

A consistent pattern of symptoms has not been demonstrable in infected patients with NUD (Table 1). For example, in an Italian study, *H. pylori* infection was present in 107 (62%) of the 174 NUD patients. The only significant symptoms associated with *H. pylori* infection were heartburn and burping (PRETOLANI et al. 1994). In a prospective German study, 149 consecutive NUD patients underwent endoscopy with biopsies taken to evaluate *H. pylori* infection using the rapid urease

Table 1. Symptoms associated with *H. pylori* infection and non-ulcer dyspepsia

Author	*n*	*H. pylori* positive (%)	Symptoms significantly associated with *H. pylori*
MARSHALL and WARREN 1984	65	58	'Burping'
ROKKAS et al. 1987	55	45	Postprandial bloating
ANDERSEN et al. 1988	33	45	Nil
BORSCH et al. 1988	69	52	Absence of flatulence
JEENA et al. 1988	69	78	Nil
LOFFELD et al. 1988	109	56	Nil
RATHBONE et al. 1988	193	54	Oesophageal reflux symptoms
DELTENRE et al. 1989	200	64	Ulcer-like symptoms
GURRE et al. 1989	96	40	Nil
SOBALA et al. 1990	186	41	Nil
STRAUSS et al. 1990	37	60	Nil
VARIA et al. 1990	107	58	Postprandial bloating
COLLINS et al. 1991	18	50	Nil
GOH et al. 1991	71	56	Nil
WALDRON et al. 1991	50	36	Nil
SCHUBERT et al. 1992	474	36	Nil
TUCCI et al. 1992	45	60	Epigastric pain, epigastric burning
HOVELIUS et al. 1994	127	35	Ulcer-like symptoms
KEMMER et al. 1994	149	51	Pain relief after food

test and histology. Seventy-six (51%) of the NUD patients were *H. pylori* positive while 73 (49%) were *H. pylori*-negative. Symptom variables associated with *H. pylori* included fasting pain and absence of diarrhoea, while symptoms of NUD were present at higher intensity in *H. pylori*-positive patients than in *H. pylori*-negative patients (KEMMER et al. 1994). LAI et al. (1996) studied symptoms in 384 NUD patients using a standard questionnaire and *H. pylori* infection was determined by scoring the density of *H. pylori* infection. Only heavy bacterial colonization of the corpus showed a significant association with ulcer-like pain. However, when adjusted for age, no association with ulcer-like pain could be found based on endoscopic findings. While some other studies have reported certain individual symptoms seemed to be associated with dyspepsia (Table 1), this most likely just reflects measurement of large number of symptoms resulting in chance associations being identified (type 1 error).

2.2.3 Dyspepsia Subgroups

The classification of dyspepsia into subgroups in order to identify the underlying pathophysiology aimed to promote identification of pathophysiological links. Early satiety, postprandial discomfort or fullness, bloating and nausea constitute dysmotility-like dyspepsia whereas epigastric pain waking the patient from sleep, worsening with hunger and improving with meals or antacids are part of ulcer-like dyspepsia (TALLEY et al. 1991). On the other hand, symptoms referrable to the esophagus alone, such as acid regurgitation or heartburn, are no longer considered to be a part of dyspepsia, although patients with epigastric distress may concurrently have typical reflux-like symptoms (KLAUSER et al. 1990; TALLEY et al. 1994).

HOLTMANN et al. (1994) evaluated 180 consecutive healthy blood donors; 32% were *H. pylori* positive on serology. They found that 26% of the subjects with *H. pylori* and 24% without *H. pylori* had pain localized to the upper abdomen. The seroprevalence of *H. pylori* was similar among dyspeptic patients who had symptoms suggestive of peptic ulcer disease versus groups with reflux-like or dysmotility-like symptoms (Fig. 1). Similarly, other community-based studies of subjects with NUD (AGREUS et al. 1995; NANDURKAR et al. 1997) have not shown any association between dyspepsia subgroups and *H. pylori* infection, although a treatment response limited to ulcer-like dyspepsia has been identified in some studies (TREPSI et al. 1994; GILVARRY et al. 1997). However, the trial results have been inconsistent, and there have been a lack of uniform methods used to define the subgroups and score the symptoms which limits the external validity of the studies (TALLEY 1994a). Dividing NUD into symptom-based subgroups has not resulted in an association appearing although this in part may be due to the considerable overlap that exists between dyspepsia categories.

2.3 Pathophysiological Mechanisms Linking Dyspepsia and *H. pylori*

If *H. pylori* causes dyspepsia in a subset of patients who are infected, how this might come about in the absence of an ulcer crater is unknown. Here we overview the possible mechanisms.

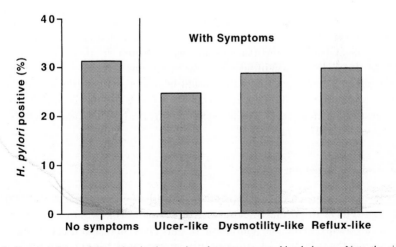

Fig. 1. Seroprevalence of *H. pylori* in dyspepsia subgroups among blood donors. Note the similar prevalence of infection among all groups (With permission from HOLTMANN et al. 1994)

2.3.1 Active Gastritis, Lymphoid Follicles and Inflammatory Mediators

An impressive gastritis characterised by a predominantly neutrophilic infiltration is present in many patients who are infected by *H. pylori*. The inflammatory response of the gastric epithelium to *H. pylori* infection is associated with release of inflammatory mediators (NOACH et al. 1994). Gastric epithelial cells release interleukin (IL) 8 and the interstitial cell adhesion molecule, ICAM1, which leads to the recruitment of neutrophils causing a further inflammatory response (CROWE et al. 1995). Neutrophils also secrete further IL-1β, IL-6 and tumour necrosis factor-■. This recruitment is *H. pylori* strain-dependent; *cagA*- and *vacA*-positive strains produce a more prominent response (CRABTREE et al. 1995). CHING et al. (1996) compared the anti-*cagA* antibody titres in patients with duodenal ulcers (84%), gastric ulcers (80%), NUD (56%) and normal subjects (29%); anti-*cagA* antibody positivity was significantly more frequent in patients with NUD than in asymptomatic healthy controls. HOLTMANN et al. (1998) however observed no such association.

Lymphoid follicles, which are not seen in the normal healthy stomach, develop during infection with *H. pylori* and are seen more frequently in the gastric antrum than the corpus and are also more common in ulcer patients (GENTA et al. 1993). Furthermore, the density of infection is correlated with the number of lymphoid follicles (EIDT et al. 1993). Whether the presence of these follicles is related to symptoms is unknown. Of interest, eradication of *H. pylori* reduces but does not lead to complete resolution of all the lymphoid follicles (GENTA et al. 1993). Could this explain the lack of symptom resolution in some patients with NUD?

If symptoms are due to the associated gastritis, they may not resolve immediately after successful eradication therapy since it may take many months for the chronic gastritis to settle, and thus long-term follow-up is needed to assess the outcome. It has been suggested that an increased neutrophilic response is required for *H. pylori* to cause symptoms (TYTGAT et al. 1991). One study found that the neutrophil density in dyspepsia was higher than in controls, but *H. pylori* status was not determined in this group (TOUKAN et al. 1985) and other studies have not observed an association (JOHNSEN et al. 1991). Moreover, this concept is oversimplistic. If NUD is a condition where the symptoms wax and wane over time it remains difficult to conceive how they could be associated with the activity of the gastritis, which is unlikely to grossly change (TALLEY 1994b). Indeed, *H. pylori*-active gastritis often exists in totally asymptomatic healthy individuals (O'MORAIN and BUCKLEY 1993).

2.3.2 Acid Dysregulation

Gastrin levels are increased in patients infected with *H. pylori* (LEVI et al. 1989) and their level returns to normal after successful treatment (PREWETT et al. 1991). The mechanism seems to be the inhibition of the D (somatostatin-producing) cell; by reducing the secretion of somatostatin, uninhibited gastrin secretion occurs (HARUMA et al. 1992).

Basal and peak acid outputs in patients with NUD, regardless of their *H. pylori* status, is comparable to healthy controls. However, an important study from Scotland demonstrated that half of the patients with NUD had an abnormal secretory response based on injecting gastrin-releasing peptide (GRP) (EL OMAR et al. 1995). GRP acts on the D cell in addition to the G (gastrin-producing) cell, and thus its use has the advantage of providing a more physiological postprandial response. The clinical relevance of acid dysregulation, however, remains to be determined.

KANEKO et al. (1993) compared somatostatin, substance P and calcitonin gene-related levels in dyspeptic patients with NUD (ulcer-like and dysmotility-like) and patients with peptic ulcers and healthy controls. They observed significantly higher somatostatin levels in the ulcer-like NUD group than in the other groups. Substance P was also higher in the ulcer-like dyspepsia group than in the peptic ulcer group, but there was no difference in the levels of calcitonin gene-related peptide. These findings suggest that different subgroups of dyspepsia may have different gastrointestinal-hormone concentrations in the gastric mucosa that might account for symptom outcome.

2.3.3 Gastroduodenal Dysmotility and Sensory Disturbances

There are a lack of convincing data that gastric motor function is related to *H. pylori* status in NUD (Table 2). While studies have disagreed, most suggest that gastric emptying is not affected. MURAKAMI et al. (1995) reported improved function and symptoms after *H. pylori* eradication in patients with delayed gastric emptying and dyspepsia, whereas QVIST et al. (1994) did not observe any changes in motility post-treatment. Follow-up and subject numbers, however, have been inadequate in the studies to date.

On the other hand, whether *H. pylori* can alter sensory function is not as well determined. A small Spanish study found no significant differences in gastric sensory thresholds between infected and uninfected dyspeptic patients using a barostat balloon placed in the gastric fundus, but there was a non-significant tendency for infected patients to be more sensitive (MEARIN et al. 1995). Duodenal sensory thresholds were also similar in infected and uninfected cases in another study although those with higher *H. pylori* antibody titres had a more sensitive duodenum (HOLTMANN et al. 1996).

3 Clinical Implications

3.1 Treatment Trials

If *H. pylori* is implicated in the pathogenesis of NUD, one would assume that there would be an improvement in symptoms among patients with *H. pylori*-positive

Table 2. Gastrointestinal motility in functional dyspepsia and *H. pylori* infection

Author	Abnormality
Delayed	
MOORE et al. 1986	Postprandial antral hypomotility in chronic gastritis. *H. pylori* not assessed
STANGHELLINI et al. 1992	Fasting and postprandial antral hypomotility in ulcer and non-ulcer dyspeptic patients. *H. pylori* not assessed
MEARIN et al. 1995	Postrprandial antral hypomotility in *H. pylori* infected patients
No difference	
CABALLERO-PLASENCIA et al. 1995	Delayed gastric emptying of solids not related to dyspepsia symptoms or *H. pylori* status
WEGNER et al. 1988	No significant difference among *H. pylori*-infected and uninfected patients
BARNETT et al. 1989	Normal gastric emptying in *H. pylori*-infected patients
TUCCI et al. 1992	Normal gastric emptying in *H. pylori*-infected patients
PIERAMICO et al. 1983	Antral motility not significantly different in *H. pylori*-infected and uninfected patients
MINOCHA et al. 1994	Gastric emptying similar in functional dyspepsia patients regardless of their *H. pylori* status
GILJA et al. 1996	Impaired postprandial proximal gastric accommodation. *H. pylori* did not influence the emptying fractions
Accelerated	
CALDWELL et al. 1992	Accelerated gastric emptying in *H. pylori*-infected patients

NUD after cure of *H. pylori* and resolution of the associated inflammation. A number of therapeutic trials now published or presented in preliminary form have tried to test the hypothesis that cure of *H. pylori* relieves symptoms. It has been surprisingly difficult to test this hypothesis. TALLEY (1994a) analysed 16 published trials; 8 reported that benefit was derived from *H. pylori* treatment, and 8 failed to detect a statistically significant benefit, but there were limitations in all of these studies. Early studies utilising bismuth compounds may have suffered from observer bias, since these compounds cause blackening of the stools and tongue; use of placebo compounds which blacken the stool may be useful in future trials (YATES et al. 1992). Furthermore, bismuth may independently reduce symptoms even in *H. pylori*-negative individuals (ROKKAS et al. 1987). Assessment of dyspeptic symptoms has been another flawed area; the symptom scores applied have not in general been validated for the relevant patient population. After eradication of *H. pylori* it may take many months for the associated gastritis to resolve (VALLE et al. 1991), and lack of adequate post-treatment follow-up may have led to failure to identify a beneficial result of treatment in patients with NUD.

Results from the most recent randomized controlled trials that applied reasonable follow-up after active *H. pylori* treatment have still produced mixed results, although currently there are more negative than positive studies (Table 3). In a preliminary study from Canada, *H. pylori*-positive patients with NUD were ran-

Table 3. Randomized controlled trials of clinical efficacy of *H. pylori* eradication in patients with non-ulcer dyspepsia with more than six months follow-up (1995–1997)

Author	Treatment	n	Time to follow up (months)	Results
VEDHUYZEN VAN ZANTEN et al. 1995	BSS+AMO+MTZ	53	6	NS[a]
LAZZARONI et al. 1996	CBS+MTZ vs CBS +Placebo	41	6	$p < 0.05$[b]
SCHUTZE et al. 1996	CLR+RAN	54	12	NS[b]
CUCCHIARA et al. 1996	CBS+TIN+AMO 1 week vs 4 weeks	64	6	NS[b]
GREENBERG et al. 1996	CLR+OME	33	12	NS[a]
SHEU et al. 1996	CBS+AMO+MTZ vs H$_2$ blocker	41	12	$p < 0.01$[c]
GILVARRY et al. 1997	CBS+MTZ+TET vs CBS+placebo	100	12	$p < 0.01$[c]
TALLEY et al. 1998	OME+CLR+AMO	275	12	NS[a]
BLUM et al. 1998	OME+CLR+AMO	328	12	NS
McCOLL et al. 1998	OME+CLR+MTZ	300	12	$p < 0.01$

[a] Patients with active treatment vs. placebo.
[b] Patients with *H. pylori* eradicated vs. those with persistent infection or with persistent and current infections.
[c] Patients with *H. pylori* eradicated vs. those receiving other active therapy.

BSS, Bismuth subsalicylate; MTZ, metronidazole; CLR, clarithromycin; RAN, ranitidine; AMO, amoxycillin; CBS, colloidal bismuth subcitrate; TIN, tinidazole; OME, omeprazole; NS, not significant.

domized to triple therapy, with an eradication rate of 96% (n = 29), or placebo (n = 24). No significant difference in symptom improvement was found over the 6-month follow-up (VEDHUYZEN VAN ZANTEN et al. 1995). SCHUTZE et al. (1996) observed symptom improvement after double therapy with clarithromycin and ranitidine, but this was independent of *H. pylori* status with return of symptoms in both infected and eradicated groups at 1-one year follow-up.

In contrast, in another randomized H_2 blocker controlled study from Hong Kong, patients who had *H. pylori* eradicated had significantly improved symptoms compared with those without eradication at two months (SHEU et al. 1996). Moreover, symptom improvement was significantly greater in patients who had *H. pylori* eradication than in patients who had *H. pylori* infection and received a H_2 blocker at 6 and 12 months after the therapy (SHEU et al. 1996). Two other studies have supported this finding. LAZZARONI et al. (1996) showed that symptoms improved at 8 weeks both in patients with and without eradication, but improvement was continued only in patients with eradication, and worsening of symptoms was reported in patients with persistent infection. No association between symptom improvement and dyspepsia subgroups (i.e. ulcer-like or dysmotility-like dyspepsia) was observed. GILVARRY et al. (1997) randomized patients with NUD to receive bismuth based triple therapy versus bismuth and placebo, and found symptom improvement at 2, 6 and 12 months after successful *H. pylori* eradication in both groups; those who remained *H. pylori* positive did not have significant symptom

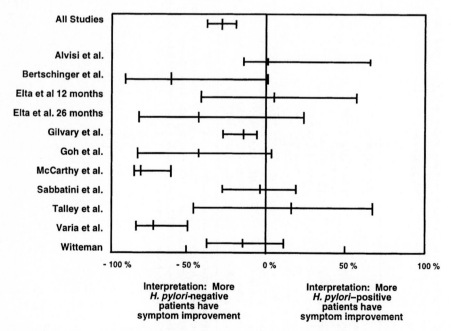

Fig. 2. Meta-analysis of eradication of *H. pylori* in non-ulcer dyspepsia. (With permission from LAHEIJ et al. 1996)

improvement. In *H. pylori* eradicated patients, symptom improvement was observed at all intervals in ulcer-like dyspepsia, but only at 2 and 6 months and not at
12 months in reflux-like or dysmotility-like dyspepsia.

A recent meta-analysis has suggested that eradication of infection does
produce a significant therapeutic gain (LAHEIJ et al. 1996). Overall, symptoms
improved in 73% or the patients who became *H. pylori*-negative and in 45% of
those with persistent infection. If eradication of *H. pylori* failed, symptoms only
improved for a short period of time, but when *H. pylori* was eradicated, symptom
improvements were more pronounced. However, only 10 our of 34 studies could be
included in this analysis for methodological reasons, and thus there is the potential
for a misleading result (Fig. 2).

4 Conclusion

It is not established that *H. pylori* is causally linked to NUD. Recent studies, which
have been the most rigorous randomized controlled trials to date and have included
12 months follow-up, have not settled the controversy; two were negative (TALLEY
et al. 1998; BLUM et al. 1998) and one was positive (McCOLL et al. 1998). Despite
the paucity of convincing evidence, the EUROPEAN HELICOBACTER PYLORI STUDY
GROUP (1997) has recently recommended *H. pylori* eradication therapy in all
infected patients with NUD who have no other obvious cause for their symptoms.
However, the optimal management for these patients is not as yet well enough
defined to support this view.

References

Agreus L, Engstrand L, Svardsudd K, Nyren O, Tibblin G (1995) *Helicobacter pylori* seropositivity
among Swedish adults with and without abdominal symptoms. A population-based epidemiologic
study. Scand J Gastroenterol 30:752–757
Andersen LP, Elsborg L, Justesen T (1988) *Campylobacter pylori* in peptic ulcer disease. III. Symptoms
and paraclinical and epidemiological findings. Scand J Gastroenterol 23:344–350
Armstrong D (1996) *Helicobacter pylori* infection and dyspepsia. Scand J Gastroenterol 31 [Suppl
215]:38–47
Barnett JL, Behler EM, Appelman HD, Etta GH (1989) *Campylobacter pylori* is not associated with
gastroparesis. Dig Dis Sci 34:1677–1680
Bernersen B, Johnsen R, Bostad L, Straume B, Sommer A-I, Burhol PG (1992) Is *Helicobacter pylori* the
cause of dyspepsia? BMJ 304:1276–1279
Bernersen B, Johnsen R, Straume B, Burhol PG, Jenssen TG, Stakkevold PA (1990) Towards a true
prevalence of peptic ulcer: the Sorreisa gastrointestinal disorder study. Gut 31(9):989–992
Blum AL, Talley NJ, O'Morain C et al. Does eradication of *H. pylori* cure dyspeptic symptoms in patients
with functional dyspepsia 12 months after cessation of treatment? Digestion 1998; 59 (Suppl 3):
A2073
Borsch G, Schmidt G, Wegner M, Sandmann M, Adamek R, Leverkus F et al. (1988) *Campylobacter
pylori*: prospective analysis of clinical and histological factors associated with colonization of the
upper gastrointestinal tract. Eur J Clin Invest 18:133–138

Caballero-Plasencia AM, Muros-Navarro MC, Martin-Ruiz JL et al. (1995) Dyspeptic symptoms and gastric emptying of solids in patients with functional dyspepsia. Scand J Gastroenterol 30:745–751

Caldwell SH, Valenzeula G, Marshall BJ et al. (1992) *Helicobacter pylori* infection and gastric emptying of solids in humans. J Gastrointest Mot 4:113–117

Ching CK, Wong BCY, Kwok E, Ong L, Covacci A, Lam SK (1996) Prevalence of CagA-bearing strains detected by the anti-CagA assay in patients with peptic ulcer disease and in controls. Am J Gastroenterol 91:949–953

Collins JSA, Hamilton PW, Watt PCH, Sloan JM, Love AHG (1989) Superficial gastritis and *Campylobacter pylori* in dyspeptic patients – a quantitative study using computer-linked image analysis. J Pathol 158:303–310

Collins JSA, Knill-Jones RP, Sloan JM et al. (1991) A comparison of symptoms between non-ulcer dyspepsia patients positive and negative for *Helicobacter pylori*. Ulster Med J 60:21–27

Crabtree JE, Covacci A, Farmery SM, Xiang Z, Tompkins DS, Perry S et al. (1995) *Helicobacter pylori* induces interleukin-8 expression in gastric epithelial cells in association with Cag A positive phenotype. J Clin Pathol 48:41–45

Crowe SE, Alvarez L, Dytoc M et al. (1995) Expression of interleukin 8 and CD54 by human gastric epithelium *Helicobacter pylori* infection in vitro. Gastroenterology 108:65–74

Cucchiara S, Salvia G, Az-Zeqeh N, D'Armiento F, DePetra MR, Rapagiolo S, Campanozzi A, Emiliano M (1996) *Helicobacter pylori* gastritis and non-ulcer dyspepsia in childhood. Efficacy of one-week triple antimicrobial therapy in eradicating the organism. Ital J Gastroenterol 28:430–435

Cupella F, Alessio I, Intropido L, Pozzi V, Einaudi E, Possi U (1991) Dyspepsia ed infezione do *Helicobacter pylori*. Studio su una popolazione di lavatori. G Ital Med Lav 13:81–84

Deltenre M, Nyst J-F, Jonas C, Glupczynski Y, Deprez C, Burette A (1989) Donnees cliniques, endoscopiques et histologiques chez 1100 patients dont 574 colonises par *Campylobacter pylori*. Gastroenterol Clin Biol 13:89–95B

Eidt S, Stolte M (1993) Prevalence of lymphoid follicles and aggregates in *Helicobacter pylori* gastritis in antral and body mucosa. J Clin Pathol 46:832–835

El Omar E, Penman ID, Ardill JES, McColl KEL (1995) A substantial proportion of non-ulcer dyspepsia patients have the same abnormality of acid secretion as duodenal ulcer patients. Gut. 36:534–538

Genta RM, Hamner HW, Graham DY (1993) Gastric lymphoid follicles in *Helicobacter pylori* infection: frequency, distribution, and response to triple therapy. Hum Pathol 26:1057–1065

Gilja OH, Hausken T, Wilhelmsen I, Berstad A (1996) Impaired accommodation of proximal stomach to a meal in functional dyspepsia. Dig Dis Sci 41:689–696

Gill HH, Desai HG, Majmudar P, Mehta PR, Prabhu SR (1993) Epidemiology of *Helicobacter pylori*: the Indian scenario. Ind J Gastroenterol 12:9–11

Gilvarry J, Buckley M, Beattie, Hamilton H, O'Morain C (1997) Eradication of *Helicobacter pylori* affects symptoms in non-ulcer dyspepsia. Scand J Gastroenterol 32:535–540

Goh KL, Parasakthi N, Peh SC, Wong NW, Lo YL, Puthucheary SD (1991) *Helicobacter pylori* infection and non-ulcer dyspepsia: the effect of treatment with colloidal bismuth subcitrate. Scand J Gastroenterol 26:1123–1131

Greenberg PD, Cello JP (1996) Prospective, double-blind treatment of *Helicobacter pylori* in patients with non-ulcer dyspepsia (abstract). Gastroenterology 110:108A

Greenberg RE, Bank S (1990) The prevalence of *Helicobacter pylori* in nonulcer dyspepsia. Importance of stratification according to age. Arch Intern Med 150:2053–2055

Gurre J, Berthe Y, Chaussade S, Merite F, Gaudric M, Tulliez M, Deslignieres S, Zone A (1989) Has *Campylobacter pylori* gastritis a specific clinical symptomatology? Klin Wochenschr 67 [Suppl XVIII]:25

Gutierrez D, Sierra F, Gomez MC, Camargo H (1988) *Campylobacter pylori* in chronic environmental gastritis and duodenal ulcer patients. Gastroenterology 94:A163

Hansen IM, Axelsson CK, Lundborg CJ (1988) Distribution of *Campylobacter pylori* in dyspeptic and non-dyspeptic gastroenterologic patients. Dan Med Bull 35:2825

Haruma K, Sumii K, Okamato S, Yoshiraha M, Tari A et al. (1992) *Helicobacter pylori* causes low antral somatostatin content: pathogenesis of inappropriate hypergastrinaemia. Gastroenterology A80

Holtmann G, Goebell H, Holtmann M, Talley NJ (1994) Dyspepsia in healthy blood donors: pattern of symptoms and association with *Helicobacter pylori*. Dig Dis Sci 39:1090–1098

Holtmann G, Talley NJ, Mitchell H, Hazell S. Antibody response to specific *H. pylori* antigens in functional dyspepsia, duodenal ulcer disease, and health. Am J Gastroenterol 1998; 93:1222–7

Holtmann G, Talley NJ, Goebell H (1996) Association between *H. pylori*, duodenal mechanosensory thresholds, and small intestinal motility in chronic unexplained dyspepsia. Dig Dis Sci 41:1285–1291

Hovelius B, Anderson SI, Hagander B, Mostad S, Reimers P, Sperlich E et al. (1994) Dyspepsia in general practice: history and symptoms in relation to *Helicobacter pylori* serum antibodies. Scand J Gastroenterol 29:506–510

Inouye H, Yamamoto I, Tanida N (1989) *Campylobacter pylori* in Japan: bacteriological features and prevalence in healthy subjects and patients with gastroduodenal disorders. Gastroenterol Jpn 24:494–504

Jeena CP, Simjee AE, Pettengall KE et al. (1988) Comparison of symptoms in *Campylobacter pylori* positive and negative patients presenting with dyspepsia for upper gastrointestinal endoscopy (abstract). S Afr Med J 73:659

Johnsen R, Bernersen B, Straume B, Forder OH, Bostad L, Burhol PG (1991) Prevalences of endoscopic and histological findings in subjects with and without dyspepsia. BMJ 302:749–752

Jorde R, Bostad L, Burhol PG (1986) Asymptomatic gastric ulcer: a follow-up study in patients with previous gastric ulcer disease. Lancet 1:119–121

Kaneko H, Mitsuma T, Uchida K, Furusawa A, Morise K (1993) Immunoreactive-somatostatin, substance p, and calcitonin gene-related peptide concentration of the human gastric mucosa in patients with nonulcer dyspepsia and peptic ulcer disease. Am J Gastroenterol 88:898–904

Katelaris PH, Tippett GHK, Norbu P, Lowe DG, Brennan R, Farthing MJG (1992) Dyspepsia, *Helicobacter pylori* and peptic ulcer in a randomly selected population in India. Gut 33:1462–1466

Kemmer TP, Domingo-Munoz JE, Klingel H, Zemmler T, Kuhn K, Malfertheiner P (1994) The association between non-ulcer dyspepsia and *Helicobacter pylori* infection. Eur J Gastroenterol Hepatol 6:571–577

Klauser AG, Schindlbeck NE, Muller Lissner SA (1990) Symptoms in gastro-oesophageal reflux disease. Lancet 335:295–298

Knill-Jones RP (1991) Geographical differences in the prevalence of dyspepsia. Scand J Gastroenterol 26 [Suppl 182]:17–24

Labenz J, Blum AL, Bayerdorffer E, Meining A, Stolte M, Borsch G (1997) Curing *Helicobacter pylori* infection in patients with duodenal ulcer may provoke reflux esophagitis. Gastroenterology 112:1442–1447

Laheij RJF, Jansen JBMJ, Van Da Lisnok EH, Severens JL, Verbeek ALM (1996) Review article: symptom improvement through eradication of *Helicobacter pylori* in patients with non-ulcer dyspepsia. Aliment Pharmacol Ther 10:843–850

Lai ST, Fung KP, Ng FH, Lee KC (1996) A quantitative analysis of symptoms of non-ulcer dyspepsia as related to age, pathology and *Helicobacter pylori* infection. Scand J Gastroenterol 31:1078–1082

Lambert JR, Dunn K, Borromeo M, Korman MG, Hansky J (1989) *Campylobacter pylori* – a role in non-ulcer dyspepsia? Scand J Gastroenterol 24 [Suppl 160]:7–13

Lazzaroni M, Bargigga S, Sangaletti O, Maconi G, Boldorini M, Bianchi Aporro G (1996) Eradication of *Helicobacter pylori* and long-term outcome of functional dyspepsia. A clinical endoscopic study. Dig Dis Sci 41:1589–1594

Levi S, Beardshall K, Swift I et al. (1989) Antral *Helicobacter pylori*, hypergastrinaemia and duodenal ulcer: effect of eradication the organism. Br Med J 299:1504–1505

Loffeld RJLF, Potters HVPJ, Arends JW, Stobberingh E, Flendrig JA (1988) Campylobacter associated gastritis in patients with non-ulcer dyspepsia. J Clin Pathol 41:85–88

Marshall BJ, Warren JR (1984) Unidentified curved bacilli in the stomach of patients with gastritis and peptic ulceration. Lancet 1:1311–1315

McColl KEL, Murray LS, El-Omar E et al. (1998) UK-MRC trial of *H. pylori* eradication therapy for non-ulcer dyspepsia. Gut 42 (Suppl):A3

Mearin F, de Ribot X, Balboa A et al. (1995) Does *Helicobacter pylori* infection increase gastric sensitivity in functional dyspepsia? Gut 37:47–51

Megraud F, Brassens-Rabbe MP, Denis F, Belbouri A, Hoa DQ (1989) Seroepidemiology of *Campylobacter pylori* infection in various populations. J Clin Micro 27:1870–1873

Minocha A, Mokshagundam S, Gallo S, Singh Rahal P (1994) Alteration in upper gastrointestinal motility in *Helicobacter pylori*-positive nonulcer dyspepsia. Am J Gastroenterol 89:1797–1800

Moore SC, Malagelada J-R, Shorter RG, Zinsmeister AR (1986) Interrelationships among gastric mucosal morphology, secretion, and motility in peptic ulcer disease. Dig Dis Sci 31:673–684

Mukhopadhyay DK, Tandon RK, Dasarathy S, Mathur M, Wali JP (1992) A study of *Helicobacter pylori* in north Indian subjects with non-ulcer dyspepsia. Ind J Gastroenterol 11:76–79

Murakami K, Fucoda T, Shiota K, Ito A, Fujiyama K, Kodama R, Kawasaki Y, Kubota T, Nasu M (1995) Influence of infection and the effect of its eradication on gastric emptying in non-ulcerative dyspepsia. Eur J Gastroenterol Hepatol 1:S93–S97

Nandurkar S, Talley NJ, Xia HH-X, Mitchell H, Hazel S, Jones M (1998) Dyspepsia in the community is linked to smoking and aspirin use but not to *Helicobacter pylori*. Infection. Arch Intern Med 158:1427–33

Noach LA, Bosma NM, Jansen J, Hock FJ, van Deventer SJH, Tytgat GNT (1994) Mucosal tumour necrosis factor-a, interleukin-1b, and interleukin-8 production in patients with *Helicobacter pylori* infection. Scand J Gastroenterol 29:425–429

O'Morain CA, Buckley M (1993) H pylori in asymptomatic people. In: Hunt RH, Tytgat GNJ (eds) *Helicobacter pylori*: basic mechanisms to clinical cure. Kluwer Academic, Dordecht, pp 423–420

Pettross CW, Appleman MD, Cohen H, Valenzuela JE, Chandrasoma P, Laine LA (1988) Prevalence of *Campylobacter pylori* and association with antral mucosal histology in subjects with and without upper gastrointestinal symptoms. Dig Dis Sci 33:649–653

Pieramico O, Ditshuneit H, Malfertheiner P (1983) Gastrointestinal motility in patients with non-ulcer dyspepsia: a role of *Helicobacter pylori* infection? Am J Gastroenterol 88:364–368

Pretolani S, Bonvicini F, Brocchi E, Baraldini M, Cilla D, Baldinelli S, Bazzocchi E, Pasini P, Gasbarrini G (1994) Nonulcer dyspepsia and *Helicobacter pylori*: effect of eradication on symptoms and gastritis. In: Gasbarrini G, Pretolani S (eds) Basic and clinical aspects of helicobacter pylori infection. Springer, Berlin Heidelberg New York

Prewett EJ, Smith JFL, Nivokolo CU, Hudson M, Sawyerr AM, Pounder RE (1991) Eradication of *Helicobacter pylori* associated 24 hour hypergastrinaemia: a prospective study in healthy subjects. Aliment Pharmacol Ther 5:283–290

Qvist N, Ramussen L, Axelsson CK (1994) Associated gastritis and dyspepsia. The influence on migrating motor complexes. Scand J Gastroenterol 29:133–137

Rathbone BJ, Wyatt J, Heatley RV (1988) Symptomatology in C pylori-positive and – negative non-ulcer dyspepsia. Gut 29:A1473

Rauws EAJ, Langenberg W, Houthoff HJ, Zanen HC, Tytgat GNJ (1988) *Campylobacter pylori* dis-associated chronic active antral gastritis. A prospective study of its prevalence and the effects of antibacterial and antiulcer treatment. Gastroenterology 94:33–40

Rokkas T, Pursey C, Uzoechina E et al. (1987) *Campylobacter pylori* and non-ulcer dyspepsia. Am J Gastroenterol 82:1149–1152

Schlemper RJ, van der Werf SDJ, Vandenbroucke JP, Biemond I, Lamers CBHW (1995) Nonulcer dyspepsia in a Dutch working population and *Helicobacter pylori*. Arch Intern Med 155:82–87

Schubert TT, Schubert AB, Ma CK (1992) Symptoms, gastritis, and *Helicobacter pylori* in patients referred for endoscopy. Gastrointest Endosc 38:357–360

Schutze K, Hentschel E, Hirschl AM (1996) Clarithromycin or amoxycillin plus high-dose ranitidine in the treatment of *Helicobacter pylori*-positive functional dyspepsia. Eur J Gastroenterol Hepatol 8:41–46

Sheu B-S, Lin C-Y, Lin X-Z, Shiesh S-C, Yang H-B, Chen C-Y (1996) Long-term outcome of triple therapy in H pylori-related nonulcer dyspepsia: a prospective controlled assessment. Am J Gastroenterol 91:441–447

Sobala GM, Dixon MF, Axon ATR (1990) Symptomatology of *Helicobacter pylori*-associated dyspepsia. Eur J Gastroenterol Hepatol 2:445–449

Stanghellini V, Ghidini C, Ricci Maccarini M et al. (1992) Fasting and postprandial gastrointestinal motility in ulcer and non-ulcer dyspepsia. Gut 33:184–190

Strauss RM, Wang TC, Kelsey PB, Compton CC, Ferraro M-J, Perez-Perez G et al. (1990) Association of *Helicobacter pylori* infection with dyspeptic symptoms in patients undergoing gastroduodenoscopy. Am J Med 89:464–469

Talley NJ (1994a) A critique of therapeutic trials in *Helicobacter pylori*-positive functional dyspepsia. Gastroenterology 106:1174–1183

Talley NJ (1994b) Why do functional gastrointestinal disorders come and go? Dig Dis Sci 39:673–677

Talley NJ, Colin-Jones D, Koch KL, Koch M, Nyren O, Stanghellini V (1991) Functional dyspepsia: a classification with guidelines for diagnosis and management. Gastroenterol Int 4:145–160

Talley NJ, Zinsmeister AR, Schleck CD, Melton LJ (1994) Smoking, alcohol, and analgesics in dyspepsia and among dyspepsia subgroups: lack of an association in a community. Gut 35:619–624

Talley NJ, Janssens J, Lauritsen K et al. Long term follow-up of patients with non-ulcer dyspepsia after *Helicobacter pylori* eradication. A randomized double-blind placebo-controlled trial. Gastroenterology 1998; 114:A305

The European *Helicobacter pylori* Study Group (1997) Current European concepts in the management of the *Helicobacter pylori* infection. The Maastricht Consensus Report. Gut 40: (in press)

Toukan AU, Kamal MF, Amr SS, Arnaout MA, Abu-Romiyeh AS (1985) Gastroduodenal inflammation in patients with non-ulcer dyspepsia: a controlled endoscopic and morphometric study. Dig Dis Sci 30:313–320

Trespi E, Broglia F, Villani L, Luinetti O, Fiocca R, Solcia E (1994) Distinct profiles of gastritis in dyspepsia subgroups. Their different clinical responses to gastritis healing after *Helicobacter pylori* eradication. Scand J Gastroenterol 29:884–888

Tucci A, Corinaldesi R, Stanghellini V, Tosetti C di Febo G, Paparo F, et al. (1992) *Helicobacter pylori* infection and gastric function in patients with chronic idiopathic dyspepsia. Gastroenterology 103:768–774

Tytgat GNJ, Noach LA, Rauws EAJ (1991) Is gastroduodenitis a cause of chronic dyspepsia? Scand J Gastroenterol 26 [Suppl 182]:33–39

Vaira D, Holton J, Osborn J et al. (1990) Endoscopy in dyspeptic patients: Is gastric mucosal biopsy useful? Am J Gastroenterol 85:701–704

Valle J, Seppala K, Sipponen O, Kosunen T (1991) Disappearance of gastritis after eradication of *Helicobacter pylori*: a morphometric study. Scand J Gastroenterol 26:1057–1065

Vedhuyzen van Zanten, Malatjilian D, Tanton R, Leddin D, Hunt RH, Blanchard W et al. (1995) The effect of eradication of H pylori on symptoms of nonulcer dyspepsia: a randomized double-blind placebo controlled trial. Gastroenterology 108:A250

Waldron B, Cullen PT, Kumar R et al. (1991) Evidence for hypomotility in non-ulcer dyspepsia: a prospective multifactorial study. Gut 32:246–251

Wegner M, Borsch G, Schaffstein J, Schulze-Flake C, Mai U, Leverkus F (1988) Are dyspeptic symptoms in patients with *Campylobacter pylori*-associated type B gastritis linked to delayed gastric emptying? Am J Gastroenterol 83:737–740

Wilhelmsen I, Tangen Haug T, Sipponen P, Berstad A (1994) *Helicobacter pylori* in functional dyspepsia and normal controls. Scand J Gastroenterol 29:522–527

Yates S, Barnett C, Peterson WL (1992) Enteric coated charcoal as a means of blinding studies comparing bismuth and H$_2$-receptor antagonist. Am J Gastroenterol 87:981–984

The Role of *Helicobacter pylori* Infection in Duodenal and Gastric Ulcer

S.J.O. Veldhuyzen van Zanten[1] and A. Lee[2]

1 Introduction

There now is unequivocal evidence that *Helicobacter pylori* is the *principal etiological factor* in duodenal ulcer disease (RABENEK 1991; VELDHUYZEN VAN ZANTEN 1994a). *H. pylori* is also recognized as an important cause of gastric ulcers (KUIPERS 1995a). In this review we evaluate the epidemiological evidence that *H. pylori* is associated with both duodenal and gastric ulcers. We also review current thinking about the pathophysiological mechanisms by which duodenal or gastric ulcers form.

[1] Division of Gastroenterology, Dalhousie University, Queen Elizabeth II Health Sciences Centre, Victoria General Hospital Site, 1278 Tower Road, Halifax, N.S., B3H 2Y9, Canada
[2] School of Microbiology and Immunology, University of New South Wales, Sydney, Australia

2 *Helicobacter* and Duodenal Ulcer

The epidemiological evidence linking *H. pylori* to duodenal ulcer is as follows:

- 90% of duodenal ulcers are *H. pylori* positive.
- Presense of gastritis is a risk factor for duodenal ulcer and for ulcer relapse.
- Cure of *H. pylori* infection leads to a dramatic reduction in ulcer relapse rate.
- Addition of antibiotics to acid suppressive thearpy increases the speed of healing of acute ulcer.
- Smoking is no longer a risk factor for ulcer recurrence after cure of *H. pylori* infection.

The prevalence of *H. pylori* in duodenal ulcer is greater than 90%, and in gastric ulcer 70%–80% (TYTGAT 1990; KUIPERS 1995a). Histological evidence of gastritis is a risk factor for duodenal and gastric ulcers and also for ulcer relapse (HUI 1991; SIPPONEN 1990). It is important to point out that *H. pylori*-negative duodenal ulcers do exist. Use of non-steroidal anti-inflammatory drug (NSAIDs) is the commonest cause of *H. pylori*-negative ulcers (BORODY 1991; LAINE 1992). *H. pylori* is a necessary but not sufficient cause of duodenal ulcer formation. Acid is clearly needed (GRAHAM 1989; FELDMAN 1991). BARON in 1963 in a meticulous study of acid secretion showed that the minimal amount of acid output that is required to develop a duodenal ulcer is 15 mEq/h in males and 18 mEq/h in females (BARON 1963). The most compelling evidence that *H. pylori* is important in duodenal ulcer development is the now accepted fact that eradication of *H. pylori* leads to cure of the disease because ulcer relapses no longer occur (GRAHAM 1991b; MARSHALL 1988; MILLER 1989; PATCHETT 1992; RAUWS 1990). This is in contrast to the control of peptic ulcer disease, which could only be achieved with anti-secretory therapy prior to the discovery of *H. pylori* (DOBRILLA 1988). GRAHAM et al. (1991a) also demonstrated that by adding acid suppression to anti-*Helicobacter* therapy the speed of ulcer healing is increased. Finally, smoking, recognized for a long time as one of the strongest risk factors for ulcer relapse, no longer causes ulcer recurrenec after cure of the infection (BORODY 1992).

3 *Helicobacter* and Gastric Ulcer

There also is strong epidemiological evidence that *H. pylori* plays a role in gastric ulcers (KUIPERS 1995a). Approximately 80% of gastric ulcers are *H. pylori* positive. The likely explanation for the lower prevalence of *H. pylori* in gastric ulcers is NSAIDs. NSAIDs cause gastric ulcers more frequently than duodenal ulcers (ratio 4:1). It has been known for a long time that prepyloric ulcers are different from high gastric ulcers (JOHNSTON 1957; MARKS 1959; DU PLESSIS 1965). Prepyloric ulcers behave more as duodenal ulcers and, in contrast to high gastric ulcers, are not associated with low acid output (WORMSLEY 1965, 1974). Although few of the gastric ulcer studies clearly specify the exact location of the ulcer, the majority of gastric ulcers in these studies appear to be located in the prepyloric area. It remains to be seen whether the prevalence of *H. pylori* in gastric ulcers located high in the body of the stomach is also in the range of 80%. A recent study showed convincingly that relapse of *H. pylori*-positive gastric ulcers is also dramatically reduced by eradication of the organism (SUNG 1995). Therefore, all gastric ulcers should be considered for anti-*Helicobacter* treatment.

4 *Helicobacter* and NSAIDs

NSAIDs are the most common cause of *H. pylori*-negative duodenal and gastric ulcers (BORODY 1991; LAINE 1992), but as the prevalence of *H. pylori* is so high in the general population, many patients may have both *H. pylori* infection and NSAID medication at the time of diagnosis of the ulcer. It is unclear whether there is synergy between NSAIDs and *H. pylori* in promoting ulcer formation, but the data thus far suggest that this either is not the case, or that the synergistic effect is small (VELDHUYZEN VAN ZANTEN 1993; HAWKEY 1996). Nevertheless, the most cost-effective strategy in patients who are on NSAIDs, and who have an ulcer is to cure of *H. pylori* infection which is what is generally recommended. Should patients with a history of ulcers still require NSAID medication following cure of *H. pylori* infection, prophylaxis to prevent NSAID-ulcer formation should be considered. Recently a clinical trial from Hong Kong was reported in which 92 *H. pylori*-positive patients who required NSAIDs therapy were randomized to either anti-*Helicobacter* therapy or no additional treatment. The patients in the *H. pylori* treatment group had a statistically significant reduction in occurrence of NSAID induced ulcers (CHAN et al. 1997). This study warrants further confirmation but raises the possibility that there may be a benefit in eradicating *H. pylori* infection in NSAIDs users.

5 How Does *Helicobacter* Cause Duodenal Ulcers?

The background prevalence of *H. pylori* in the general population is high. The best known risk factors for infection are age and lower socioeconomic status. Although it is hard to give exact figures the life-time risk of ever developing an ulcer in the general population (which includes both *H. pylori* infected and non-infected individuals) is probably 3%–5%. This risk is increased two- to threefold, to 10%–15% *H. pylori*-infected individuals.

5.1 Acid Secretion

Few studies using pentagastrin stimulation to measure acid output have found differences between *H. pylori* infected and non-infected patients (POUNDER 1996). In older studies considerable overlap of basal acid output and peak acid output was seen among patients with and without duodenal ulcers (WORMSLEY 1974). On average, duodenal ulcer patients tend to have acid output in the upper range. It is very difficult to study acid output in humans in the in-vivo situation for several reasons; first pH measurement is only an indication of average H^+ ion concentrations, not the total amount of acid which is produced in the stomach or, more importantly, passes the duodenal cap; second, it is difficult to measure acid secretion when patients are eating normally throughout the day.

McCOLL and co-workers published several studies of the effect of *H. pylori*-infection on gastrin-mediated acid secretion (EL-OMAR 1995; McCOLL 1991). To overcome the technical difficulty of reliably determining acid output in response to a meal they measured gastrin-mediated acid secretion after intravenous infusion of gastrin-releasing peptide (GRP). GRP stimulates the release of endogenous gastrin, which in turn stimulates acid secretion. Their argument is that this technique makes it possible to measure accurately the combined functional response of the antrum and body of the stomach as would be produced by a meal.

The McCOLL group studied duodenal ulcer patients, *H. pylori*-positive healthy volunteers and *H. pylori*-negative healthy volunteers. Duodenal ulcer patients had a threefold increase in basal acid output. The increase in basal acid output in *H. pylori*-infected individuals is probably a direct reflection of the fasting serum gastrin levels and is reversed following eradication of *H. pylori*.

The median acid output to gastrin releasing peptides infusion in the *H. pylori*-positive healthy volunteers was 15 mmol/h, three times that of *H. pylori*-negative healthy volunteers (median 5.5 mmol/h). The median acid output in *H. pylori*-positive duodenal ulcers was 37 mmol/h, which was six times that of the *H. pylori*-negative healthy volunteers. Finally, McCOLL et al. also showed that duodenal ulcer patients had an increased maximal response to exogenous gastrin and increased ratio of basal acid output to maximal gastrin-stimulated acid output. Eradication of *H. pylori* in the duodenal ulcer patients lowered basal acid output to normal levels. It also decreased GRP-stimulated acid secretion by a median of 66% but this was still higher than values obtained in non-infected non-ulcer control patients (EL-OMAR 1995).

5.2 Gastrin

It is generally accepted that *H. pylori*-infection affects the antral mucosa more than the body mucosa in most infected individuals. In the antrum the G-cells are located which release gastrin, a major stimulant of the parietal cell. There is consensus that the antral inflammation caused by *H. pylori* results in an increase in gastrin release from the G-cells both in the basal state and following a meal (LEVI 1989; EL-OMAR

1995). The increase in basal serum gastrin and exaggerated gastrin response in relation to a meal is seen both in patients infected with *H. pylori* who have duodenal ulcers but also in *H. pylori*-positive non-ulcer dyspepsia patients and in healthy *H. pylori*-infected asymptomatic volunteers.

In the McColl studies the median plasma gastrin concentration during stimulation with GRP were similar in *H. pylori*-positive duodenal ulcer patients and *H. pylori*-positive healthy volunteers but higher than *H. pylori*-negative volunteers (El-Omar 1995). Given that the GRP-stimulated acid output was higher in *H. pylori*-positive duodenal ulcer patients than in *H. pylori*-positive non-duodenal ulcer patients, the duodenal ulcer patients appear to be more sensitive to gastrin stimulation. Eradication of *H. pylori* lowered the plasma gastrin in duodenal patients to values equivalent to the *H. pylori*-negative volunteers.

In summary, the findings showed a threefold increase in acid secretion in *H. pylori*-positive healthy volunteers that is explained by *H. pylori*-induced hypergastrenemia and a sixfold increase in acid secretion in the duodenal ulcer patients that is explained by the combination of *H. pylori*-induced hypergastrenemia and an exaggerated acid response to stimulation by gastrin. McColl et al.(1991) therefore believe that increased gastrin mediated acid secretion is the key factor in the pathophysiology of duodenal ulceration. Recently, Gillen and coworkers (1998) reported on further studies of gastrin in duodenal ulcer patients. They found that there was an increased maximal acid secretory capacity in response to gastrin in *H. pylori*-positive duodenal ulcer patients indicating that these patients are more sensitive to gastrin. In contrast, there was a decreased sensitivity to gastrin in infected healthy volunteers who did not have ulcers.

5.3 Somatostatin

Somatostatin is a peptide produced by the D-cells which is also present in the antral mucosa. Somatostatin is known to have an inhibitory effect on gastrin secretion. A few studies have shown that the density of somatostatin-containing cells is reduced in *H. pylori*-infected patients (Moss 1992; Graham 1993). Eradication of *H. pylori* results in an increase in antral somatostatin-containing cells. Therefore, the exaggerated gastrin response may be the result of increased gastrin-release from the G-cells, possibly in combination with a decrease in mucosal somatostatin concentration produced by the D-cells. There is agreement that the *Helicobacter*-induced inflammation in the antrum is the trigger for these abnormalities.

6 Duodenal Gastric Metaplasia

H. pylori organisms thrive only in mucus adjacent to gastric type epithelium. Although the infection is commonly found in the antrum and to a lesser extent body and fundus, it is much less frequently seen in the duodenum. One defence mechanism that the duodenum appears to have against an increased acid load is the development of gastric metaplasia. It is unclear whether the prevalence of gastric metaplasia is increased in *H. pylori*-infected individuals. WYATT et al. (1990) showed that gastric metaplasia is more extensive in *H. pylori*-positive duodenal ulcers patients, even though the prevalence of gastric metaplasia in their study was *not increased*, both an increase in prevalence of gastric metaplasia and/or an increase in surface area of gastric type epithelium in the duodenal cap make it easier for the *H. pylori* organisms to move from the antrum into the duodenal cap. Presense of *H. pylori* in the duodenum can produce duodenitis and set the stage for the formation of a duodenal ulcer as the result of the combination of an inflammatory response and gastric acid. Indeed it has been shown that the combination of antral *H. pylori* gastritis, duodenal gastric metaplasia and duodenal *H. pylori* markedly increases the risk of duodenal ulcer formation (CARRICK 1989).

7 Abnormal Gastrin Response in Response to Antral Distension

Recently OLBE et al. (1996) described another pathophysiological mechanism by which *H. pylori* infection may contribute to duodenal ulcer formation. In *H. pylori*-positive and -negative duodenal ulcer patients and healthy volunteers the effect of antral distension on gastrin release and GRP- and pentagastrin-stimulated acid output was measured. Antral distension was performed using a balloon which was positioned in the antrum and which could be inflated to a volume of 150 cc. In *H. pylori* uninfected duodenal ulcer patients and healthy volunteers but not in *H. pylori* infected duodenal ulcer patients antral distension resulted in a decrease in GRP-stimulated gastrin release and decrease in pentagastrin-stimulated acid output. Both these abnormalities normalized following cure of the *H. pylori* infection. The interpretation of these findings is that *H. pylori* both affects the response of antral and body mucosa. The abnormal antral response is an increase in the gastrin release in relationship to antral distension, i.e. a meal. The abnormal response of the body mucosa is a prolonged production of gastric acid. Both these abnormalities produce an increased acid load, which promotes the formation of a duodenal ulcer.

8 The Unifying Duodenal Ulcer Hypothesis

A hypothesis which unifies these data is as follows. *H. pylori* infection leads to an antral predominant gastritis, which causes an exaggerated gastrin response especially in relationship to meals. This possibly could lead to an increase in overall acid secretion, although this link in the hypothesis has been shown only for GRP and not, for example, for pentagastrin stimulation (EL-OMAR 1995; POUNDER 1996). In addition, there also is an abnormal response of the antrum to distension which also contributes to the abnormal gastrin response and increased acid production. The duodenal cap responds to an increased acid load by formation of gastric metaplasia. This in turn makes it possible for the *H. pylori* organisms to move from the antrum into the duodenal cap resulting in duodenitis and possibly formation of a duodenal ulcer if the noxious stimuli are sufficiently severe. Once a duodenal ulcer forms it may be difficult to find *H. pylori* organisms in the duodenum as the gastric type epithelial cells may be destroyed. Needless to say, other factors may still be important, including genetic predisposition, blood group, smoking, and possibly NSAIDs.

9 Why Do Some Patients Develop Duodenal and Others Gastric Ulcers?

There are probably many factors which determine whether an individual develops a duodenal ulcer or a gastric ulcer. Acid output possibly is one of the important determinants (DIXON 1993; LEE 1995). It has been known for a long time that duodenal ulcer patients have an antral predominant gastritis. Gastric ulcer patients, especially individuals with a high gastric ulcer, have a pangastritis affecting both the antrum and body. Patients who genetically are at the high end of gastric acid output at the time of *H. pylori* colonization of the stomach develop an antral predominant gastritis. This antral gastritis does not extend easily into the body as it has been shown that *H. pylori* organisms actually do not thrive well at low pH. As gastric acid is produced by the parietal cells located in the body and fundus the microenvironment here is not conducive to growth of *H. pylori*. In those patients with genetically low or low normal gastric output it may be easier for the *H. pylori* organisms gastritis to move up into the body and the fundus, and in these patients a pan-gastritis develops. There now is good evidence that presence of *H. pylori* infection in the body leads to the development of atrophic gastritis (KUIPERS 1995b), which may over many years result in a lowering of the gastric acid output. The development of atrophic gastritis is also associated with the formation of intestinal metaplasia. Both atrophic gastritis and intestinal metaplasia are recognized risk factors for development of gastric ulcers and gastric cancer; CORREA 1980. Patients who at the time of the acquisition of the *H. pylori* infection are at the intermediate (normal) level of acid output develop a gastritis pattern that involves the antrum more than the body but have some progressive gastritis in the body mucosa. Such patients are at low risk for duodenal or gastric ulcer development. In reality there are likely other factors that come into play. These may include genetic or environmental factors, smoking or differences in virulence factors of *H. pylori*.

10 Who Should Be Treated?

Given the overwhelming evidence of the role of *H. pylori* in duodenal and gastric ulcer, there now is worldwide consensus that all patients diagnosed with an ulcer should be investigated for *H. pylori* and treated if positive. Treatment is also recommended in patients who are *H. pylori*-positive and are taking NSAIDs at the time of ulcer diagnosis. Treatment options are discussed in a separate chapter of this volume ("Antibiotic Treatment of *Helicobacter pylori* Infection"). The largest group of patients that needs to be targetted are those who are currently taking acid suppression maintenance therapy for proven peptic ulcer disease in the past.

11 Is Cure of *H. pylori* Infection Associated with an Increased Risk of Gastroesophageal Reflux Disease?

Recent reports have suggested that patients who are successfully treated for *H. pylori* are at increased risk of developing gastroesophageal reflux disease (GERD) (O'CONNOR 1994; LABENZ and MALFERTHEINER 1997; LABENZ et al. 1997). However, it is important to stress that the most often quoted study of LABENZ et al. (1997) was not a truly randomized trial and was not set up to address this particular question. A careful analysis of patients enroled in the DU-MACH and GU-MACH studies has not shown an increase in GERD during a 6-month follow-up (MALFERTHEINER et al. 1997). On the contrary, there was a tend in the duodenal ulcer patients, in whom the infection was cured, towards less frequent development of GERD compared to patients with persistent infection. Clearly the issue of GERD needs more study. It is certianly possible that *H. pylori*-positive patients without ulcers behave differently than DU or GU patients as their pattern of gastritis is different.

References

Baron JH (1963) Studies of basal and peak acid output with an augmented histamine test. Gut 4:136 144
Borody TJ, George LL, Brandl S et al (1991) *H. pylori*-negative duodenal ulcer. Am J Gastroenterol 86:1154 1157
Borody TJ, George LL, Brandl S, Andrews P, Jankiewicz E, Ostapowicz N (1992) Smoking does not contribute to duodenal ulcer relapse after H pylori eradication. Am J Gastroenterol 87:1390 1393
Carrick J, Lee A, Hazell S et al (1989) Campylobacter pylori, duodenal ulcer, and gastric metaplasia: possible role of functional heterotopic tissue in ulcerogenesis. Gut 30:790 797
Chan FKL, Sung JJY, Sydney Chung SC, To KF, Ynug MY, Leung VKS, Lee Y, Chan CSY, Li EKM, Woo J (1997) Randomised trial of eradication of *H. pylori* before NSAID therapy to prevent peptic ulcers. Lancet 350:975 979

Correa P (1980) The epidemiology and pathogenesis of chronic gastritis: three etiologic entities. Front Gastro Intest Res 6:98–108

Dixon MF (1993) Acid, ulcers and H pylori. Lancet ii:384–385

Dobrilla G, Vallaperta P, Amplatz S (1988) Influence of ulcer healing on ulcer relapse after discontinuation of acute treatment: a pooled estimate of controlled trials. Gut 29:181–187

du Plessis DJ (1965) Pathogenesis of gastric ulcer. Lancet I:974–978

El-Omar EM, Penman ID, Ardill JES et al (1995) *H. pylori* infection and abnormalities of acid secretion in patients with duodenal ulcer disease. Gastroenterology 109:681–691

Feldman M (1991) *H. pylori* and the etiology of duodenal ulcer: necessary but not sufficient. Am J Med 91:563–565

Gillen D, El-Omar EM, Wirz AA, Ardill S, McColl KEL (1998) The acid response to gastrin distinguishes duodenal ulcer patients from *H. pylori*-infected healthy subjects. Gastroenterology 114:50–57

Graham DY (1989) Campylobacter pylori and peptic ulcer disease. Gastroenterology 96:615–625

Graham DY, Lew GM, Evans DG, Evans DJ, Klein P (1991) Effect of triple therapy (antibiotics plus bismuth) on duodenal ulcer healing. A randomized controlled trial. Ann Intern Med 115:266–269

Graham DY, Lew GM, Klein PD et al (1991) Effect of treatment of *H. pylori* infection on the long-term recurrence of gastric or duodenal ulcer. A randomized controlled study. Ann Intern Med 116:705–708

Graham DY, Lew GM, Lechage J (1993) Antral G-cell and D-cell numbers in *H. pylori* infection: effect of *H. pylori* eradication. Gastroenterology 104:1655–1660

Hawkey CJ (1996) Are NSAIDs and *H. pylori* separate risk factors? In: Hunt RH, Tytgat GNJ et al (eds) *H. pylori*: basic research to clinical cure, chap 32. Kluwer Academic, London

Hui WM, Ho J, Lam SK (1991) Pathogenetic role of *H. pylori* in duodenal ulcer disease. Multivariate analysis of factors affecting relapse. Dig Dis Sci 36:424

Johnson HD (1957) The clasification and principles of treatment of gastric ulcers. Lancet ii:518–520

Kuipers EJ (1995) *H. pylori* and peptic ulcer disease. Aliment Pharmacol Ther 9 [Suppl 2]:59–69

Kuipers EJ, Uyterlinde AM, Pena AS et al (1995) Long term sequelae of *H. pylori* gastritis. Lancet 345:1525–1528

Labenz J, Malfertheiner P (1997) *H. pylori* in gastroesophageal reflux disease: causal agent, independent or protective factor? Gut 41:277–280

Labenz J, Blum AL, Bayerdorffer E, Maining A, Stolte M, Borsch G (1997) Curing *H. pylori* infection in patients with duodenal ulcer may provoke reflux esophagitis. Gastroenterology 112:1442–1447

Laine L, Martin-Sorensen M, Weinstein W (1992) NSAID-associated gastric ulcers do not require *H. pylori* for their development. Am J Gastroenterol 87:1398–1402

Lee A, Dixon MF, Danon SJ, Kuipers E, Megraud F, Larsson H, Mellgard B (1995) Local acid production and *H. pylori*: a unifying hypothesis of gastroduodenal disease. Eur J Gastroenterol Hepatol 7:461–465

Levi S, Beardshall K, Haddad G, Playford R, Ghosh P, Calam J (1989) *Campylobacter pylori* and duodenal ulcers: the gastrin link. Lancet i:1167–1168

Marks IN, Shay H (1959) Observations on the pathogenesis of gastric ulcer. Lancet i:1107–1111

Marshall BJ, Goodwin CS, Warren JR et al (1988) Prospective double-blind trial of duodenal ulcer relapse after eradication of *Campylobacter pylori*. Lancet ii:1437–1442

Malfertheiner P, Veldhuyzen van Zanten SJO, Dent J, Bayerdorffer E, Lind T, O'Morain C, Spiller RC, Unge P, Zeijlon L (1997) Does cure of *H. pylori* infection induce heartburn? Gastroenterology (AGA abstract)

McColl KEL, Fullarton GM, Chittajalu R et al (1991) Plasma gastrin, daytime intragastric pH, and nocturnal acid output before and at 1 and 7 months after eradication of *H. pylori* in duodenal ulcer subjects. Scand J Gastroenterol 26:339–346

Miller JP, Faragher EB (1989) The potential impact of *Campylobacter pylori* on the treatment of duodenal ulcer disease. Scand J Gastroenterol 24(S160):39–45

Moss SF, Legon S, Bishop AE, Polak JM, Calam J (1992) Effect of *H. pylori* on gastric somatostatin in duodenal ulcer disease. Lancet 340:930–932

O'Connor HJ, Cunnane K (1994) *H. pylori* and gastroesophageal reflux disease – a prospective study. Ir J Med Soc 163:369–373

Olbe L, Hamlet A, Dalenback J, Fandriks L (1996) A mechanism by which *H. pylori* infection of the antrum contributes to the development of duodenal ulcer. Gastroenterology 110:1386–1394

Patchett S, Beattie S, Leen E, Keane C, O'Morain C (1992) *H. pylori* and duodenal ulcer recurrence. Am J Gastroenterol 87:24–27

Pounder RE (1996) *H. pylori* and gastroduodenal secretory function. Gastroenterology 110:947–950

Rabeneck L, Ransohoff DF (1991) Is *H. pylori* a cause of Duodenal Ulcer? A methodologic critique of current evidence. Am J Med 91:566–572

Rauws EJ, Tytgat GNJ (1990) Cure of duodenal ulcer disease associated with eradication of *H. pylori*. Lancet 335:1233–1235

Sipponen P, Varis K, Fraki O, Korri UM, Seppala K, Siurala M (1990) Cumulative 10 year risk of symptomatic duodenal and gastric ulcer in patients with or without gastritis. Scand J Gastroenterol 25:966–973

Sung JJY, Chung SCS, Ling TKW et al (1995) Antibacterial treatment of gastric ulcers associated with *H. pylori*. N Engl J Med 332:139–142

Tytgat GNJ, Rauws EAJ (1990) *Campylobacter pylori* and its role in peptic ulcer disease. Gastroenterol Clin North Am 19:183–196

Veldhuyzen van Zanten SJO, Sherman PM (1994) *H. pylori* infection as a cause of gastritis, duodenal ulcer, gastric cancer and nonulcer dyspepsia: a systematic overview. Can Med Assoc J 150:177–185

Veldhuyzen van Zanten SJO (1994) *H. pylori* and NSAIDS: a meta-analysis on interactions of acute gastroduodenal injury, gastric and duodenal ulcers and upper gastrointestinal symptoms. In: Hunt RH, Tytgat GNJ et al (eds) *H. pylori*: basic research to clinical cure, chap 42. Kluwer Academic, London

Wormsley KG, Grossman MI (1965) Maximal histalog test in control subjects and patients with peptic ulcer. Gut 6:427–435

Wormsley KG (1974) Progress report. The pathophysiology of duodenal ulcer. Gut 15:59–81

Wyatt JI, Rathbone BJ, Sobala GM et al (1990) Gastric epithelium in the duodenum: its association with *H. pylori* and inflammation. J Clin Pathol 43:981–986

Gastric Cancer and Lymphoma

P. Mukhopadhyay

1 Introduction

In 1983 WARREN and MARSHALL discovered a spiral urease-producing organism in the human stomach, later classified as *Helicobactor pylori*. The prevalence of *H. pylori* infection varies worldwide, but higher infection rates are seen in developing countries compared with developed ones (MEGRAUD et al. 1989; DOOLEY et al. 1989; MITCHELL et al. 1988; ANONYMOUS 1990). It may be the most common infection worldwide. In developed countries infection with *H. pylori* occurs in more than 50% of adults, while developing countries have infection rates reaching 90% (HOPKINS and MORRIS 1994). *H. pylori* are gram-negative microaerophilic spiral bacteria that can colonize the gastric mucosa for years (MORRIS et al. 1991), and in most cases they probably persist for life. *H. pylori* has been shown to be strongly associated with peptic ulcer disease, and antibiotic therapy to eradicate this organism is an important treatment for duodenal and gastric ulcers (ANONYMOUS 1994). *H. pylori* infection is now considered a risk factor for gastric adenocarcinoma and for primary gastric non-Hodgkin's lymphoma.

2 Gastric Carcinoma

Gastric carcinoma is estimated to be the world's second most common cancer and is second only to lung cancer as a cause of cancer death worldwide (PARKIN et al.

Department of Internal Medicine, Division of Hematology-Oncology, Texas A&M University College of Medicine, and Central Texas Veterans Health Care System, Medical Service (111-H), 1901 S. First Street, Temple, TX 76504, USA

1988). At the beginning of the century, gastric cancer was the leading cause of cancer death in the United States, but the annual incidence of gastric cancer has decreased significantly from 33 of 100,000 persons in 1935 to 9 of 100,000 in the last decade.

Although the dramatic decline in the incidence of gastric carcinoma in the United States and Western Europe over the past 50 years has led some to proclaim an "unplanned triumph" (Howson et al. 1986), in much of Latin America and Asia the incidence remains very high (Parkin 1986; Muir et al. 1987). In Japan, Eastern Europe, and South America, especially in Chile and Costa Rica, gastric cancer is epidemic. In Japan the incidence is highest (100:100,000), and stomach cancer represents the leading cause of death from all malignant diseases, the number one cause of death nationally (Mishima and Hirayama 1987). Although gastric cancer afflicts fewer than 10 per 100,000 persons per year in the United States and Western Europe (Young 1981), there are ethnic groups with increased risk. In the United States, for example, the incidence of gastric cancer among African-Americans, Asian-Americans, and Hispanics is almost double that among whites (Young 1981).

The study of migrant populations who moved from regions of high gastric cancer risk to regions of lower risk has given clues to the events that resulted in the decline in gastric cancer incidence (Hotz and Goebell 1989; Correa et al. 1970; Staszewski 1972; Haenszel et al. 1972; Correa 1985; Boeing 1997). For instance, persons who moved from Japan, a high-risk country, to regions of lower risk in the United States only moderately decreased their cancer risk, even if they immigrated at a younger age. The risk among the second-generation migrants, however, decreased much closer to that of their new country. Similar results have been found in European immigrants to Australia and Puerto Rican migrants to New York. In Polish migrants living in the United States for 10 years, the incidence of gastric cancer decreased and became intermediate between the countries of origin and adoption (Staszewski 1972). Among Japanese migrants the high risk of stomach cancer was observed in second-generation offspring who continued to consume a Japanese diet but was low in those adopting a western diet (Haenszel et al. 1972). From these studies it has been inferred that environmental factors initiate malignant transformation and exert a major portion of their influence in childhood but that other environmental or cultural factors may continually influence the predisposition to cancer. Many factors predispose to gastric malignancy. Epidemiological studies suggest that diet high in salted meats or fish and nitrates or nitrites, high in complex carbohydrates, low in animal protein and fat, contribute to gastric cancer risk. Diets rich in Vitamin A and C are associated with a low risk for gastric cancer (Hotz and Goebell 1989).

Consumption of raw vegetables, fruit, citrus fruit, and high fiber bread are inversely related to gastric cancer risk (Hotz and Goebell 1989; Boeing 1997; Chyou et al. 1990; Nomura et al. 1990). Other factors associated with increased risk of developing gastric cancer include smoked foods, poor drinking water, low socio-economic status, smoking, prior gastric surgery, gastric atrophy and gastritis.

The possibility that a bacterial infection may predispose to gastric malignancy has renewed interest in the geographic clustering of gastric carcinoma observed worldwide. The epidemiological features of gastric carcinoma and *H. pylori* infection are similar (SITAS et al. 1991). Chronic infection has been causally linked with diverse malignancies. A few examples include bladder carcinoma following vesicular schistosomiasis, hepatic carcinoma with chronic hepatitis B infection, and squamous cell carcinoma following chronic osteomylitis.

Several lines of evidence link infection with *H. pylori* and development of gastric cancer. It has been known for decades that chronic gastritis and subsequent atrophy are precancerous conditions. The cumulative and relative risk of gastric cancer is clearly increased in atrophic gastritis, particularly when atrophy is severe and extensive (SIPPONEN et al. 1985). In studies of patients with and without gastric cancer, the relative risk of gastric cancer has been calculated to be 80–90 times higher in patients with severe antral atrophy or with severe panatrophy than in those with a normal stomach (SIPPONEN et al. 1985).

In 1965 LAUREN proposed two main histological types for gastric cancer: intestinal and diffuse. Persons in areas of high risk of gastric carcinoma tend to have the intestinal type of histological appearance while persons living in low-risk areas are more likely to have the diffuse type (MUNOZ et al. 1968). CORREA et al. (1976, 1990b) prospectively studied the premalignant changes that occurred in a cohort of patients at high risk of developing gastric carcinoma. Normal mucosa first progressed to nonspecific chronic gastritis, then progressed to chronic atrophic gastritis. Finally, intestinal metaplasia and dysplasia developed and this progressed to gastric cancer of the intestinal type. The association of premalignant lesions and the diffuse type of gastric cancer has not been prospectively studied. *H. pylori* infection is causally an etiological factor in at least 80% of the cases with chronic gastritis. It has been hypothesized that with time this will result in mucosal atrophy and intestinal metaplasia in a proportion of affected subjects, which will favor the development of gastric cancer (SIPPONEN 1992).

Evidence linking infection with *H. pylori* and gastric cancer comes from other types of studies. Histopathological studies have demonstrated that *H. pylori* is commonly present in histological specimens adjacent to gastric cancer (LOFFELD et al. 1990). *H. pylori* has affinity for normal gastric mucosa but not for metaplastic, dysplastic or malignant tissue (HAZELL et al. 1987). As such, studies correlating histological changes to infection need either to focus on tissue from normal section of stomach or to use nonbiopsy based tests for determination of infection status (LOFFELD et al. 1990).

Cross-sectional studies reveal rates of infection between 50% and 100% in persons with gastric carcinoma (LOFFELD et al. 1990; CHENG et al. 1987; JASKIEWICZ et al. 1989). In addition, a statistically significant positive correlation between *H. pylori* infection and gastric carcinoma has been shown for cancer patients compared with blood donors (FORMAN et al. 1990). In the study by JASKIEWICZ et al. (1989) in a high risk population of South Africa, all six patients with gastric malignancy were found to have infection on biopsy, compared with 34% of the persons with normal gastric mucosa ($p = 0.003$). In the study by LOFFELD et al. (1990) 61% of patients with gastric cancer were found to be infected on biopsy or gastric resection compared with 34% of the age-matched blood donor controls (risk ratio 4.2, $p < 0.001$). Similar strong correlation between *H. pylori* infection and gastric cancer has been reported by other studies (PARSONNET et al. 1991b; TALLEY et al. 1991). In the study by TALLEY et al. (1991) patients with adenocarcinoma of the antrum, fundus, or body of the stomach had an odds ratio of 2.7 for concomitant infection with *H. pylori* when compared with the healthy controls. In this study control subjects included patients with esophageal, colorectal and lung malignancies, none of which were linked to *H. pylori* infection.

In addition to these cross-sectional studies, many other epidemelogic studies show a striking parallel between *H. pylori* infection and incidence of gastric cancer (FORMAN et al. 1990; CORREA et al. 1990a; BURSTEIN et al. 1991; DEHESA et al. 1991). Several populations with extremely high rates of gastric cancer, notably in South America, have endemic *H. pylori* infection at a young age (CORREA et al. 1990a; ANONYMOUS 1990). Within rural China, there was a significant geographical correlation between gastric cancer mortality and *H. pylori* infection (FORMAN et al. 1990). The long-established association between poor socioeconomic conditions and gastric cancer (HOWSON et al. 1986) has been reflected in a similar association with *H. pylori* infection (SITAS et al. 1991; GRAHAM et al. 1991), and it is plausible that the worldwide decline in gastric cancer mortality (KURIHARA et al. 1989) could, at least partly, be due to secular changes in bacterial infection (MARSHALL 1990).

Lastly three prospective case control studies have shown similarly strong evidence that *H. pylori* infection increases risk for later development of gastric cancer (FORMAN et al. 1991; NOMURA et al. 1991). In these prospective studies, all cohort subjects had banked serum at the onset of a clinical observation period. Cases of gastric cancer that were identified within the cohorts in subsequent years were matched to controls by age and date of serum collection, and the sera was tested in a blinded fashion for *H. pylori* infection. In all three studies, cancer subjects had significantly higher risk of prior infection with *H. pylori* than did controls with odds ratio varying between 2.8 and 6.0. In the study by NOMURA (1991), as the level of antibody to *H. pylori* increased, there was a progressive increase in the risk of gastric carcinoma. In one of these studies (PARSONNET et al. 1991a) the odds ratio was particularly high in women (odds ratio, 18) and blacks (odds ratio, 9).

There is therefore impressive evidence linking *H. pylori* infection and risk of gastric cancer. TALLEY et al. (1991) have added to this evidence the observation that *H. pylori* infection has a specific association with gastric cancer in so far as other groups of patients with colorectal, lung, and esophageal cancers did not have significantly increased infection rates. In addition it has been shown that the risk is high only with noncardia gastric cancer (TALLEY et al. 1991; PARSONNET et al. 1991a). Patients with cancers of the cardia and the gastroesophageal junction did not have higher infection rates than their controls. There was, however, no difference in risk between patients with cancers in the gastric antrum or corpus or between patients with intestinal or diffuse forms of cancer.

It is clear, however, that infection with *H. pylori* alone cannot explain the pathogenesis of gastric carcinoma. *H. pylori* infection is extraordinarily common, affecting approximately 50% of North American adults who are older than 50 years, and in some developing nations it affects almost all adults (PARSONNET

1989). Only a very small percentage of infected persons will ever have gastric carcinoma. In addition some gastric carcinoma occur in subjects who are not infected. There must be other critical cofactors affecting risk, cofactors that may also explain the difference in risk between blacks and whites and between men and women. It is certain, however, that *H. pylori* infection is at least a marker for increased gastric adenocarcinoma risk. Definitive proof of causality will depend on randomized intervention trials on the long-term effects of *H. pylori* eradication on the risk of gastric cancer or precancerous lesions. It has been postulated that even if future clinical trials demonstrate that it is possible to prevent gastric cancer through *H. pylori* eradication, screening programs may only be cost-effective among high risk groups (HOPKINS and MORRIS 1994). Such a long-term prospective treatment trial is currently being undertaken and until results of such trials are available, the role of *H. pylori* screening and treatment in prevention of gastric cancer remains uncertain.

3 Gastric Lymphoma

Primary non-Hodgkin's Lymphoma of the stomach is an uncommon cancer, accounting for only 10% of lymphomas and 3% of gastric neoplasms (SPIRO 1983). There are only 7.1 cases of gastric non-Hodgkin's lymphoma per million population per year in the United States (SEVERSON and DAVIS 1990). Gastric non-Hodgkin's lymphoma remains, however, the most common extranodal form accounting for 20% of primary extranodal lymphomas (RUBIN and FARBER 1990). Although relatively rare in the United States, it occurs with extraordinarily high frequency in certain parts of Europe (DOGLIONI et al. 1992), such as the Veneto region of Italy, where its incidence equals that of non-Hodgkin's lymphoma of the lymph nodes. In contrast to gastric adenocarcinoma, the incidence of gastric lymphoma may be increasing in the United States (HAYES and DUNN 1989; HOLFORD et al. 1992).

Studies of gastric lymphomas have suggested that their clinicopathological features are more closely related to the structure and function of so-called mucosa-associated lymphoid tissue (MALT) than of peripheral lymph nodes (ISAACSON and WRIGHT 1983; ISAACSON and SPENCER 1989; ISAACSON and NORTON 1994). In contrast to peripheral lymph nodes, which are adapted to respond to antigens carried to the node in afferent lymphatics, MALT appears to have evolved to protect mucosal tissue directly in contact with antigens in the external environment. The most thoroughly characterized MALT has been in the gastrointestinal tract, where it comprises four lymphoid compartments which include Peyer's patches, lamina propria, the intraepithelial lymphocytes, and the mesentric lymph nodes.

The concept of mucosa associated lymphoid tissue derived lymphoma, introduced by ISSACSON and WRIGHT in 1983 (1983), now is well established in the classification of non-Hodgkin's lymphomas as a distinct subtype of lymphoma (HARRIS et al. 1994). These lymphomas arise from a wide variety of extranodal sites, most frequently from the gastrointestinal (GI) tract, stomach being the most common site. Other sites include conjunctiva (HARDMAN-LEA et al. 1994), thyroid gland (HYJEK and ISAACSON 1988), skin (SLATER 1994), lung (WOTHERSPOON et al. 1990), urinary bladder (PAWADE et al. 1993), kidney (PARVEEN et al. 1993), gallbladder (MOSNIER et al. 1992), breast (MATTIA et al. 1993), thymus (ISAACSON et al. 1990), salivary glands (HYJEK et al. 1988), and lacrimal glands.

Many of the sites where MALT lymphomas occur lack any native lymphoid tissue. Before a lymphoma can arise, therefore, lymphoid tissue must be acquired. This is clearly the case in the salivary gland and thyroid, where lesions characterized by the accumulation of lymphoid tissue – namely, myoepithelial sialadenitis and Hashimoto's thyroiditis are necessary precursors of the development of MALT lymphoma.

Although MALT is normally present in the small intestine and colon, such tissue is never found in healthy gastric mucosa (DUKES and BUSSEY 1926). Prior to 1988, prominent lymphoid hyperplasia found in the gastric mucosa was designated as lymphofollicular lymphoma or pseudolymphoma, with the pathogenesis of such conditions being mostly speculative. However, in 1988, WYATT and RATHBONE first reported a propensity of gastric mucosa to form lymphoid follicles in gastritis where *H. pylori* organisms were detected. Lymphoid follicles were present in 64 of 171 gastric mucosa samples from patients with *Helicobacter*-associated gastritis, as compared with 0 of 25 samples from patients with *Helicobacter*-negative gastritis. In 1989 STOLTE and EIDT also made the same association between lymphoid follicles and *H. pylori* gastritis. In their study, 54% of patients with *H. pylori* gastritis had lymphoid follicles (1297/2544) as compared with 0% in patients with reflux gastritis (104) and normal patients (220). Indeed, the presence of lymphoid follicles in gastric mucosa is virtually pathognomonic of *H. pylori* infection (GENTA et al. 1993).

Several lines of evidence support the notion that gastric lymphoma arises from this acquired MALT. The first is that in over 90% of cases of gastric MALT lymphoma, *H. pylori* can be demonstrated in the gastric mucosa (WOTHERSPOON et al. 1991; EIDT et al. 1994). Other evidence include a case-control study by Parsonnet and colleagues (PARSONNET et al. 1994) which showed that non-Hodgkin's lymphoma affecting the stomach, but not other sites is associated with previous *H. pylori* infection. Finally in Veneto region of Italy, where there is a very high incidence of gastric lymphoma, there is an accompanying high prevalence of *H. pylori* infection (DOGLIONI et al. 1992).

More direct evidence comes from in vitro studies as well as clinical studies showing progression of gastritis to monoclonal B-cell lymphoma and regression of gastric MALT lymphoma after antibiotic therapy and eradication of *H. pylori* infection. Multiple publications have now reported regression of localized stage I gastric MALT lymphomas after antibiotic therapy and eradication of *H. pylori* infection. STOLTE (1992) initially reported that treatment to eradicate *H. pylori* organisms resulted in resolution of lymphoid follicles but not MALT lymphomas. However, the initial report had a limited 4-week follow-up, and a subsequent follow-up reported regression of the lymphomas in six patients (STOLTE and EIDT

1993). Wotherspoon reported regression of MALT lymphoma after eradication of *H. pylori* in five of six patients who received antibiotic therapy (WOTHERSPOON et al. 1993). In a prospective cohort study by ROGGERO and colleagues (1995) there was disappearance or almost total regression of the lymphomatous tissue in 15 of 25 (60%) evaluable patients with MALT lymphoma. In a case reported by CARLSON and colleagues (1996), a progression from *H. pylori*-associated gastritis through lymphoid hyperplasia to a monoclonal B-cell lymphoma was observed and a resolution of the lymphoma was documented on eradication of *H. pylori* organisms (CARLSON et al. 1996). In the study by PINOTTI and colleagues (1995), eradication of *H. Pylori* resulted in complete regression of MALT lymphoma in 21 of 31 (67%) of the cases. In the largest reported series 35 of 50 (70%) patients had complete regression of their gastric MALT lymphoma following eradication of *H. pylori* after a median follow-up of 24 months (NEUBAUER et al. 1997). However, 22 of 31 tested patients in remission had evidence of monoclonal B-cells by PCR. Whether these patients are truly cured of their lymphomas remains to be determined.

The relationship of *H. pylori* with invasive and high grade gastric lymphoma is uncertain. It is has been suggested that *H. pylori* is more likely to be associated with the early or initial states of primary gastric lymphoma than advanced tumors, and that *H. pylori* may also disappear during the progression of gastric lymphoma (NAKAMURA et al. 1997). Almost all reported cases of gastric lymphoma successfully treated by eradication of *H. pylori* have been flat mucosal lesions. A single case was reported in which a large ulcerated gastric lymphoma that penetrated the submucosa was successfully treated by eradication of *H. pylori* (WEBER et al. 1994). In the series by Neubauer and associates (NEUBAUER et al. 1997), in 6 out of 50 patients there was no change in the gastric lymphoma after eradication of *H. pylori*. All six patients underwent surgery and in four of the six transition into high-grade lymphoma was found on histological review.

The mechanism by which *H. pylori* infection leads to the development of B-cell MALT lymphoma has not been completely elucidated. HUSSELL et al. (1993) co-cultured gastric MALT lymphoma tumor cells with 12 isolates of *H. pylori* in an attempt to investigate the immunological response of the tumor cells. When unsorted cells from cases of low-grade primary B-cell gastric lymphoma are cultured under standard conditions, they characteristically die within the first 5 days. However, in three cases studied, when heat-killed whole cell preparations of certain strains of *H. pylori* were added to these cultures, clustering and proliferation of tumor cells were observed. Interestingly, neoplastic B-cell proliferation was prevented by T-cell depletion, suggesting that either the MALT lymphoma B-cells were directly responsive to *H. pylori* but required help of T-cell to make a proliferative response, or *H. pylori* is antigenically stimulating nonneoplastic T-cells to release cytokines that stimulate the proliferation and transformation of the B-cells. Recently CALVERT et al. (1995) studied gastrectomy specimens from 12 patients with B-cell gastric lymphoma, although only five had documented *H. pylori* infection. In some of these patients they detected an allele imbalance at loci for tumor-suppressor genes that were present in sections containing MALT lymphomas, but not present in sections containing only gastritis. They suggest that this

64   P. Mukhopadhyay

difference between the two sections reflects ongoing genetic damage to the cells, possibly caused by *H. pylori* organisms.

Gastric MALT lymphomas are B-cell neoplasms. Primary gastric T-cell lymphoma is very rare (NAKAMURA et al. 1995). There is a possibility that *H. pylori* may also influence the development of gastric T-cell lymphoma (NAKAMURA et al. 1997). MALT lymphoma is an indolent disease, that usually presents as localized extranodal tumor without accompanying adverse prognostic factor for nearly all patients. These patients have a high response rate to treatment and a long survival (THIEB- LEMONT et al. 1997). In the series reported by COGLIATTI et al. (1991) the survivals following a variety of treatment protocols, all of which included surgical resection of the stomach, were 91% at 5 years and 75% at 10 years. The 5-year survival was considerably better for stage I E disease (95%) than for stage II E (82%).

The best therapy for patients with gastric MALT lymphoma who fail to respond or progress after antibiotic eradication of *H. pylori* is unknown. The optimal management has not been clearly defined with regard to the role of surgery, chemotherapy, and radiotherapy. Traditional therapy for localized gastric MALT lymphoma has been largely surgical, with patients receiving partial or total gastrectomy. In the series by COGLIATTI et al. (1991), in which MALT lymphomas were considered separately from higher grade lymphomas, 5-year survival rates of 95% for stage I E and 82% for stage II E had been obtained with surgery. However, the true survival rate associated with surgical therapy alone is difficult to discern, as adjuvant chemotherapy or radiation therapy was frequently used. Because of relapses in the gastric remnant after partial gastrectomies and the multifocal nature of gastric MALT lymphomas, most treatment recommendations are to perform total gastrectomy to eradicate lymphoma when it is confined to the stomach, and chemotherapy for disseminated cases (MONTALBAN et al. 1995; COGLIATTI et al. 1991; RADASZKIEWICZ et al. 1992). However, HAMMEL et al. (1995) consider total gastrectomy an aggressive treatment that is not justified because of the indolent behavior of MALT lymphoma and because it did not prevent relapses outside the GI tract. In the series by Hammel et al. single agent chemotherapy with oral cyclophosphamide or chlorambucil given for a median of 18 months in patients with stage I E or stage IV gastric MALT lymphoma resulted in complete remission in 18 or 24 patients (75%). Of 17 patients treated with stage I E disease, two relapsed (12%) and three (18%) had partial remission.

At present the natural history as well as the best therapeutic approach of gastric MALT lymphoma remains poorly defined as most of the publications are retrospective, involve select populations, ancedotal, small sample sizes, short follow-up and widely varying treatment protocols. The Lymphoma Committee of the Southwest Oncology Group plans to determine in a prospective clinical trial, the response rate associated with antibiotic eradication of *H. pylori* in stage I E or II E gastrointestinal MALT lymphoma (VOSE et al. 1997). Patients who do not achieve a complete response after antibiotic therapy will receive aggressive locoregional therapy with three cycles of cyclophosphamide, doxorubicin, vincristine, and prednisone chemotherapy plus involved-field radiation therapy to obviate the morbidity of total gastrectomy.

In conclusion, clinical and experimental studies indicate that gastric MALT lymphoma is a B-cell neoplasm which is an indolent disease that presents in a localized extranodal location without any associated adverse prognostic factor for nearly all patients and that the first step in the pathogenesis of this lymphoma is accumulation of lymphoid tissue (MALT) in response to infection of the stomach by *H. pylori*. Only rarely is there a monoclonal B-cell proliferation from the MALT which results in a monoclonal lymphoproliferative lesion that is responsive to *H. pylori*-driven T-cell help and *H. pylori* is considered to be more closely associated with the early or initial states of primary gastric lymphoma than the advanced states. An understanding of the biological mechanisms underlying the link between *H. pylori* infection and gastric lymphoma is of profound importance not only in primary gastric lymphoma, but also for the management of the more common, low-grade B-cell lymphomas of lymph nodes.

4 Conclusions

There is now overwhelming evidence to implicate *H. pylori* in the development of both gastric adenocarcinoma and gastric MALT lymphoma. However, the exact role that *H. pylori* plays in carcinogenesis remains to be defined. While infection with *H. pylori* can clearly be a risk factor, the low percentage of infected individuals that actually develop these malignancies indicates that *H. pylori* must act in concert with one or several environmental or genetic cofactors. Large-scale, appropriately controlled, studies that might elucidate these cofactors or further define the influence of *H. pylori* on the host need to be performed before this picture becomes complete. Additionally, the existence of appropriate animal models employing either *H. pylori* or other gastric Helicobacter species that mimic gastric adenocarcinoma and/or MALT lymphoma progression would greatly facilitate research in this area. Such advances would not only increase our understanding about carcinogenesis in general, but would better enable us to identify individuals for appropriate preventative treatment. Currently, there does not appear to be enough information to warrant the screening of asymptomatic individuals for the presence of *H. pylori* infection. However, because *H. pylori* has been identified as a carcinogen by the World Health Organization, the prudent course of action for now would be to treat any individual who for clinical reasons has been screened and identified as being infected with *H. pylori*.

References

Anonymous (1990) *Helicobacter pylori* and gastritis in Peruvian patients: relationship to socioeconomic level, age, and sex. The Gastrointestinal Physiology Working Group. Am J Gastroenterol 85:819
Anonymous (1994) *Helicobacter pylori* in peptic ulcer disease. NIH Consensus Statement 12:1

Boeing H (1997) Epidemiological research in stomach cancer: Progress over the last ten years. J Cancer Res Clin Oncol 117:133

Burstein M, Monge E, Leon-Barua R, Lozano R, Berendson R, Gilman RH, Legua H, Rodriguez C (1991) Low peptic ulcer and high gastric cancer prevalence in a developing country with a high prevalence of infection by *Helicobacter pylori*. J Clin Gastroenterol 13:154

Calvert R, Randerson J, Evans P, Cawkwell L, Lewis F, Dixon MF, Jack A, Owen R, Shiach C, Morgan GJ (1995) Genetic abnormalities during transition from *Helicobacter-pylori*-associated gastritis to low-grade MALToma. Lancet 345:26

Carlson SJ, Yokoo H, Vanagunas A (1996) Progression of gastritis to monoclonal B-cell lymphoma with resolution and recurrence following eradication of *Helicobacter pylori*. JAMA 275:937

Cheng SC, Sanderson CR, Waters TE, Goodwin CS (1987) *Campylobacter pyloridis* in patients with gastric carcinoma. Med J Aust 147:202

Chyou PH, Nomura AMYH, Hankin JH, Stemmermann GN (1990) A case-cohort study of diet and stomach cancer. Cancer Res 50:7501

Cogliatti SB, Schmid U, Schumacher U (1991) Primary B-cell gastric lymphoma: a clinicopathological study of 145 patients. Gastroenterology 101:1159

Correa P, Cuello C, Duque E (1970) Carcinoma and intestinal metaplasia in the stomach in Colombian migrants. J Natl Cancer Inst 44:297

Correa P, Cuello C, Duque E (1976) Gastric cancer in Colombia: III. Natural history of precursor lesions. J Natl Cancer Inst 57:1027

Correa P (1985) Clinical implications of recent developments in gastric cancer pathology and epidemiology. Semin Oncol 12:2

Correa P, Fox J, Fontham E, Ruiz B, Lin YP, Zavala D, Taylor N, Mackinley D, de Lima E, Portilla H et al. (1990a) *Helicobacter pylori* and gastric carcinoma. Serum antibody prevalence in populations with contrasting cancer risks. Cancer 66:2569

Correa P, Haenszel W, Cuello C (1990b) Gastric precancerous process in a high risk population: cross-sectional studies. Cancer Res 50:4731

Dehesa M, Dooley CP, Cohen H, Fitzgibbons PL, Perez-Perez GI, Blaser MJ (1991) High prevalence of *Helicobacter pylori* infection and histologic gastritis in asymptomatic Hispanics. J Clin Microbiol 29:1128

Doglioni C, Wotherspoon AC, Moschini A, de Boni M, Isaacson PG (1992) High incidence of primary gastric lymphoma in northeastern Italy. Lancet 339:834

Dooley CP, Cohen H, Fitzgibbons PL, Bauer M, Appleman MD, Perez-Perez GI, Blaser MJ (1989) Prevalence of *Helicobacter pylori* infection and histologic gastritis in asymptomatic persons. N Engl J Med 321:1562

Dukes C, Bussey HJR (1926) The number of lymphoid follicles of the human large intestine. J Pathol Bacteriol 29:111

Eidt S, Stolte M, Fischer R (1994) *Helicobacter pylori* gastritis and primary gastric non-Hodgkin's lymphomas. J Clin Pathol 47:436

Forman D, Sitas F, Newell DG, Stacey AR, Boreham J, Peto R, Campbell TC, Li J, Chen J (1990) Geographic association of *Helicobacter pylori* antibody prevalence and gastric cancer mortality in rural China. Int J Cancer 46:608

Forman D, Newell DG, Fullerton F, Yarnell JW, Stacey AR, Wald N, Sitas F (1991) Association between infection with *Helicobacter pylori* and risk of gastric cancer: evidence from a prospective investigation. BMJ 302:1302

Genta RM, Hamner HW, Graham DY (1993) Gastric lymphoid follicles in *Helicobacter pylori* infection: frequency, distribution, and response to triple therapy. Hum Pathol 24:577

Graham DY, Malaty HM, Evans DG, Evans DJ Jr, Klein PD, Adam E (1991) Epidemiology of *Helicobacter pylori* in an asymptomatic population in the United States. Effect of age, race, and socioeconomic status. Gastroenterology 100:1495

Haenszel W, Kurihara M, Segi M, Lee RKC (1972) Stomach cancer among Japanese in Hawaii. J Natl Cancer Inst 49:969

Hammel P, Haioun C, Chaumette MT (1995) Efficacy of single-agent chemotherapy in low-grade B-cell mucosa-associated lymphoid tissue lymphoma with prominent gastric expression. J Clin Oncol 13:2524

Hardman-Lea S, Kerrmuir M, Wotherspoon AC (1994) Mucosal-associated lymphoid tissue lymphoma of the conjunctiva. Arch Ophtalmol 112:1207

Harris NL, Jaffe ES, Stein H (1994) A revised European-American classification of lymphoid neoplasms: a proposal from the International Lymphoma Study Group. Blood 84:1361

Hayes J, Dunn E (1989) Has the incidence of primary gastric lymphoma increased? Cancer 63:2073

Hazell SL, Hennessy WB, Borody TJ, Carrick J, Ralston M, Brady L, Lee A (1987) Campylobacter pyloridis gastritis II: distribution of bacteria and associated inflammation in the gastroduodenal environment. Am J Gastroenterol 82:297

Holford TR, Zheng T, Mayne ST, Mckay LA (1992) Time trends of non-Hodgkin's lymphoma: Are they real? What do they mean? Cancer Res 52:5443S

Hopkins RJ, Morris JG Jr (1994) *Helicobacter pylori*: the missing link in perspective. Am J Med 97:265

Hotz J, Goebell H (1989) Epidemiology and pathogenesis of gastric carcinoma. In: Meyer HJ, Schmoll HJ, Hotz J (eds) Gastric carcinoma. Springer, Berlin Heidelberg New York

Howson CP, Hiyama T, Wynder EL (1986) The decline in gastric cancer: epidemiology of an unplanned triumph. Epidemiol Rev 8:1

Hussell T, Isaacson PG, Crabtree JE, Spencer J (1993) The response of cells from low-grade B-cell gastric lymphomas of mucosa-associated lymphoid tissue to *Helicobacter pylori*. Lancet 342:571

Hyjek E, Smith WJ, Isaacson PG (1988) Primary B-cell lymphoma of salivary glands and its relationship to myoepithelial sialadenitis. Hum Pathol 19:766

Hyjek E, Isaacson P (1988) Primary B-cell lymphoma of the thyroid and its relationship to Hashimoto's thyroiditis. Hum Pathol 19:1315

Isaacson P, Wright DH (1983) Malignant lymphoma of mucosa-associated lymphoid tissue: A distinctive type of B-cell lymphoma. Cancer 52:1410

Isaacson PG, Chan JKC, Tang C (1990) Low grade B-cell lymphoma of mucosa-associated lymphoid tissue arising in the thymus: a thymic lymphoma mimicking myoepithelial sialadenitis. Am J Surg Pathol 14:342

Isaacson PG, Norton AJ (1994) Extranodal lymphomas. Churchill Livingstone, Edinburgh

Isaacson PG, Spencer J (1989) Malignant lymphoma of mucosa associated lymphoid tissue. Histopathology 11:445

Jaskiewicz K, Louwrens HD, Woodroof CW, van Wyk MJ, Price SK (1989) The association of *Campylobacter pylori* with mucosal pathological changes in a population at risk for gastric cancer. S Afr Med J 75:417

Kurihara M, Aoki K, Hisamichi S (1989) Cancer mortality statistics in the world 1950–. University of Nagoya Press. Nagoya

Lauren P (1965) The two histological main types of gastric carcinoma: diffuse and so-called intestinal-type carcinoma. Acta Pathol Microbiol Scand 64:31

Loffeld RJ, Willems I, Flendrig JA, Arends JW (1990) *Helicobacter pylori* and gastric carcinoma. Histopathology 17:537

Marshall BJ (1990) *Campylobacter pylori*: its link to gastritis and peptic ulcer disease. Rev Infect Dis 12 Suppl 1:S87–S93

Mattia AR, Ferry JA, Harris NL (1993) Breast lymphoma: A B-cell spectrum including the low grade B-cell lymphoma of mucosa-associated lymphoid tissue. Am J Surg Pathol 17:574

Megraud F, Brassens-Rabbe MP, Denis F, Belbouri A, Hoa DQ (1989) Seroepidemiology of *Campylobacter pylori* infection in various populations. J Clin Microbiol 27:1870

Mishima Y, Hirayama R (1987) The role of lymph node surgery in gastric cancer. World J Surg 11:406

Mitchell HM, Lee A, Berkowicz J, Borody T (1988) The use of serology to diagnose active *Campylobacter pylori* infection. Med J Aust 149:604

Montalban C, Manzanal A, Boixeda D, Redondo C, Bellas C (1995) Treatment of low-grade gastric MALT lymphoma with *Helicobacter pylori* eradication. Lancet 345:798

Morris AJ, Ali MR, Nicholson GI, Perez-Perez GI, Blaser MJ (1991) Long-term follow-up of voluntary ingestion of *Helicobacter pylori*. Ann Intern Med 114:662

Mosnier JF, Brousse N, Sevestre C (1992) Primary low grade B-cell lymphoma of the mucosa-associated lymphoid tissue arising in the gallbladder. Histopathology 20:273

Muir C, Waterhouse J, Mack T (1987) Cancer incidence in five continents. vol 5, IARC, Lyon, no 88

Munoz N, Correa P, Cuello C, Duque E (1968) Histologic types of gastric carcinoma in high and low risk areas. Int J Cancer 3:809

Nakamura S, Akazawa K, Yao T (1995) Primary gastric lymphoma: A clinicopathologic study of 233 cases with special reference to evaluation with the MIB-index. Cancer 76:1313

Nakamura S, Yao T, Aoyagi K, Iida M, Fujishima M, Tsuneyoshi M (1997) *Helicobacter pylori* and primary gastric lymphoma. A histopathologic and immunohistochemical analysis of 237 patients. Cancer 79:3

Neubauer A, Thiede C, Morgner A, Alpen B, Ritter M, Neubauer B, Wundisch T, Ehninger G, Stolte M, Bayerdorffer E (1997) Cure of *Helicobacter pylori* infection and duration of remission of low-grade gastric mucosa-associated lymphoid tissue lymphoma. J Natl Cancer Inst 89:1350

Nomura A, Grove JS, Stemmermann GN, Severson RK (1990) A prospective study of stomach cancer and its relation to diet, cigarettes, and alcohol consumption. Cancer Res 50:627

Nomura A, Stemmermann GN, Chyou PH, Kato I, Perez-Perez GI, Blaser MJ (1991) *Helicobacter pylori* infection and gastric carcinoma among Japanese Americans in Hawaii. N Engl J Med 325:1132

Parkin DM (1986) Cancer occurrence in developing countries. IARC, Lyon, no 75

Parkin DM, Laara E, Muir CS (1988) Estimates of the worldwide frequency of sixteen major cancers in 1980. Int J Cancer 41:184

Parsonnet J (1989) The epidemiology of *C. pylori*. In: Blaser MJ (ed) Campylobacter pylori in gastritis and peptic ulcer disease. Igaku-Shoin, New York

Parsonnet J, Friedman GD, Vandersteen DP, Chang Y, Vogelman JH, Orentreich N, Sibley RK (1991a) *Helicobacter pylori* infection and the risk of gastric carcinoma. N Engl J Med 325:1127

Parsonnet J, Vandersteen D, Goates J, Sibley RK, Pritikin J, Chang Y (1991b) *Helicobacter pylori* infection in intestinal-and diffuse-type gastric adenocarcinomas. J Natl Cancer Inst 83:640

Parsonnet J, Hansen S, Rodriguez L, Gelb AB, Warnke RA, Jellum E, Orentreich N, Vogelman JH, Friedman GD (1994) *Helicobacter pylori* infection and gastric lymphoma. N Engl J Med 330:1267

Parveen T, Navarro-Roman L, Medeiros LJ (1993) Low-grade B-cell lymphoma of mucosa-associated lymphoid tissue arising in the kidney. Arch Pathol Lab Med 117:780

Pawade J, Banerjee SS, Harris M (1993) Lymphoma of mucosa-associated lymphoid tissue arising in the urinary bladder. Histopathology 23:147

Pinotti G, Roggero E, Zucca E (1995) Primary low-grade gastric MALT lymphoma (abstract). Proc Am Soc Clin Oncol 14:393

Radaszkiewicz T, Dragosics B, Bauer P (1992) Gastrointestinal malignant lymphomas of the mucosa-associated lymphoid tissue: factors relevant to prognosis. Gastroenterology 102:1628

Roggero E, Zucca E, Pinotti G, Pascarella A, Capella C, Savio A, Pedrinis E, Paterlini A, Venco A, Cavalli F (1995) Eradication of *Helicobacter pylori* infection in primary low-grade gastric lymphoma of mucosa-associated lymphoid tissue. Ann Intern Med 122:767

Rubin E, Farber JL (1990) The gastrointestinal tract. In: Rubin E, Farber JL (eds) Essential pathology. Lippincott, Philadelphia

Severson RK, Davis S (1990) Increasing incidence of primary gastric lymphoma. Cancer 66:1283

Sipponen P, Kekki M, Haapakoski J (1985) Gastric cancer risk in chronic atrophic gastritis: Statistical calculations of cross-sectional data. Int J Cancer 35:173

Sipponen P (1992) *Helicobacter pylori* infection – a common worldwide environmental risk factor for gastric cancer? Endoscopy 24:424

Sitas F, Forman D, Yarnell JW, Burr ML, Elwood PC, Pedley S, Marks KJ (1991) *Helicobacter pylori* infection rates in relation to age and social class in a population of Welsh men. Gut 32:25

Slater DN (1994) MALT and SALT: The clue to cutaneous B-cell lymphoproliferative disease. Br J Dermatol 131:557

Spiro HM (1983) Clinical gastroenterology, 3rd edn. Macmillan, New York

Staszewski J (1972) Migrant studies in alimentary tract cancer: Recent results. Cancer Res 39:85

Stolte M (1992) *Helicobacter pylori* gastritis and gastric MALT-lymphoma. Lancet 339:745

Stolte M, Eidt S (1989) Lymphoid follicles in antral mucosa: immune response to Campylobacter pylori? J Clin Pathol 42:1269

Stolte M, Eidt S (1993) Healing gastric MALT lymphomas by eradicating H pylori? Lancet 342:568

Talley NJ, Zinsmeister AR, Weaver A, DiMagno EP, Carpenter HA, Perez-Perez GI, Blaser MJ (1991) Gastric adenocarcinoma and *Helicobacter pylori* infection. J Natl Cancer Inst 83:1734

Thieblemont C, Bastion Y, Berger F (1997) Mucosa-associated lymphoid tissue gastrointestinal and nongastrointestinal lymphoma behavior: analysis of 108 patients. J Clin Oncol 15:1624

Vose JM, Fisher RI, Lister AA (1997) Unusual lymphoma entities: Evaluation and management. In: Education book – 33rd Annual Meeting, spring 1997. American Society of Clinical Oncology, pp 365

Warren JR, Marshall B (1983) Unidentified curved bacilli on gastric epithelium in active chronic gastritis. Lancet 1:1273

Weber DM, Dimopoulos MA, Anandu DP, Pugh WC, Steinbach G (1994) Regression of gastric lymphoma of mucosa-associated lymphoid tissue with antibiotic therapy for *Helicobacter pylori*. Gastroenterology 107:1835

Wotherspoon AC, Soosay GN, Diss TC (1990) Low grade primary B-cell lymphoma of the lung: An immunohistochemical, molecular, and cytogenetic study of a single case. Am J Clin Pathol 94:655

Wotherspoon AC, Ortiz-Hidalgo C, Falzon MR, Isaacson PG (1991) *Helicobacter pylori*-associated gastritis and primary B-cell gastric lymphoma. Lancet 338:1175

Wotherspoon AC, Doglioni C, Diss TC, Pan L, Moschini A, de Boni M, Isaacson PG (1993) Regression of primary low-grade B-cell gastric lymphoma of mucosa-associated lymphoid tissue type after eradication of *Helicobacter pylori*. Lancet 342:575

Wyatt JI, Rathbone BJ (1988) Immune response of the gastric mucosa to Campylobacter pylori. Scand J Gastroenterol Suppl 142:44

Young JL (1981) Surveillance, epidemiology, and end results: incidence and mortality data 1973– . National Cancer Institute, Bethesda, monograph no 57

Pediatric *Helicobacter pylori* Infection: Clinical Manifestations, Diagnosis, and Therapy

B.D. Gold

1 Introduction

Peptic ulcer disease causes significant morbidity and mortality in adults (SONNEN-BERG et al. 1996; SONNENBERG 1988, 1995). However, studies have yet to be performed that evaluate both the overall prevalence of peptic ulcer disease in large pediatric populations and the health care impact of this condition on the care of children. Gastritis, the "precursor" lesion to mucosal ulceration (i.e., peptic ulcer disease) is an important clinical entity and may be an important cause of abdominal

Division of Pediatric Gastroenterology and Nutrition, Department of Pediatrics, School of Medicine, Emory University, 2040 Ridgewood Dr. NE, Atlanta, GA 30322, USA pain in children (DRUMM et al. 1988; LOOF et al. 1985). Anectdotal reports suggest that ulcer frequency in children is higher than previously reported, and multicenter studies may contribute to a better understanding of the prevalence and economic impact of these entities in the pediatric population (KURATA et al. 1984; EASTHAM et al. 1991; MACARTHUR et al. 1995; GOLD 1996).

Gastritis and ulcers of the duodenum or stomach have historically been classified either as primary or secondary (Table 1) (GOLD 1996; DRUMM et al. 1996). It was previously believed that the majority of children with gastritis and ulcers in the stomach or duodenum have secondary inflammation or mucosal ulceration. Secondary gastroduodenal ulcers generally occur due to a systemic condition such as overwhelming sepsis or as a result of drug ingestion (i.e., nonsteroidal anti-inflammatory agents; SILEN 1987; KURATA et al. 1997). Secondary gastric or duodenal ulcers can also occur in specific diseases such as Zollinger-Ellison syndrome and Crohn's disease (HIRSCHOWITZ 1996; MOONKA et al. 1993; RUUSKA et al. 1994). Although uncommon, secondary ulcers have been reported occurring in other diseases such as cystic fibrosis and sickle cell disease (SERJEANT et al. 1973; RAO et al. 1990; OPPENHEIMER et al. 1975; ROSENSTEIN et al. 1986). A distinguishing factor of secondary compared to primary ulcers can be determined by taking a good patient history on initial evaluation. Careful historical information obtained from children with secondary ulcers rarely reveals a family history of peptic ulcer disease (BOURKE et al. 1996; SHERMAN 1994).

Studies also indicate that children presenting with duodenal or gastric ulcers who are less than 18 years of age and have no other identified causes have primary gastroduodenal ulceration (SHERMAN 1994; MITCHELL et al. 1993). An easily elicited family history of peptic ulcer disease is a frequent positive finding in these patients (MURPHY et al. 1987; JACKSON 1972). In virtually all of these patients mucosal inflammation and, if present, ulceration is caused by a spiral-shaped,

Table 1. Classification and causes of gastritis and ulcers in children (classification/category etiology)

Primary	*Helicobacter pylori*
Secondary	
Excessive acid production	Zollinger Ellison syndrome Antral gastrin (G) cell hyperplasia Antral G cell hyperfunction Systemic mastocytosis Renal failure, hyperparathyroidism
Stress	Infants: traumatic delivery, neonatal sepsis, perinatal asphyxia
	Children: shock, trauma, sepsis, head injury, burns
Other conditions	Eosinophilic gastroenteritis Menetrier's disease, hypertrophic gastritis Lymphocytic (varioliform) gastritis Autoimmune (atrophic) gastritis Gastroduodenal Crohn's disease
Drug-related	Nonsteriodal anti-inflammatory agents (NSAIDS; with or without *H. pylori*) Aspirin Ethanol (alcohol)

gram-negative, microaerobic rod, *Helicobacter pylori* (DRUMM et al. 1987; GOOD-WIN et al. 1989).

Further evidence for the "familial" nature of primary gastritis and peptic ulceration occurring in children are the findings of *H. pylori* clustering among family members of affected individuals (DRUMM et al. 1990; WANG et al. 1993). *H. pylori* infects almost 50% of the world's population; however, the majority of individuals do not experience symptoms that they deem reportable to their physician and most are unaware of their infection. *H. pylori* colonizes the gastric antrum and has satisfied Koch's postulates as human pathogen causing primary, chronic-active gastritis in children (DRUMM 1993; CZINN et al. 1986) as well as adults (BLASER 1992; MARSHALL et al. 1995). Many investigations provide compelling evidence that this organism is associated with a significant proportion (90%–100%) of duodenal ulcers and, to a lesser extent, gastric ulcers in children (PRIETO et al. 1992; YEUNG et al. 1990). Evidence also indicates that the more significant the gastroduodenal inflammation, the earlier *H. pylori* infection was acquired (PARSONNET 1995; VELDHUYZEN VAN ZANTEN et al. 1994). Furthermore, epidemiological data have linked chronic *H. pylori* infection (likely beginning in childhood) with the development of gastric carcinomas (MITCHELL et al. 1992; FORMAN et al. 1991; CORREA 1995).

Both host and bacterial factors have been identified as potentially playing a role in gastroduodenal inflammation associated with *H. pylori* infection (BLASER 1997). However, there are still many features of *H. pylori* associated disease in humans that remain undefined. An understanding of *H. pylori* as the etiological agent in gastroduodenal inflammation and neoplasia is critical to define the pathogenesis of gastritis and peptic ulcer disease.

2 Epidemiology

Most epidemiological studies of *H. pylori* infection have been performed in adults who likely were infected for decades before diagnosis (WEBB et al. 1994; VELDHUYZEN VAN ZANTEN et al. 1994). In addition, there are numerous studies of the prevalence of *H. pylori* infection, yet a notable lack of investigations which characterize the incidence of this infection (SONNENBERG et al. 1996; PARSONNET 1995). These types of incidence studies are difficult to perform for a variety of reasons. Large natural history studies in children are logistically difficult to carry out due to the lower prevalence rates in the younger age group and to the necessity for multiple centers. In addition, there is a lack of clear markers (i.e., clinical correlates) to determine the exact time of initial infection acquisition, further confounding investigators abilities to both design and carry out proper incidence studies.

Throughout the world the incidence of *H. pylori* infection appears to be higher in children than adults (PARSONNET 1995). Data on the incidence of *H. pylori* infection in children are limited (STAAT et al. 1996; ASHORN et al. 1996; MALATY et al. 1994). The incidence of *H. pylori* infection in industrialized countries has been estimated at approx. 0.5% of the susceptible population per year. This incidence appears to be decreasing; thus infected adults are more likely to have been infected in childhood (MALATY et al. 1996; VELDHUYZEN VAN ZANTEN et al. 1994). In addition, the incidence of *H. pylori* infection continues to be high in developing countries, estimated at 3%–10% per year. For example, data from author's laboratory demonstrate that the seroprevalence rate of *H. pylori* in Bolivian children (70% seropositive by age 9 years) compared to Alaska Native children (69% seropositive by age 9 years) is quite high; this is evidence that infections occur quite early in populations living in developing countries or developing regions, respectively (FRIEDMAN et al. 1997; YIP et al. 1997). Conversely, seroprevalence rates for *H. pylori* in children living in the southeastern United States are much lower (12%–15% by age 9 years) (CHONG et al. 1997); however, rates are highly variable depending on a child's ethnicity even in a developed country.

Although not clearly characterized in humans, the route of transmission of *H. pylori* is postulated to be person to person via fecal-oral or oral-oral routes (MEGRAUD 1995; GOODMAN et al. 1995). The fecal-oral route of transmission has been definitively characterized in an animal model of *H. pylori* infection, the ferret (Fox et al. 1993). Studies in this model demonstrate that gastric colonization of ferret stomachs by *H. mustelae* results in similar pathology as humans infected with *H. pylori* (Fox et al. 1990). Moreover, ferrets have been shown to get chronic gastritis, duodenal and gastric ulcers and to develop gastric carcinoma as the end result of long-term *H. mustelae* infection (LEE 1995; PERKINS et al. 1996; YU et al. 1995). Molecular studies provide further support of the fecal-oral or oral-oral route of transmission in humans. Several studies have identified *H. pylori* DNA in the dental plaque and saliva of adults and children with polymerase chain reaction (PCR) techniques (CHOW et al. 1995; LUZZA et al. 1995; BANATVALA et al. 1995). Interpretation of these data suggests that the mouth may be either an initial site of *H. pylori* colonization prior to seeding the stomach and colonizing the gastric epithelia or an actual reservoir for this infection.

Humans appear to be the primary natural reservoir of *H. pylori* infection, although others have been proposed, including water, domestic cats, and houseflies (KLEIN et al. 1991; HANDT et al. 1994, 1995; ENROTH et al. 1995; GRUBEL et al. 1997). Water, as an environmental source of *H. pylori* infection, was first described in a study of Peruvian infants. These authors used ^{13}C-breath testing as the measure of infection in young children and made an epidemiological association with contaminated water and the high prevalence of this infection. The specific viability of *H. pylori* in water has not yet been definitively confirmed. However, the methods used to identify organisms in water (immunomagnetic beads, fluorescent microscopy, and PCR), and the epidemiology that associate "contaminated" water and the presence of infection in humans have been well designed (ENROTH et al. 1995). Domestic cats have been shown to harbor *H. pylori* (HANDT et al. 1995; EL-ZAATARI et al. 1997), although this was not found in stray cats. The housfly, which has been postulated but not confirmed to be a definitive vector for other enteric pathogens (e.g., *Salmonella* spp.) has been proposed as a transmission vehicle for

H. pylori infection in humans. However, the data regarding this route remain equivocal. Recent investigations from two different groups have proposed contradicting theories regarding the housefly as a potential vector for *H. pylori* transmission (GRUBEL et al. 1997; OSATO et al. 1997).

H. pylori primarily infects children, and the risk factors that have been described include persons residing in a developing country, living in conditions of poor socioeconomic circumstances and/or familial overcrowding, and being of certain ethnicities. In particular, in the United States the prevalence rates among African-Americans and Hispanics are similar to those among populations in developing countries (STAAT et al. 1996). Little is known, however, about the phenotype and genotype of *H. pylori* strains infecting children, and in particular, the epidemiology of infecting pediatric *H. pylori* strains.

3 Pathogenesis

3.1 Host Factors

The outcome of gastroduodenal disease after *H. pylori* colonization is believed to be a result of both host and bacterial determinants. Acid secretion for many years has been described as the critical factor for the development of mucosal ulceration in the stomach or duodenum. However, the effect of *H. pylori* on gastric acid secretion is a rather controversial subject. In particular, the effect of *H. pylori* on acid secretion in children remains poorly defined. One recent study demonstrated that there may be a difference between acid secretion in children with gastric ulcers as compared with those with duodenal ulcers (NAGITA et al. 1996). In a study of 82 subjects – 10 children with gastric ulcers, 9 with duodenal ulcers, 58 nonulcer patients, and 5 healthy adults – the authors looked at 24-h pH measurements as a determination of acid secretion. Gastric acidity was significantly reduced in patients with primary gastric ulcers (i.e., *Helicobacter pylori*-associated). However, gastric acidity was increased or above adult levels in those children with duodenal ulcers (NAGITA et al. 1996).

Other studies in children demonstrated a 24-h acid output distinctly different in ulcer patients than in normal controls (YAMASHIRO et al. 1995). This study was performed in each subject with intragastric pH monitoring over a 48-h period, the first 24h untreated and the second 24h with three doses of the acid suppressing H_2 receptor antagonist, cimetidine. Children with duodenal ulcers lacked the "intragastric pH inversion" that occurs in normals around midnight, and had persistent hypergastric acidity for most of the 24h period. Unfortunately however, the majority of adult studies are equivocal; in maximal acid output (MAO) the acid output values over a 24-h period or even basal acid output (BAO) are not predictive of the likelihood of ulcer development.

Evidence suggests that the pathogenesis of gastritis and gastroduodenal ulceration due to *H. pylori* infection is also mediated by disturbances in bicarbonate secretion and the mucus layer over gastric and duodenal epithelium. The mucus layer serves as a barrier to luminal pepsin and hydrochloric acid, preventing access of pepsin to the apical surface of gastric epithelial cells and by neutralizing the acid through the presence of bicarbonate secreted into the mucus layer. The mucus layer also provides protection for the epithelial cell turnover both in normal and perturbed states, as well as from mechanical damage during the hypermotile state of the digestive and intestinal phases of digestion. Mucosal production of bicarbonate secretion can be stimulated by prostaglandins, but inhibited by nonsteriodal anti-inflammatory agents (McQUEEN et al. 1983). Recent studies demonstrate that there are impaired rates of proximal duodenal bicarbonate production in patients with duodenal ulceration (ISENBERG et al. 1987; MERTZ-NIELSON et al. 1996). Clearly, further studies of gastric acid and duodenal bicarbonate secretion in *H. pylori* infected compared to uninfected children are critically needed.

It has been demonstrated that when there is inflammation in the stomach and duodenum in both humans and ferrets as a result of *Helicobacter* infection, there is a concurrent decrease in gastroduodenal mucosal surface hydrophobicity. This is believed to be due to a disturbance in the mucus layer (GOLD et al. 1996; LICHTENBERGER et al. 1994; Go et al. 1993). It is postulated that the mucus confers hydrophobicity to the stomach, and its decreased production and erosion leads to exposure of gastric epithelial cells to pepsin, acid, and other aggressive factors. Adult studies have demonstrated that a decreased polymerization of the component glycoproteins of mucus contribute to the deficient structure of duodenal ulcer patient mucus (YOUNAN et al. 1982). Evidence points to disturbances in the gastroduodenal mucus layer and bicarbonate secretion as factors in ulcer pathogenesis, but no studies have been carried out in children.

Gastric hormones, specifically gastrin (TAYLOR et al. 1984) and pepsinogens I and II (DEFIZE et al. 1987), may also play an important role in *H. pylori* associated inflammation, as "ulcer-causing factors." Early studies suggested an inheritable pattern of increased serum pepsinogen levels. These investigations showed that children with duodenal ulcers and their parents had increased levels of serum pepsinogen I (ROTTER et al. 1979). Subsequent studies of *H. pylori* infected demonstrate that chronic infection is associated with elevated levels of serum pepsinogen (ODERDA et al. 1990). Since this organism clusters in families, this observation has been felt to be evidence for the "inheritable" nature of peptic ulcer disease (DRUMM et al. 1990).

A vigorous local and systemic host immune response is observed after gastric colonization by *H. pylori* organisms (WYATT 1995). However, spontaneous clearance of *H. pylori* without antimicrobial-based therapeutic regimens is a rare occurrence. A monocyte and macrophage response can be seen in infected gastric mucosa, with both polymorphonuclear cells and plasma cells also present in the inflammatory infiltrate of adults (ASHORN et al. 1995; WHITNEY et al. 1996). Although definitive data are still lacking, a number of reports describe a lack of neutrophils in the *H. pylori* infected child's gastric mucosa (WHITNEY et al. 1996,

1998). It is still not clear whether T-cells play a major role in the inflammation associated with *H. pylori* infection, yet elevated levels of interleukin (IL)-1, IL-2, IL-6, and IL-8, as well as tumor necrosis factor-α are detectable in the gastric epithelium of infected individuals (ANDERSON et al. 1994). Circulating immuno-globulin G antibodies are easily detectable in *H. pylori* infected individuals, and it is based on these circulating IgG antibodies that many of the diagnostic assays have been developed (CUTLER 1995).

3.2 Bacterial Factors

Bacteria cause host disease by using one or more of three basic mechanisms called virulence determinants (GOTSCHLICH 1983): adhesion, invasion, and toxin elabo-ration. *H. pylori* is a gram-negative organism that resides under microaerobic conditions (~80% N_2, 10% CO_2, 5% H_2, and 5% O_2), in a neutral microenvi-ronment away from the gastric acidity, in the mucus layer and adherent to the epithelial cells primarily in the gastric antrum (MCGOWAN et al. 1996; DEKIGAI et al. 1995). Two primary morphological shapes, bacillary, and coccoid have been de-scribed for this organism (CHAN et al. 1994). Although it is believed that the bacillary form is the more virulent morphology, the biological relevance of each morphological form is not clearly understood.

H. pylori is highly motile, with multiple unipolar flagella, and the genetic basis for this virulence determinant has been well characterized (SCHMITZ et al. 1995). Biochemically, *H. pylori* produces catalase, oxidase, and urease enzymes. The ur-ease enzyme enables this organism to metabolize the urea present in the gastric mucus and establish the neutral microenvironment in which it lives and replicates. The production of the urease enzyme is what biochemically separates *H. pylori* from the intestinal *Campylobacter* spp. (OWEN et al. 1994; KARITA et al. 1995). The urease enzyme has received much attention and provides a useful, rapid diagnostic tool both in the endoscopy suite and by noninvasive carbon-13 or ^{14}C-labeled breath testing (STEEN et al. 1995; GRAHAM et al. 1987). Additionally, the urease enzyme is the specific virulence determinant towards which the development of vaccine constructs against *H. pylori* infection has been focused (CORTHESY-THELEUZ 1996).

At least 15 other species of *Helicobacter* that have been identified (Fox 1995). For example, *H. fennellieae* and *H. cinaedi* are both human pathogens that reside in the lower gastrointestinal tract and cause diarrheal disease in immunocompromised patients. Most of the other *Helicobacter* spp. are animal pathogens. Much attention has been given to *H. felis*, an organism that infects domestic and wild cats, and which causes chronic gastritis in the feline stomach (LEE et al. 1988). *H. felis* has been employed in recent investigations of a mouse model of chronic and acute gastritis in the development of vaccine against gastric *Helicobacter* infection (CZINN et al. 1991). Another *Helicobacter* of great interest is *H. hepaticus*, which infects certain strains of mice and has satisfied Koch's postulates as a causative agent of hepatocellular carcinoma in these murine strains (FOX et al. 1996). Studies of this bacteria as an etiological factor in the pathobiology of murine hepatocellular carcinoma may provide great insight into the biological plausibility and relationship of *H. pylori* to gastric cancer in humans. *Gastrospirillum hominis*, or *H. helmanii*, has been observed by histological staining of gastric biopsies obtained at upper endoscopy performed on patients with chronic-active gastritis. However, primary culture of these organisms has not been successfully performed, and the clinical relevance of these gastric spirochetes remains unclear.

A proposed schematic of the natural history of *H. pylori* infection is depicted in Fig. 1. However, the interrelationship between bacterial virulence properties and the host immune response that results in mucosal disease is still not clearly characterized. Many bacterial virulence factors have been described for *H. pylori*. (FIGURA et al. 1996). Specifically, urease (*ureA*, *ureB*, *ureC* genes) is produced in large quantities by all *H. pylori* isolates, as well as the other gastric *Helicobacter* spp. identified (MOBLEY et al. 1995). As mentioned above, this organism utilizes its flagella (*flaA*, *flaB* genes) to navigate through the gastric mucus to reach the apical surface of gastric epithelial cells where it adheres, replicates, and occupies its biological niche (O'TOOLE et al. 1994). More recent attention has been given to the vacuolating cytotoxin produced by more than 50% of isolated *H. pylori* strains. This

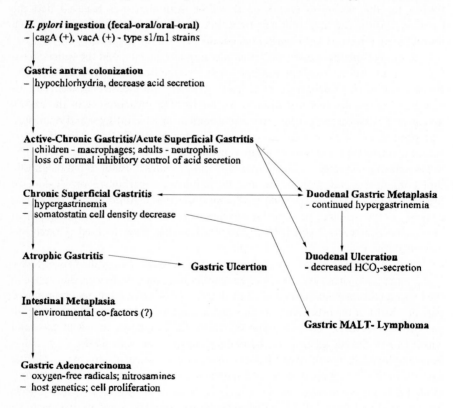

Fig. 1. Proposed schematic of *H. pylori* infection and gastroduodenal disease

cytotoxin was first described in the late 1980s and produces vacuoles in the cyto-plasm of eukaryotic cells in vitro (FIGURA et al. 1989; LEUNK et al. 1988). The gene (*vacA*) for this vacuolating cytotoxin, an 87-kDa protein, has at least two alleles and is quite variably expressed among *H. pylori* isolates (ATHERTON et al. 1995).

In addition to cytotoxin activity, *H. pylori* strains also differ in a high mo-lecular weight protein, designated as CagA, with a range of 105–140kDa (TUM-MURU et al. 1993). About 60% of *H. pylori* isolates produce this protein, and its presence is thought to be strongly correlated with the expression of the vacuolating cyototoxin activity. The *cagA* gene has been shown to be absent from those strains lacking the CagA protein product. The presence or absence of the cyotoxin pro-duction has led researchers to classify *H. pylori* strains into type I, those that are cyotoxin positive, and type II strains, those that are cytotoxin negative (XIANG et al. 1995). Type I strains appear to be associated with more severe gastroduodenal pathology than the gastric or duodenal disease associated with type II strains. However, no studies have been performed in children, and therefore the definitive relationship of bacterial genotype to gastroduodenal disease phenotype remains to be determined. More recently, shortly before the *H. pylori* genome was sequenced (TOMB et al. 1997), it was determined that there may be a major part of the *H. pylori* genome that confers pathogenicity to the organism, and this pathogenicity island, as it is now been called, may contain a number of different genes that confer virulence to the particular organism in a susceptible host (CENSINI et al. 1996; ATHERTON et al. 1997; BLASER et al. 1995).

4 Clinical Manifestations

4.1 Gastritis

The presence of *H. pylori* in the gastric mucosa and antral gastritis in adults was first reported by WARREN and MARSHALL in 1983, and shortly thereafter this finding was also described in children (DRUMM et al. 1987). Studies in adults established the presence of the organism in nearly all cases of chronic gastritis (PETERSON 1991). It was initially suggested that *H. pylori* colonizes inflamed tissue rather than causing the inflammation, since gastritis is a common finding in adults (PETERSON 1991). However, the prevalence of gastritis is less frequent in children, thereby enabling the investigations of *H. pylori* as a cause for gastritis rather than an opportunistic colonizer of inflamed tissue (DRUMM et al. 1987). Subsequent studies have shown that *H. pylori* colonization is not a common finding on the gastric mucosa of children with secondary causes of gastritis, for example, eosin-ophilic gastroenteritis and Crohn's disease (DRUMM et al. 1990). However, bacteria were clearly present in the majority of children with gastritis (DRUMM et al. 1987). This observation is strong evidence for the pathogenic role of *H. pylori* in the development of chronic antral gastritis in children.

In 1986 HILL et al. (1986) reported that four children with chronic gastritis were infected with *H. pylori*. Later that year CADRANEL and colleagues found the organism to be present in a group of eight patients with chronic gastritis. Shortly thereafter DRUMM et al. (1988) observed the bacteria in 70% of 67 pediatric patients with chronic active gastritis. Similar observations that year were also made by MAHONY and colleagues in 38 pediatric patients and CZINN and CARR (CZINN et al. 1986) in 25. Numerous additional studies confirm that *H. pylori* colonization of the gastric mucosa is virtually always associated with chronic gastritis in children (DRUMM et al. 1990; KILBRIDGE et al. 1988; YEUNG et al. 1990). Despite the well-known predominance of gastrointestinal pathology in males, *H. pylori*-associated gastritis has been shown to be equally frequent in boys as in girls (BLECKER et al. 1994). Finally, eradication of *H. pylori* from the gastric mucosa is associated with healing of the antral gastritis, another finding in favor of *H. pylori* as the cause of primary gastritis in children (YEUNG et al. 1990).

H. pylori associated gastritis in children is often not apparent at endoscopy, thereby making biopsy essential for definitive diagnosis (DRUMM et al. 1987; CZINN et al. 1987). In a prospective study the endoscopic findings were normal in eight of ten children who had histological antral gastritis. A nodularity of the antral mucosa has also been described to occur in association with *H. pylori* gastritis in children (BUJANOVER et al. 1990). Although less common an occurrence, this finding has also been observed in adults (MARSHALL et al. 1986; SBEIH et al. 1996).

4.2 Ulcers

Although there is a notable lack of good large population-based pediatric studies, rates of peptic ulcer disease in childhood seems to be low. Large pediatric endoscopy centers have reported an incidence of five to seven children with gastric or duodenal ulcers per year (DRUMM et al. 1988). Almost all peptic ulcers in children are located in the duodenum, and gastric ulcers are extremely rare in children (CHONG et al. 1995). A strong correlation has been demonstrated between duodenal ulceration and *H. pylori* gastritis in children (DRUMM et al. 1990). In fact *H. pylori* gastritis has been found in 90%–100% of pediatric duodenal ulcer disease patients (KILBRIDGE et al. 1988). Similarly, as in adults (BLASER et al. 1995), duodenal ulcerations in the absence of *H. pylori* are extremely rare in children. It has also been demonstrated that duodenal ulcer disease in children does not relapse if *H. pylori* is eradicated from the gastric mucosa (DOOLEY et al. 1988). YEUNG and colleagues (1990) treated 23 children with *H. pylori* gastritis associated with duodenal ulcer disease, using either cimetidine alone or a combination of cimetidine and amoxicillin. Although only a small portion of the children in this study remained uninfected, when the gastric mucosa remained free of *H. pylori* (combination therapy), no recurrence of duodenal ulcer disease was detected 6 months after the end of treatment. In contrast, 50% of patients whose ulcers were originally healed, but who remained colonized by *H. pylori* (cimetidine only therapy) had a recurrence of their ulcer by 6 months.

4.3 Gastric Cancer

Support for the role of *H. pylori* in gastric cancer comes from a variety of sources: studies paralleling the epidemiological features of cancer with those of *H. pylori* infection (RECAVARREN-ARCE et al. 1991; CORREA et al. 1990), cross-sectional studies of *H. pylori* infection in patients with cancer (PARSONNET et al. 1991a,b), and prospective studies of *H. pylori* infections (FORMAN et al. 1991; PARSONNET et al. 1991a,b).

Gastric cancer prevalence is higher in areas of poverty; afflicting persons in developing nations and lower socioeconomic classes of the industrialized world (Fox et al. 1989). In many countries of Latin America and Asia, gastric cancer remains the most common malignancy among men and the second most common among women (JOLY 1977; PARKIN 1986). Incidence rates as high as 80 per 100,000 population have been reported in Colombia and Japan. In contrast, gastric cancer affects less than 10 per 100,000 persons per year in the United States and Western Europe (YOUNG et al. 1981). However, within low-risk countries there are certain ethnic groups with increased risk. In the United States, for example, the prevalence of gastric cancer among blacks, Asians, and Hispanics is almost double that among whites (YOUNG et al. 1981).

Clues to the decline in gastric cancer incidence come from studies of persons who have moved from a region of high gastric cancer risk to one of low risk. Those immigrating from Japan, a high-risk country, to regions of lower risk in the United States have only moderately decreased cancer risk, even if they immigrated at a young age (HAENZEL et al. 1972). Second-generation immigrants, however, show a gastric cancer risk much closer to that of their new country. Similar results have been found in European immigrants to Australia (McMICHAEL et al. 1980) and Puerto Rican immigrants to New York (ROSENWAIKE 1984). From these studies it has been concluded that environmental factors initiate malignant transformation in the stomach.

H. pylori infection can therefore be called a marker of increased gastric adenocarcinoma risk. Definite proof of cause, however, would be established only if controlled trials demonstrate that elimination or prevention of infection prevents malignancy. As mentioned above, studies of *H. hepaticus* as a cause of liver cancer in mice and *H. mustelae* as an etiological agent in gastric adenocarcinoma in ferrets add biological plausibility to the role of *H. pylori* in gastric cancer in humans. Moreover, WATANABE et al. (WATANABE et al.) have recently shown that long term infection (26–62 weeks) of Mongolian gerbils by *H. pylori* results in the development of gastric adenocarcinoma in >37% of the animals. This provides even more compelling evidence to support the biologic plausibility for *H. pylori*'s role in human stomach cancer. In addtion, short-term studies documenting reversal of *pre*neoplastic conditions with anti-*H. pylori* therapy lend support to the association of of *H. pylori* and cancer. However, whether intestinal metaplasia and, in particular, gastric epithelial cell dysplasia as a result of *H. pylori* infection, are irreversible remains to be determined (CORREA et al. 1990; LANSDOWN et al. 1990).

4.4 Gastric Lymphomas

In infancy and early childhood, the stomach lacks a significant number of immunocompetent lymphocytes and plasma cells. Chronic inflammation can develop as the child becomes older, leading lymphocytes to accumulate in the submucosa and gradually increase their depth of penetration. With the eradication of *H. pylori*, chronic inflammation decreases, and the density of submucosal lymphocytes dramatically declines (ROBERT et al. 1993; KOSUNEN et al. 1992). Since most gastric lymphomas arise in areas of chronic inflammation (BROOK et al. 1983), it seems plausible that prior *H. pylori* infection and gastric lymphomas are linked. Primary non-Hodgkin's lymphoma of the stomach is an uncommon cancer, accounting for only 10% of lymphomas and 3% of gastric neoplasms (SPIRO 1983). Gastric non-Hodgkin's lymphoma remains, however, the most common extranodal form of this lymphoma, accounting for 20% of primary extranodal disease (RUBIN et al. 1990). In addition, immunological studies have shown these tumors to be of B-cell lineage (VILLAR et al. 1991).

Low-grade B-cell lymphomas that arise in the stomach, lung, salivary gland, and thyroid are similar to the structural features of mucosa-associated lymphoid tissue (MALT) as typified in Peyer's patches (ISAACSON et al. 1987). These lymphomas, together with the high-grade lesions that may evolve from them (CHAN et al. 1990), are known collectively as MALT lymphomas (ISAACSON et al. 1987). MALT lymphomas were first described in the early 1980s when ISAACSON and WRIGHT (1983) noted that the histology of certain low grade, B-cell gastrointestinal lymphomas was unlike that of comparable low-grade nodal lymphomas but was similar to that of MALT. Paradoxically, however, MALT is not present in either the normal stomach or other sites in which MALT lymphomas arise.

In the stomach, lymphoid tissue is acquired as a result of colonization of the gastric mucosa by *H. pylori* (STOLTE et al. 1989). WOTHERSPOON and colleagues (1991) demonstrated that this *H. pylori*-associated lymphoid tissue is of MALT type. They subsequently suggested that MALT acquired in response to *H. pylori* infection provides the background on which other, yet unidentified factors act, and that this leads to the development of lymphoma in a small proportion of cases. Very recently HUSSELL and colleagues (1993) demonstrated that cellular proliferation of low-grade B-cell gastric MALT lymphomas to *H. pylori* is dependent on *H. pylori* specific T-cells and their products rather than on the bacteria themselves. Multiple serological studies provide evidence suggesting that infection with *H. pylori* increases the risk of gastric non-Hodgkin's lymphoma (PARSONNET et al. 1991a,b; DOGLIONI et al. 1992; FORMAN et al. 1990; PARSONNET et al. 1994).

Specific colonization of lymphoid follicle centers by neoplastic cells (ISAACSON et al. 1991) and the binding of specific antibodies (GRIENER er al. 1994) suggest that MALT tumors are immunologically responsive. Given the close association between gastric MALT lymphoma and *H. pylori*, this organism might evoke the immunological response, and eradication of *H. pylori* might thereby inhibit the tumor. Studies have suggested that anti-*H. pylori* therapy eradicates MALT lymphoma in some cases (WOTHERSPOON et al. 1993; BAYERDORFFER et al. 1994).

5 Methods of Detection

5.1 Indications for Diagnostic Testing

At present there are no reliably defined indications or guidelines for the clinician to follow in deciding whether a child should undergo testing for *H. pylori* infection. Indiscriminate testing for *H. pylori* could consume a tremendous amount of health care resources, and in asymptomatic patients, particularly children, ethical concerns are an important issue to consider. Therefore, from one perspective, neither the costs of treatment nor the risk of testing is justified in asymptomatic children. However, the primary pediatrician and pediatric gastroenterologist must also consider the parent's fears of the presence of an infection that could in the long run result in significant morbidity (e.g., ulcers) and potentially mortality (e.g., gastric cancer). Thus, on the contrary, refusal to test for the infection if the specific clinical situation suggests that testing might be reasonable, may in fact be detrimental to the patient's health and well being. Consensus has not necessarily been reached for this infection in the pediatric population despite three large recently published consensus conferences. Therefore testing for *H. pylori* should be considered as appropriate only if treatment is planned and should have an impact on the management of the child (LEE et al. 1997). At present there is no evidence of benefit from *H. pylori* eradication in individuals without gastrointestinal symptoms (e.g., dyspepsia); asymptomatic adults and especially asymptomatic children. Therefore the clinician should use a carefully documented history of abdominal complaints and related symptoms (e.g., anorexia, weight loss) as well as family history to determine the indications for diagnosis on the presumption that if *H. pylori* is found by a validated and reliable test for children, the infection will be treated.

5.2 Diagnostic Testing

The reference method for the diagnosis of active *H. pylori* infection is esophago-gastro-duodenoscopy with gastric biopsies. However, there are numerous other, reasonably accurate detection assays that recently have become commercialized and available for clinical use. Invasive techniques are based on upper endoscopy and multiple biopsies for the detection of *H. pylori*. Histological demonstration of the *H. pylori* upon staining or its identification by microbiological means (i.e., culture) constitute direct evidence of the presence of this micro-organism. Most noninvasive techniques rely on detecting a feature of *H. pylori* (e.g., the ability to hydrolyze urea) or the response of the immune system to its colonization of the gastric epithelium (i.e., specific antibodies).

5.3 Invasive Techniques

5.3.1 Histological Identification

The characteristic histological appearance of *H. pylori* is a 3.0×0.5mm spiral rod located adjacent to the gastric epithelium. Although the modified silver stain (Warthin-Starry or Steiner stain) is considered the best method for the identification of *H. pylori* organisms, a trained pathologist can readily see the curved, spiral organisms on a Giemsa stain of the gastric biopsy sections.

In addition to the stain used, a second factor that influences the histological detection of *H. pylori* is the uneven distribution of the organism throughout the gastric mucosa. A considerable variation in the numbers of bacteria can be observed in biopsy specimens from a single source, and in 10% of all cases there are sections from a positive case completely free of organisms (DIXON et al. 1996; WYATT et al. 1988). Two biopsies taken from within 2–5cm of the pylorus are generally considered to be sufficient for diagnosis (EL-ZIMAAITY et al. 1995) in infected adults. Unlike investigations in *H. pylori* infected adults, in whom systematic gastric mapping studies have determined the appropriate number of biopsies necessary for optimal yeild of positive culture and/or histological staining, comparable studies have not been performed in children and are critically needed to better devise guidelines for endoscopic diagnosis of active pediatric *H. pylori* infection.

Because histological gastritis may be present in the absence of macroscopic mucosal abnormalities, particularly in children, this examination permits a better correlation between the presence of *H. pylori* and its pathological result (ELTA et al. 1987; SAUERBACH et al. 1984). The observation of histological chronic (active) gastritis without evidence of *H. pylori* should prompt a careful reexamination of the sections to exclude the bacterium. Histological examination of gastric biopsies can provide important information about the presence of *H. pylori* and the condition of the mucosa.

5.3.2 Culture

H. pylori is obligately microaerophilic, and the observation of uneven distribution of the organism may contribute to falsely negative cultures. Other factors that have been implicated in unsuccessful culturing of *H. pylori* include recent antibiotic use, ingestion of a topical anesthetic or simethicone during endoscopy, and contamination of the biopsy forceps with other organisms or glutaraldehyde. Due to increasing resistance rates to metronidazole and clarithromycin both in the United States and in Europe, an important application for culture is the determination of the antibiotic susceptibility profile of treatment-resistant organisms (McNULTY et al. 1988).

The ability of the organism to produce urease in a significantly (approx. 1000×) higher concentration than any other known bacteria that might inhabit the human stomach is an important characteristic of *H. pylori* that forms the basis of several diagnostic tests (HAZELL et al. 1986; ABDALLA et al. 1989). Urease catalyzes the degradation of urea to ammonia and bicarbonate. This reaction causes an increase in the pH of the surrounding medium, which can be detected with a pH indicator, resulting in a color change (ABDALLA et al. 1989). A number of tests have been developed, ranging from simple "homemade" solutions of urea, water, and phenol, to the various commercially produced tests, of which the CLO test (Trimed, Kansas, MO, USA) is one of the more frequently used. Positive results are obtained with good sensitivity and specificity within a few hours after addition of the biopsy specimen to the medium. Urease tests are also dependent on the density of the bacteria and the patient who is on acid suppressing agents such as the proton pump inhibitor omeprazole.

5.4 Noninvasive Techniques

One of the most promising noninvasive methods with great potential for application in the pediatric population is based on urease enzyme production by *H. pylori* organisms and involves the administration of a ^{13}C- or ^{14}C-labeled urea meal and then testing expired breath samples over a 2-h period. In *H. pylori*-colonized patients the urea is metabolized to ammonia and labeled bicarbonate, and the latter is carried to the lungs and excreted in the expired breath as labeled carbon dioxide. The labeled carbon excreted can then be quantified. This test is semiquantitative, measuring the approximate bacterial load in the entire stomach, and of all the noninvasive tests it may be the best predictor of treatment success. Analysis of the amount of labeled carbon dioxide in single, pooled, or serial breath samples is directly related to the extent of urea hydrolysis and the presence or absence of *H. pylori*. The original description of this technique in humans used the stable, naturally occurring isotope ^{13}C (GRAHAM et al. 1987). Although ^{13}C has the advantage of being nonradioactive, its measurement requires an expensive and complicated gas isotope ratio mass spectrometer. Because this equipment is not widely available, an adaptation of this method, using ^{14}C, has been devised (DEBOGNIE et al. 1991; HENZE et al. 1990; MARSHALL et al. 1988). ^{14}C can be easily quantified by using a scintillation counter. It has been estimated that a single upper gastrointestinal series produces more bone marrow exposure than a 100 ^{14}C-urea breath tests (MARSHALL et al. 1991). While this noninvasive technique has the disadvantage of not being able to actually culture the bacteria, the urea breath test detects *H. pylori* over a much greater surface area of the stomach.

5.4.1 Serology

It is clear that virtually all *H. pylori* infected subjects develop a local and a systemic immune response against this organism (NEWELL et al. 1989, 1992). Several sero-immunological techniques have been used to determine the antibody response to *H. pylori*, including hemagglutination, bacterial agglutination, complement fixation, indirect immunofluorescence, immunoblotting, and enzyme-linked immuno-sorbent assays (ELISA) (CULTER et al. 1995). In general, these assays have been found to be more sensitive in detecting *H. pylori* antibodies than bacterial agglutination or complement fixation (CHONG et al. 1995). Commercially available serological assays, based primarily on IgG antibody levels against *H. pylori* antigens, have reasonable accuracy in detecting the "presence" of *H. pylori* infection (CUTLER et al. 1995). However, caution must be used when depending on these assays for patient management, particularly in the pediatric population. The assays are limited in their accuracy when applied in populations different from those in which the assays were developed (e.g., a developing country such as Peru as compared to the United States). In addition, most commercially available assays have been standardized and validated (against esophago-gastroduo-denoscopy with biopsy) in adult populations, therefore have different cutoff values than those which may be appropriate for use in children. It has been demonstrated that results obtained for serological tests for the detection of *H. pylori* in adults cannot necessarily be extrapolated to children (WESTBLOM et al. 1992; MEGRAUD 1993). Although the reason for this discrepancy between pediatric and adult age groups is not yet fully understood, it has been suggested that a difference in *H. pylori* antigen recognition is responsible for the decreased sensitivity and specificity in children. Conversely, due to the variable immune response in children, a significant difference in cutoff values between the adult and pediatric populations might be the causative factor (CZINN et al. 1987; KHANNA et al. 1997). Finally, the IgG response to *H. pylori* infection persists for at least 3 months and by some reports more than 1 year in the face of successful antimicrobial treatment of the infection; thus the use of serology for posttreatment monitoring may be limited.

5.4.2 Polymerase Chain Reaction

Performing PCR techniques in a laboratory, usually research, with considerable expertise is exquisitely sensitive, but can be fraught with false positives, such as from contaminated forceps or endoscopy equipment. This technique has been able to detect *H. pylori* in biopsy specimens (BICKLEY et al. 1993; KOOISTRA-SMID et al. 1993), gastric juice and saliva (WESTBLOM et al. 1993), dental plaque (BICKLEY et al. 1993; NGUYEN et al. 1993), and feces (MAPSTONE et al. 1993). However, because of the relatively high cost and time consumption of PCR as a diagnostic tool for the detection of *H. pylori*, this technique does not yet belong to the routine diagnostic possibilities in clinical practice.

6 Treatment and Vaccine Development

6.1 Indications for Treatment

An area for critically needed studies is treatment for *H. pylori* infection in the pediatric age group; in particular, indications for treatment and the appropriate treatment regimen. Of all the "consensus" conferences convened to develop guidelines for the diagnosis and management of *H. pylori* infection, no recommendations have been reached regarding the *H. pylori* infected child (HOWDEN 1997). In 1994 the NIH Consensus Conference recommended that a person should be treated if there is evidence of a gastric or duodenal ulcer (NIH 1994). In 1997 the American Digestive Health Conference (ADHF) recommended that an *H. pylori* infected individual should be treated if there is an active or past history of duodenal or gastric ulcer, and if there is resection of an early gastric cancer or MALT lymphoma. The ADHF also recommended retesting after treatment for patients with bleeding or otherwise complicated peptic ulcer disease (FENNERTY 1997). The Canadian Consensus Conference recommendations are similar except for the following; (a) routine testing for *H. pylori* in patients with gastroesophageal reflux disease (GERD) is not recommended due to the lack of data on a relationship between *H. pylori* infection and GERD; (b) eradication should be considered in high-risk populations for gastric cancer development (i.e., those of Japanese origin), although the benefits are still unproven; (c) eradication should be attempted in patients with *H. pylori* infection and severe histological gastritis and absence of ulcer as eradication clearly reverses inflammation; and (d) patients with chronic persistent (> 3 months) dyspepsia (pain or discomfort in the upper abdomen) and without alarm features (anemia, weight loss) can be considered on a case-by-case basis for eradication if *H. pylori* positive by noninvasive testing (breath test, serology) (HUNT et al. 1998).

Finally, the European *Helicobacter pylori* Study Group (EHPSG) held a consensus conference in 1996 involving 19 European countries, with observers from the United States, Canada, and Japan (EHPSG 1997). The EHPSG conference guidelines agree with the above recommendations for eradication therapy in the face of peptic ulcer disease, MALT lymphoma, early gastric carcinoma and in individuals with a strong family history or endemic country with gastric carcinoma. They also agree with the North American guidelines (i.e., ADHF and Canadian) for the eradication of *H. pylori* infection in severe gastritis, but there is considerable debate and controversy regarding indications for therapy in the *H. pylori* infected individual with nonulcer dyspepsia, GERD and in particular in asymptomatic subjects. Overall, however, the European guidelines are to treat if one intends to test for *H. pylori* – "test and treat" strategy.

Thus the guidelines for children remain undefined. This author believes that it is reasonable to recommend that a child with refractory abdominal symptoms and documented *H. pylori* infection with histopathological findings (i.e., chronic-active gastritis) should be treated with antimicrobial agents. Patients who have failed empiric acid-blockade therapy (i.e., H$_2$ receptor antagonists), should be evaluated for *H. pylori* infection before initiation of antimicrobial therapy. Evaluation should be performed by upper endoscopy and biopsies with at least histological evaluation and appropriate staining employed by the evaluating pathologist (i.e., Giemsa, Warthin-Starry). Urea breath testing could be used as a screen until appropriate controlled trials of breath testing with establishment of proper cutoff values in children are performed. If using serology as a screening method, the clinician *must* have a careful understanding of the assay chosen, the study population used for validation (age, diagnosis, geographic location) taken into account before subjecting the patient to the test and charge. Children who are undergoing maintenance antisecretory therapy and are subsequently diagnosed with *H. pylori* associated peptic ulcer disease should be treated for their infection regardless of whether they are suffering from the initial disease presentation or from a recurrence. Controlled prospective studies are needed to assess the benefits of treating nonulcer dyspeptic children with *H. pylori* infection (NIH 1994; ROWLAND et al. 1997; HUNT et al. 1998).

6.2 Treatment

The recurrence of duodenal ulcers can be dramatically reduced and prevented by a single course of antimicrobial therapy directed at the eradication of *H. pylori* organisms infecting the gastric mucosa. Because of the economic impact of peptic ulcer disease (i.e., treatment costs, morbidity and mortality) approx. $U.S.13 billion (1993 dollars) annually for the management of acute and chronic ulcers, approx. 6500 annual deaths, as well as the prevalence of *H. pylori* worldwide, it can be easily determined that all patients with ulcers who are also infected by *H. pylori* should receive antimicrobial therapy. As mentioned above, there is a notable lack of consensus on which patients should receive therapy when infected by *H. pylori* and manifesting other gastroduodenal disease (i.e., gastritis). Reports of reinfection rates vary in the literature, but cross-infection may occur and can be quite high in families with small children (ROWLAND et al. 1997).

   H. pylori is a difficult organism to treat, and success of therapy requires the concurrent administration of two or more antimicrobial drugs. In treatment trials the success of therapy has often been arbitrarily defined as the absence of detectable organisms by tissue sampling or carbon-labeled urea breath tests, 1 month or more after discontinuation of treatment. The clear majority of treatment trials have been performed in adults, with a notable lack of available information on treating *H. pylori* infected children. None of the drug regimens currently used to treat *H. pylori* eradicates the organism successfully 100% of the time, and some regimens are associated with a relatively high frequency of side effects. In addition, *H. pylori* is resistant to only a few antimicrobial agents, (i.e., vancomycin, nalidixic acid), but it can become readily resistant to metronidazole and to a lesser extent clarithromycin. Therefore the success of the therapeutic regimen depends highly upon patient compliance, the resistance that may develop in *H. pylori* strains colonizing the infected individual, and adverse reactions.

   Successful *combination therapies* for *H. pylori* are based on a antibacterial agent that acts luminally to cause significant suppression of the bacterium. In this scenario, a second agent acting both topically and systematically is more efficacious and less likely to cause selection of resistant isolates. Amoxicillin has been widely used to treat *H. pylori*, especially in combination with bismuth (BIANCHI et al. 1993; ROSIORU et al. 1993). A disadvantage of amoxicillin is a 5% incidence of *Clos-*

tridium difficile induced colitis, which may be prevented by combining the drug with metronidazole (MARSHALL 1993). This regimen was advocated as a 7-day treatment by LOGAN et al. (1994a), with an overall eradication rate of 74%.

Others have observed *H. pylori* eradication in 60%–70% of patients given combination dual therapy with amoxicillin and omeprazole (UNGE et al. 1989); due to previous studies demonstrating treatment failure with monotherapy of amoxicillin. It has been proposed that omeprazole would enhance antibiotic penetration into a pH neutral location (i.e., between parietal cells where *H. pylori* tend to colonize). Preliminary results from a larger study using the combination amoxicillin-omeprazole demonstrated an eradication rate of 80% (BAYERDORFFER et al. 1994). In addition, ulcer relapse was virtually nonexistent (< 2%) in the patients in whom *H. pylori* had been eradicated. A recent trial investigated the effect of a clarithromycin-omeprazole combination therapy in 73 patients with *H. pylori* associated gastroduodenal pathology (LOGAN et al. 1994b). As defined by a negative [^{13}C]urea breath test, *H. pylori* was cleared after 2 weeks of treatment in 95.9% of the patients and eradicated in 78.1%.

Triple therapies have the advantage of both luminal and systemic activity. Luminally active agents against *H. pylori* are bismuth, tetracycline, amoxicillin, clarithromycin, and furazolidone (GRAHAM et al. 1989). Most triple therapies contain a nitroimidazole (i.e., metronidazole), appearing to be the most active component against *H. pylori*, provided that bacterial suppression with the other agents has occurred (Table 2). The combination of bismuth, tetracycline, and metronidazole seems to be particularly effective (HOSKING et al. 1994; ISER et al. 1994; MCCARTHY et al. 1993; THIJS et al. 1993; WILHELMSEN et al. 1994). One investigation demonstrated a 90% eradication rate, suggesting that more than 50% of the metronidazole-resistant forms are eradicated by this triple therapy (BORODY et al. 1992, 1994). Further support is provided by a recent comparison of various combination therapies for metronidazole-resistant organisms, in which the eradication rate exceeded 50% even if *H. pylori* infection was retreated with the same triple therapy (BORODY et al. 1992, 1994). Since the eradication rate with dual tetracycline-bismuth therapy is very low, it appears that synergism exists between metronidazole and the other two drugs (GRAHAM et al. 1993).

BAZZOLI and colleagues (1993) reported an *H. pylori* eradication rate of 100% in 36 patients with a 1-week regimen utilizing omeprazole, clarithromycin, and tinidazole triple therapy. These results were later confirmed with follow-up eradication rates of 95% (BAZZOLI et al. 1994; MOAYYEDI et al. 1994). Furthermore, the bacterial eradication rate decreased markedly after substitution of nitroimidazole by tetracycline, suggesting that tinidazole or metronidazole are important for implementation of treatment options that confer sufficiently high bacterial eradication (LABENZ et al. 1994).

A recent multicenter adult study, using clarithromycin, omeprazole, and amoxicillin for 1 week, obtained an eradication rate of 96% with this short-term triple therapy (LIND et al. 1996). Because of the short duration and excellent eradication rate of this triple therapy, the treatment should be considered as a potential first choice for the initial treatment and eradication of *H. pylori* in both

Table 2. Triple-therapy combinations (from BLECKER and GOLD 1997)

	n	Days	Eradication rate (%)
Tetracycline-bismuth-metronidazole			
LABENZ et al. (1994)	19	14	84.2
CUTLER et al. (1995)	118	28	96.6
GRAHAM et al. (1992)	93	14	87.0
WILHELMSEN et al. (1994)	152	14	89–98
HOSKING et al. (1994)	76	7	94.0
ISER et al. (1994)	101	14	90.0
THIJS et al. (1993)	100	15	93.0[a]
			50.0[c]
			98.4[b]
BELL et al. (1993)	43	14	90.9[b]
			33.3[c]
Amoxicillin-bismuth-metronidazole			
BURETTE et al. (1992)	36	14	63.0[c]
			95.0[b]
SEPPALA et al. (1992)	93	14	84.0
RAUTELIN et al. (1992)	86	14	91.0
Amoxicillin-bismuth-tinidazole			
BIANCHI PORRO et al. (1993)	17	14	83.0
DI NAPOLI et al. (1992)	50	10	69.0
Omeprazole-tetracycline-metronidazole			
MCCARTHY et al. (1993)	43	7	58.0
Omeprazole-amoxicillin-metronidazole			
BELL et al. (1992)	127	14	96.4[b]
			75.0[c]
Omeprazole-clarithromycin-tinidazole			
BAZZOLI et al. (1994)	65	7	95.0
Omeprazole-clarithromycin-metronidazole			
LABENZ et al. (1994)	80	7	95.0
Tetracycline-bismuth-amoxicillin			
GRAHAM et al. (1993)	16	14	43.0
Amoxicillin-furazolidone-metronidazole			
COELHO et al. (1992)	47	5	75.0
Omeprazole-clarithromycin-amoxicillin			
LIND et al. (1996)	787	7	96.0

[a] Overall eradication.
[b] Metronidazole-sensitive strains.
[c] Metronidazole-resistant strains.

adults and children. However, it is important to understand that at most institutions, antibiotic sensitivity testing of *H. pylori* strains is unavailable; therefore, current recommendations suggest triple therapy as a logical practical first choice for *H. pylori* eradication (BLANCO et al. 1988).

Another difficulty in devising an optimal treatment for the eradication of *H. pylori* infection is the acquisition of resistance. *H. pylori* appears to easily acquire resistance to certain antimicrobial drugs, such as imidazole derivatives (GOODWIN et al. 1988), quinolones (GLUPCZYNSKI et al. 1987; STONE et al. 1988), and erythromycin (MARSHALL 1993). Therefore these drugs should no longer be used as monotherapy. This is of special importance in certain underdeveloped areas with a high prevalence of *H. pylori* infection, where these drugs are frequently used for many other conditions and *H. pylori* strains have been shown to develop increasing resistance (EHPSG 1992).

Adverse effects are primarily caused by antibiotics, not acid-suppressing agents, employed in the anti-*H. pylori* therapy regimens (MARSHALL et al. 1988). Despite the increased success at *H. pylori* eradication, triple therapy combinations of a bismuth compound, metronidazole, and either amoxicillin or tetracycline produce an increased risk of adverse reactions (AXON et al. 1991; RAUWS et al. 1990). Adverse reactions in turn lead to noncompliance, which results in treatment failure and/or antibiotic resistance. The most commonly reported reactions are gastrointestinal complaints that may lead to discontinuation of therapy. The risk of commonly reported adverse reactions to the antibiotics explains the reluctance by so many practitioners to use triple therapy despite the well-documented long-term effect on ulcer healing (MALFERTHEIMER et al. 1993). In therapeutic trials for duodenal ulcer disease the use of a single antibiotic (e.g., tinidazole) combined with a bismuth compound cause adverse events in up to 16% of patients (MARSHALL et al. 1988). Triple therapy, however, increases the incidence of adverse events (RAUWS et al. 1990; GRAHAM et al. 1992), with up to 21% of study patients withdrawing from treatment (RAUWS et al. 1990). Bismuth compounds may also cause adverse reactions, although less commonly than antibiotics (MALFERTHEIMER et al. 1993). Bismuth toxicity with compounds such as bismuth subsalicylate and colloidal bismuth subcitrate is rare and can be avoided by proper use; intake limited to a period of no more than 4 weeks, and no treatment in the presence of renal insufficiency (MALFERTHEIMER et al. 1993).

Patient compliance in taking prescribed medications depends on a number of factors. Numerous studies have listed the following as being of primary importance in the determination of compliance: severity of symptoms, number and quantity of drugs taken, duration of treatment, complexity of the treatment regimen, and drug-related adverse effects are of crucial importance (MALFERTHEIMER et al. 1993). Thus patient compliance can be a significant problem with triple therapy. GRAHAM et al. (1992), demonstrated lack of compliance as the main cause for eradication failure by triple therapeutic regimens. In this study, age, gender, type of gastrointestinal disease, duration of therapy, and the amount of bismuth had no effect on the eradication rate. However, *H. pylori* was eradicated in 96% of the patients who took more than 60% of the prescribed medication, and only in 69% of the patients who took less than 60% of the drugs.

In addition, compliance may be significantly reduced by the rapid resolution of abdominal pain, as a consequence of antiulcer therapy (MALFERTHEIMER et al. 1993). The patients discontinue the prescribed medications when symptoms disappear, thereby not completing the treatment course and potentially failing to clear or eradicate their *H. pylori*. Since compliance seems to be a major factor in the successful treatment of *H. pylori* infection, it is of no surprise that longer courses of therapy do not seem to offer any advantage over treatments of short duration. It may be suggested that good compliance for 7 days is better than mediocre compliance for 14 days or longer. For this reason, several investigators have tried to eradicate *H. pylori* with short courses of combination therapy, even attempting single-day therapy (Tucci et al. 1993). However, to date, the optimal duration of therapy has still not been determined.

6.3 Vaccines

The most promising treatment and possible prevention of *H. pylori* infection and its significant gastroduodenal disease sequelae lie in the development of an efficacious vaccine. Given the long-term risk of gastric cancer associated with *H. pylori* infection and the varied rates of eradication with antimicrobial regimens, a vaccination approach to prevent the late and life-threatening manifestations of *H. pylori* infection should be considered. Extensive efforts in many laboratories are currently underway worldwide. Prophylaxis by vaccination seems essential since host natural immunity is inadequate to clear this infection despite a seemingly vigorous local and systemic immune response (Wyatt et al. 1988).

It has been shown in many studies that host natural immunity is inadequate to clear this infection despite a seemingly vigorous local and systemic immune response (Wyatt et al. 1988; Jaskiewicz et al. 1993). Recently Czinn and colleagues (1993) and Chen et al. (1993) demonstrated in a mouse model that oral immunization with a crude lysate of *H. felis* induces protection against gastric infection by *H. pylori* and associated this protection with high concentrations of secretory IgA antibodies. Further studies have shown that gastric infection in a mouse model infected with *H. pylori* can be prevented by the administration of a recombinant urease oral vaccine with *E. coli* heat-labile toxin given as adjuvant (Marchetti et al. 1995).

Preliminary studies have shown that cats can be infected by *H. pylori* (Wang et al. 1994). This observation raises the possibility that this animal may be used as a model to test vaccines. Moreover, other animal models such as the cat (Lee et al. 1988) and the ferret (Fox et al. 1986), which have their own naturally occurring *Helicobacter* infection, may prove useful for further vaccine development.

Negrini and colleagues (1994) demonstrated the presence of antibodies that cross-reacted with the gastric mucosa as a result of human *H. pylori* infection. There was also a heterogeneity in these cross-reactive humoral responses. These authors found that strains from patients with atrophic gastritis induce more cross-reactive responses in mice than strains from patients with mild gastritis. These results underscore the need to identify the optimal *H. pylori* antigens in order to design an effective vaccine which will not induce a cross-reactive immune response.

Finally, in addition, the initial steps of vaccine development showed that prophylactic immunization is possible, and it now appears that a vaccine is capable of serving as treatment of active *H. pylori* infection and gastritis in animal models (Corthesy-Theulaz et al. 1995; Doidge et al. 1994). Time will tell to what extent this possibility of preventing and treating major gastroduodenal diseases associated with *H. pylori* is realistic.

References

Abdalla SFM, Perez RM (1989) Rapid detection of *Campylobacter pylori* colonization by a simple biochemical test. J Clin Microbiol 27:2604–2605

Anderson LP, Crabtree JI (1994) Immunological aspects of *Helicobacter pylori*. Curr Opin Gastroenterol 10:26–29

Ashorn M (1995) What are the specific features of *Helicobacter pylori* gastritis in children. Ann Med 27:617–620

Ashorn M, Miettinen A, Ruuska T, Laippala P, Maki M (1996) Seroepidemiological study of *Helicobacter pylori* infection in infancy. Arch Dis Child Fetal Neonatal Edn 74:141–142

Atherton JC, Cao P, Peek JRM, Tummuru KR, Blaser MJ, Cover TL (1995) Mosaicism in vacuolating cytotoxin alleles of *Helicobacter pylori*. Association of vacA types with cytotoxin production and peptic ulceration. J Biol Chem 270:17771–17777

Atherton JC, Peek JCR, Tham KT, Cover TL, Blaser MJ (1997) Clinical and pathological importance of heterogeneity in vacA, the vacuolating cytotoxin gene of *Helicobacter pylori*. Gastroenterology 112:92–99

Axon ATR (1991) *Helicobacter pylori* therapy: effect on peptic ulcer disease. J Gastroenterol Hepatol 6:131–137

Banatvala NYA, Clements L, Herbert A, Davies J, Bagg J, Shephard JP, Feldman RA, Hardie JM (1995) *Helicobacter pylori* infection in dentists: a case-control study. Scand J Infect Dis 27:149–151

Bayerdörffer E, Simon T, Bästlein C, Ottenjann R, Kasper G (1987) Bismuth/ofloxacin combination for duodenal ulcer (letter). Lancet 2:1467–1468

Bayerdörffer E, Neubauer A, Eidt S et al (1994) Double-blind treatment of early gastric malt-lymphoma patients by *H. pylori* eradication (abstract). Gastroenterology 106:370

Bazzoli F, Zagari RM, Fossi S, Pozzato P, Roda A, Roda E (1993) Efficacy and tolerability of a short term, low dose triple therapy for eradication of *Helicobacter pylori* (abstract). Gastroenterology 104:A40

Bazzoli F, Zagari RM, Fossi S et al (1994) Short-term, low dose triple therapy for eradication of *Helicobacter pylori*. Eur J Gastroenterol Hepatol 6:773–777

Bell GD, Powell KV, Burridge SM, Bowden AN et al. (1993) *Helicobactor pylori* eradication. Efficacy and side effects profile of a combination of Omeprazole, amoxicillin and metronidazole compared with four alternative regimens. Quarterly J Med 86:743–750

Bianchi Porro G, Parente F, Lazzaroni M (1993) Short and long term outcome of *Helicobacter pylori* positive resistant duodenal ulcers treated with colloidal bismuth subcitrate plus antibiotics or sucralfate alone. Gut 34:466–469

Bickley J, Owen RJ, Fraser AJ, Pounder RE (1993) Evaluation of the polymerase chain reaction for detecting the urease C gene of *Helicobacter pylori* in gastric biopsy samples and dental plaque. J Med Microbiol 39:338–344

Blanco M, Pajares JM, Jimenez ML, Lopez-Brea M (1988) Effect of acid inhibition on *Campylobacter pylori*. Scand J Gastroenterol Suppl 142:107–109

Blaser MJ (1992) *Helicobacter pylori*: its role in gastroduodenal disease. Clin Infect 15:386–393

Blaser MJ (1995) Intrastrain differences in *Helicobacter pylori*: a key question in mucosal damage? Ann Med 27:559–563

Blaser MJ (1997) Not all *Helicobacter pylori* strains are created equal: should all be eliminated? Lancet 349:1020–1022

Blaser MJ, Chyou PH, Normura A (1995) Age at establishment of *Helicobacter pylori* infection and gastric carcinoma, gastric ulcer and duodenal ulcer risk. Cancer Res 55:562–565

Blecker U, Gold BD (1997) Treatment of *Helicobacter pylori* infection: a review. Pediatr Infect Dis J 16:391–399

Blecker U, Mehta DI, Vandenplas Y (1994) Sex-ratio of *Helicobacter pylori* infection in childhood. Am J Gastroenterol 89:293

Borody TJ, Brandl S, Andrews P, Ferch N, Jankiewicz E, Hyland L (1994) Use of high efficacy, lower dose triple therapy to reduce side effects of eradicating *Helicobacter pylori*. Am J Gastroenterol 89:33–38

Borody TJ, Brandl S, Andrews P, Jankiewicz E, Ostapowicz N (1992) *Helicobacter pylori* eradication failure – further treatment possibilities (abstract). Gastroenterology 102:A43

Bourke B, Jones N, Sherman P (1996) *Helicobacter pylori* infection and peptic ulcer disease in children. Pediatr Infect Dis J 15:1–13

Brooks JJ, Enterline HT (1983) Primary gastric lymphomas: a clinicopathologic study of 58 cases with long-term follow-up and literature review. Cancer 51:701–711

Bujanover Y, Konikoff F, Baratz M (1990) Nodular gastritis and *Helicobacter pylori*. J Pediatr Gastroenterol Nutr 11:41–44

Burette A, Glupcyznski Y, Deprez C (1992) Two weeks triple therapy overcomes metronidazole resistance: results of a randomized double blind study. Gastroenterology 102:A46

Cadranel S, Goossens H, De Boeck M, Malengreau A, Rodesch P, Butzler JP (1986) *Campylobacter pylori*dis in children. Lancet 1:735–736

Censini S, Lange C, Xiang ZY, Crabtree JE, Ghiara P, Borodovsky M, Rappuoli R, Covacci A (1996) cag, a pathogenicity island of *Helicobacter pylori*, encodes type I-specific and disease-associated virulence factors. Proc Natl Acad Sci USA 93:14648–14653

Chan JKC, CS NG, Isaacson PG (1990) Relationship between high-grade lymphoma and low-grade B-cell mucosa associated lymphoid tissue lymphoma (MALToma) of the stomach. Am J Pathol 136:1153–1164

Chan WY, Hui PK, Leung KM, Chow J, Kwok F, Ng CS (1994) Coocoid forms of *Helicobacter pylori* in the human stomach. Clin Micribiol Infect Dis 102:503–507

Chen MH, Lee A, Hazell S, Hu PJ, Li YY (1993) Immunisation against gastric infection with Helicobacter species – first step in the prophylaxis of gastric cancer? Int J Microbiol Virol Parasitol Infect Dis 280:155–165

Chong SK, Lou Q, Asnicar MA, Zimmerman SE, Croffie JM, Lee CH (1995) *Helicobacter pylori* infection in recurrent abdominal pain in childhood: comparison of diagnostic tests and therapy. Pediatrics 96:211–215

Chong SKF, Lou QY, Tolia V, Rosenberg AJ, Rabinowitz S, Elitsur Y, Gold B, Peacock JS (1997) A preliminary report on a multi-site investigation of seropositivity for *Helicobacter pylori* in children of the US. Gastroenterology 112(4):A89

Chow TKF, Lambert JR, Wahlqvist ML, Hsu-Hage BHH (1995) *Helicobacter pylori* in Melbourne Chinese immigrants: evidence for oral-oral transmission via chopsticks. J Gastroenterol Hepatol 10:562–569

Coelho LGV, Passos MCF, Chausson Y, Viera WIS, et al. (1992) One week $12.00 therapy heals duodenal ulcer and eradicates *H. pylori*. Gastroenterology 102:A51

Correa P, Fox J, Fontham E, Ruiz B, Lin YP, Zavala D, Taylor N, Mackinley D, de Lima E, Portilla H et al (1990) *Helicobacter pylori* and gastric carcinoma: Serum antibody prevalence in populations with contrasting cancer risks. Cancer 66:2569–2574

Correa P, Haenszell W, Cuello C, Zavala D, Fontham G, Tannenbaum S, Collazos T, Ruiz B (1990) Gastric precancerous process in a high risk population: Cohort follow-up. Cancer Res 50:4737–4740

Correa P (1995) *Helicobacter pylori* and gastric carcinogenesis. Am J Surg Pathol 19:S37–S43

Corthésy-Theulaz I, Porta N, Glauser M, Saraga E, Vaney AC, Haas R, Kraehenbuhl JP, Blum AL, Michetti P (1995) Oral immunization with *Helicobacter pylori* urease B subunit as a treatment against *Helicobacter pylori* infection in mice. Gastroenterology 109:115–121

Corthesy-Theulaz I, Ferrero RL (1996) Vaccines. Clin Opin Gastroenterol 12:41–44

Cutler AF, Havstad S, Ma CK, Blaser MJ, Perez-Perez GI, Schubert TT (1995) Accuracy of invasive and noninvasive tests to diagnose *Helicobacter pylori* infection. Gastroenterology 109:136–141

Czinn S, Dahms B, Jacobs G, Kaplan B, Rothstein F (1986) *Campylobacter*-like organisms in association with symptomatic gastritis in children. J Pediatr 109:80–83

Czinn SJ, Carr HS (1987) Rapid diagnosis of *Campylobacter pylori*dis associated gastritis. J Pediatr 110:569–570

Czinn SJ, Nedrud JG (1991) Oral immunization against *Helicobacter pylori*. Infect Immun 59:2359–2363

Czinn SJ, Cai A, Nedrud JG (1993) Protection of germ-free mice from infection by *Helicobacter felis* after active oral or passive IgA immunization. Vaccine 11:637–642

Debognie JC, Pauwels S, Raat A, de Meeus Y, Haot J, Mainguet P (1991) Quantification of *Helicobacter pylori* infection in gastritis and ulcer disease using a simple and rapid carbon-14 urea breath test. J Nucl Med 32:1192–1198

Defize J, Meuwissen SG (1987) Pepsinogens: an update of biochemical, physiological, and clinical aspects. J Pediatr Gastroenterol Nutr 6:493–508

Dekigai H, Murakami M, Kita T (1995) Mechanism of *Helicobacter pylori* associated gastric mucosa injury. Dig Dis Sci 40:1332–1339

Di Napoli A, Petrino R, Bocro M, Bellis M et al. (1992) Quantitative assessment of histologic changes in chronic gastritis after eradication of *Helicobacter pylori*. J Clin Pathol 45:796–798

Dixon MF, Genta RM, Yardley JH, Correa P and the participants of the International Workshop on the Histopathology of gastritis, Houston, 1994 (1996) Classification and grading of gastritis: the updated Sydney system. Am J Surg Pathol 20:1161–1181

Doglioni C, Wotherspoon AC, Moschini A, de Boni M, Isaacson PG (1992) High incidence of primary gastric lymphoma in northeastern Italy. Lancet 339:834–835

Doidge C, Gust I, Lee A, Buck F, Hazell S, Manne U (1994) Therapeutic immunization against *Helicobacter pylori* infection (letter). Lancet 343:914–915

Dooley CP, Cohen H (1988) The clinical significance of *Campylobacter pylori*. Ann Intern Med 108:70–79

Drumm B (1993) *Helicobacter pylori* in the pediatric patient. Gastroenterol Clin North Am 22:169–182

Drumm B. PS, Cutz E, Karmali M (1987) Association of *Campylobacter pylori* on the gastric mucosa with antral gastritis in children. N Engl J Med 316:1557–1561

Drumm BD, Rhoades JM, Stringer DA, Sherman PM, Ellis LE, Durie PR (1988) Peptic ulcer disease in children: etiology, clinical findings, and clinical course. Pediatrics 82:410–414

Drumm B, Perez-Perez GI, Blaser MJ, Sherman PM (1990) Intrafamilial clustering of *Helicobacter pylori* infection. N Engl J Med 322:359–363

Drumm B, Gormally S, Sherman PM (1996) Gastritis and peptic ulcer disease. In: Walker AW, Durie PR, Hamilton JR, Walker-Smith J (eds) Pediatric gastrointestinal disease: pathophysiology, diagnosis and management, vol 1. Decker, St Louis, pp 506–518

Eastham EJ (1991) Peptic ulcer. In: Walker WA, Durie PR, Hamilton JR, Walker-Smith JA, Watkins JB (eds) Pediatric gastrointestinal disease: pathophysiology, diagnosis and management, vol 1. Decker, Toronto, pp 438–451

Elta GH, Appelman HD, Behler EM, Wilson JA, Nostrant TJ (1987) A study of the correlation between endoscopic and histological diagnoses in gastroduodenitis. Am J Gastroenterol 82:749–753

El-Zaatari FA, Woo JS, Badr A, Osato MS, Serna H, Lichtenberger LM, Genta RM, Graham DY (1997) Failure to isolate *Helicobacter pylori* from stray cats indicates that H pylori in cats may be an anthroponosis – an animal infection with a human pathogen. J Med Microbiol 46:372–376

El-Zimaity HMT, Al-Assi MR, Genta RM, Graham DY (1995) Confirmation of successful therapy of *Helicobacter pylori* infection: number and site of biopsies or a rapid urease test. Am J Gastroenterol 90:1962–1964

Enroth H, Engstrand L (1995) Immunomagnetic separation and PCR for detection of *Helicobacter pylori* in water and stool specimens. J Clin Microbiol 33:2162–2165

European *Helicobacter pylori* study group (1997) Current European concepts in the management of *Helicobacter pylori* infection. The Maastricht consensus report. Gut 41:8–13

European Study Group on Antibiotic Susceptibility of *Helicobacter pylori* (1992) Results of a multicentre survey in 1991 of metronidazole resistance in *Helicobacter pylori*. Eur J Clin Microbiol 11:777–781

Fennerty MB (1997) What are the treatment goals for *Helicobacter pylori*? Gastroenterology 113: S120–S125

Figura N, Tabaqchali S (1996) Bactertial pathogenic factors. Curr Opin Gastroenterol 12:11–15

Figura N, Guglielmetti P, Rossolini A, Barberi A, Cusi G, Musmanno RA, Russi M, Quaranta S (1989) Cytotoxin production by *Campylobacter pylori* strains isolated from patients with peptic ulcers and from patients with chronic gastritis only. J Clin Microbiol 27:225–226

Forman D, Sitas F, Newell DG, Stacey AR, Boreham J, Peto R, Campbell TC, Li J, Chen J (1990) Geographic association of *Helicobacter pylori* antibody prevalence and gastric cancer mortality. Int J Cancer 46:608–611

Forman D, Newell DG, Fullerton F, Yarnell JW, Stacey AR, Wald N, Sitas F (1991) Association between infection with *Helicobacter pylori* and risk of gastric cancer: evidence from a prospective investigation. Br Med J 302:1302–1305

Fox JG, Blanco MC, Yan L, Shames B, Polidoro D, Dewhirst FE, Paster BJ (1993) Role of gastric pH in isolation of *Helicobacter mustelae* from the feces of ferrets. Gastroenterology 104:86–92

Fox JG, Correa P, Taylor NS, Lee A, Otto G, Murphy JC, Rose R (1990) *Helicobacter mustelae*-associated gastritis in ferrets. An animal model of *Helicobacter pylori* gastritis in humans. Gastroenterology 99:352–362

Fox JG, Correa P, Taylor NS, Zavala D, Fontham E, Janney F, Rodriguez E, Hunter F, Diavoltsis S (1989) *Campylobacter pylori*-associated gastritis and immune response in a population at increased risk of gastric carcinoma. Am J Gastroenterol 84:775–781

Fox JG, Edrise BM, Cabot EB, Beaucage C, Murphy JC, Prostak KS (1986) *Campylobacter*-like organisms isolated from gastric mucose of ferrets. Am J Vet Res 47:236–239

Fox JG (1995) Non-human reservoirs of *Helicobacter pylori*. Aliment Pharmacol Ther 9:93–103

Fox JG, Li X, Yan L, Cahill RJ, Hurley R, Lewis R, Murphy JC (1996) Chronic proliferative hepatitis in A/JCr mice associated with persistent *Helicobacter hepaticus* infection: a model of *Helicobacter*-induced carcinogenesis. Infect Immun 64:1548–1558

Friedman CR, Quick R, Khanna B, Salcido A, Iihoshi N, Gironaz M, Ganzales O, Hutwagner L, Tauxe R, Mintz E, Gold BD (1997) Epidemiology of *Helicobacter pylori* infection in rural Bolivian children. J Pediatr Gastro Nutr 25(4):466

Glupczynski Y, Labbe M, Burette A, Deltenre M, Avesani V, Bruck C (1987) Treatment failure of Ofloxacin in *Campylobacter pylori* infection. Lancet 1:1096

Go MF, Lew GM, Lichtenberger LM, Genta RM, Graham DY (1993) Gastric mucosal hydrophobicity and *Helicobacter pylori*: response to antimicrobial therapy. Am J Gastroenterol 88:1362–1365

Gold BD (1996) *Helicobacter pylori* infection and peptic ulcer disease. Semin Pediatr Infect Dis 7: 265–271

Gold BD, Islur P, Policova Z, Czinn S, Neumann AW, Sherman PM (1996) Surface properties of *Helicobacter mustelae* and ferret gastrointestinal mucosa. Clin Invest Med 19:92–100

Goodman KJ, Correa P (1995) The transmission of *Helicobacter pylori*: a critical review of the evidence. Int J Epidemiol 24:875–887

Goodwin CS, Marshall BJ, Blincow ED, Wilson DH, Blackbourn S, Phillips M (1988) Prevention of nitroimidazole resistance in *Campylobacter pylori* by coadministration of colloidal bismuth subcitrate: clinical and in vitro studies. J Clin Pathol 41:207–210

Goodwin CS, Armstrong JA, Chilvers T, Peters M, Collins MD, Sly L, McConnell, W, Harper WES (1989) Transfer of *Campylobacter pylori* and Campylobacter mustelae to Helicobacter gen. nov. as *Helicobacter pylori* comb. nov. and Helicobacter mustelae comb. nov., respectively. Int J Syst Bacteriol 39:397–405

Gotschlich EC (1983) Thoughts on the evolution of strategies used by bacteria for evasion of host defenses. Rev Infect Dis 5:S778–S783

Graham DY, Klein PD, Evans DJ Jr, Graham DY, Klein PD, Evans DY, Alpert LC, Opekum AR, Boutton TW (1987) *Campylobacter pylori* detected noninvasively by the ^{13}C-urea breath test. Lancet 1:1174–1177

Graham DY, Klein PD, Opekun AR, Smith KE, Polasani RR, Evans DJ Jr, Evans DG, Alpert LC, Michaletz PA, Yoshimura HH, Adam E (1989) In vivo susceptibility of *Campylobacter pylori*. Am J Gastroenterol 84:233–238

Graham DY, Lew GM, Malaty HM, Evans DG, Evans DJ, Klein PD, Alpert LC, Genta RM (1992) Factors influencing the eradication of *Helicobacter pylori* with triple therapy. Gastroenterology 102:493–496

Graham DY, Lew GM, Ramirez FC, Genta RM, Klein PD, Malaty HM (1993) Short report: a non-metronidazole trriple therapy for eradication of *Helicobacter pylori* infection – tetracycline, amoxicillin, bismuth. Alim Pharmacol Ther 7:111–113

Greiner A, Marx A, Schausser B, Muller-Hermelink HK (1994) The pivotal role of the immunoglobulin receptor of tumor cells from B-cell lymphomas of mucosa associated lymphoid tissue (MALT). Adv Exp Med Biol 355:189–193

Grubel P, Hoffman JS, Chong FK, Burstein NA, Mepani C, Cave DR (1997) Vector potential of Houseflies (Musca domestica) for *Helicobacter pylori*. J Clin Microbiol 35:1300–1303

Haenszel W, Kurihara M, Segi M, Lee RK (1972) Stomach cancer among Japanese in Hawaii. J Natl Cancer Inst 49:969–988

Handt LK, Fox JG, Dewhirst FE, Fraser GJ, Paster BJ, Yan LL, Rozmiarek H, Rufo R, Stalis IH (1994) *Helicobacter pylori* isolated from the domestic cat: public health implications. Infect Immun 62: 2367–2374

Handt LK, Fox JG, Stalis IH, Rufo R, Lee G, Linn J, Li X, Kleanthous H (1995) Characterization of feline *Helicobacter pylori* strains and associated gastritis in a colony of domestic cats. J Clin Microbiol 33:2280–2289

Hazell SL, Lee A (1986) *Campylobacter pylori*, urease, hydrogen ion back diffusion, and gastric ulcers. Lancet 2:15–17

Henze E, Malfertheiner P, Clausen M, Burkhardt H, Adam WE (1990) Validation of a simplified carbon-14-urea breath test for routine use for detecting *Helicobacter pylori* noninvasively. J Nucl Med 31:1940–1944

Hill R, Pearman J, Worthy P, Caruso V, Goodwin S, Blincow E (1986) *Campylobacter pyloridis* and gastritis in children. Lancet 1:387

Hirschowitz BI (1996) Zollinger-Ellison syndrome: pathogenesis, diagnosis and management. Am J Gastroenterol 92 [Suppl 4]:445–85

Hosking SW, Ling TK, Chung SC, Yung MY, Cheng AF, Sung JJ, Li AK (1994) Duodenal ulcer healing by eradication of *Helicobacter pylori* without anti-acid treatment: randomised controlled trial. Lancet 343:508–510

Howden CW (1997) For what conditions is there evidence-based justification for treatment of *Helicobacter pylori* infection? Gastroenterology 113:S107–S112

Hunt R, Thompson BR (1998) Canadian *Helicobacter pylori* Consensus Conference. Can J Gastroenterol 12:31–41

Hussel T, Isaacson PG, Crabtree JE, Spencer J (1993) The response of cells from low-grade B-cell gastric lymphomas of mucosa-associated lymphoid tissue to *Helicobacter pylori*. Lancet 342:571–574

Isaacson PG, Spencer J (1987) Malignant lymphoma of mucosa-associated lymphoid tissue. Histopathology 11:445–462

Isaacson PG, Wright DH (1983) Malignant lymphoma of mucosa-associated lymphoid tissue. A distinctive type of B-cell lymphoma. Cancer 52:1410–1416

Isaacson PG, Wotherspoon AC, Diss T, Pan LX (1991) Follicular colonization in B-cell lymphoma of mucosa-associated lymphoid tissue. Am J Surg Pathol 15:819–828

Isenberg JI, Selling JA, Hogan DL, Koss MA (1987) Impaired proximal duodenal mucosal bicarbonate secretion in patients with duodenal ulcer. N Engl J Med 316:374–379

Iser JH, Buttigieg RJ, Iseli A (1994) Low dose, short duration therapy for the eradication of *Helicobacter pylori* in patients with duodenal ulcer. Med J Aust 160:192–196

Jackson RH (1972) Genetic studies of peptic ulcers disease in children. Paediatr Scand 61:493–494

Jaskiewicz K, Louw JA, Marks IN (1993) Local cellular and immune response by antral mucosa in patients undergoing treatment for eradication of *Helicobacter pylori*. Dig Dis Sci 38:937–943

Joly DJ (1977) Resources for the control of cancer in Latin America: preliminary survey. Bol Sanit Panam 83:330–345

Karita M, Tsuda M, Nakazawa T (1995) Essential role of urease in vitro and in vivo *Helicobacter pylori* colonisation study using a wild-type and isogenic mutant strain. J Clin Gastroenterol 21:S160–S163

Khanna B, Cutler A, Perry M, Lastovica A, Gold BD (1997) Sensitivity of commercially available serology tests to detect *Helicobacter pylori* infection in children. Gastroenterology 112:A172

Kilbridge PM, Dahms BB, Czinn SJ (1988) *Campylobacter pylori* associated gastritis and peptic ulcer disease in children. Am J Dis Child 142:1149–1152

Klein PD, Graham DY, Opekun AR, O'Brian-Smith E (1991) Water as a risk factor for *Helicobacter pylori* infection in Peruvian children. Lancet 337:1503–1506

Kooistra-Smid AM, Schirm J, Snijder JA (1993) Sensitivity of culture compared with that of polymerase chain reaction for detection of *Helicobacter pylori* from antral biopsy samples. J Clin Microbiol 31:1918–1920

Kosunen TU, Seppala K, Sarna S, Sipponen P (1992) Diagnostic value of decreasing IgG, IgA, and IgM antibody titres after eradication of *Helicobacter pylori*. Lancet 339:893–895

Kurata JH, Haile BM (1984) Epidemiology of peptic ulcer disease. Clin Gastroenterol 13:289–307

Kurata JH, Nogawa AN (1997) Meta-analysis of risk factors for peptic ulcer disease: nonsteroidal antiinflammatory drugs, *Helicobacter pylori*, and smoking. J Clin Gastroenterol 24:2–17

Labenz J, Stolte M, Rühl GH, Becker T, Tillenburg B, Sollböhmer, Börsch G (1994) One week low dose triple therapy for cure of *Helicobacter pylori*. Eur J Gastroenterol Hepatol 7:9–11

Lansdown M, Quirke P, Dixon MF, Axon AT, Johnston D (1990) High grade dysplasia of the gastric mucosa: a marker for gastric carcinoma. Gut 31:977–983

Lee A, Hazell SL, O'Rourke J, Kouprach S (1988) Isolation of a spiral-shaped bacterium from the cat stomach. Infect Immun 56:2843–2850

Lee A (1995) Helicobacter infections in laboratory animals: a model for gastric neoplasia. Ann Medi 27:575–582

Lee J, O'Morain C (1997) Consensus or confusion: a review of existing national guidelines on *Helicobacter pylori*-related disease. Eur J Gastroenterol Hepatol 8:537–531

Leunk RD, Johnson PT, David BC, Kraft WG, Morgan DR (1988) Cytotoxic activity in broth culture filtrates of *Campylobacter pylori*. J Med Microbiol 26:93–99

Lichtenberger LM, Romero JJ (1994) Effect of ammonium ion on the hydrophobic and barrier properties of the gastric mucus gel layer: implications on the role of ammonium in *H. pylori* induced gastritis. J Gastroenterol Hepatol 9:S13–S19

Lind T, Veldhuyzen van Zanten SJO, Unge P, Spiller R, Bayerdorffer E, O'Morain C, Bardhan KD, Bradette M, Chiba N, Wrangstadh M, Cederberg C, Idstrom JP (1996) Eradication of *Helicobacter pylori* using one-week triple therapies combining omeprazole with two antimicrobials: the MACH 1 study. Helicobacter 1:138–144

Logan RP, Gummett PA, Misiewicz JJ, Karim QN, Walker MM, Baron JH (1994a) One week's anti-*Helicobacter pylori* treatment for duodenal ulcer. Gut 35:15–18

Logan RP, Gummett PA, Schaufelberger HD, Greaves RR, Mendelson GM, Walker MM, Thomas PH, Baron JH, Misiewicz JJ (1994b) Eradication of *Helicobacter pylori* with clarithromycin and omeprazole. Gut 35:323–326

Loof L, Adami HO, Agenas I, Gustavsson S, Nyberg A (1985) The Diagnosis and Therapy Survey October 1978-March 1983, health care and consumption and current durg therapy in Sweden with respect to the clinical diagnosis with gastritis. Scand J Gastroenterol [Suppl] 109:35–39

Luzza F, Maletta M, Imeneo M, Fabiano E, Doldo P, Biancone L, Pallone F (1995) Evidence against an increased risk of *Helicobacter pylori* infection in dentists: a serological and salivary study. Eur J Gastroenterol Hepatol 7:773–776

Macarthur C, Saunders N, Feldman W (1995) *Helicobacter pylori*, gastroduodenal disease, and recurrent abdominal pain in children. JAMA 273:729–734

Mahony MJ, Wyatt JI, Littlewood JM (1988) *Campylobacter pylori* gastritis. Arch Dis Child 63:654–655

Malaty HM, Graham DY (1994) Importance of childhood socioeconomic status on the current prevalence of *Helicobacter pylori* infection. Gut 35:742–745

Malaty HM, Kim JG, Kim SD, Graham DY (1996) Prevalence of *Helicobacter pylori* infection in Korean children: inverse relation to socioeconomic status despite a uniformly high prevalence in adults. Am J Epidemiol 143:257–262

Malfertheiner P (1993) Compliance, adverse events and antibiotic resistance in *Helicobacter pylori* treatment. Scand J Gastroenterol 28[Suppl 196]:34–37

Malfertheiner P, Nilius M (1993) Bismuth salts. In: Goodwin CS, Worsley B (eds) *Helicobacter pylori*: biology and clinical practice. CRC Press, Boca Raton

Mapstone NP, Lynch DA, Lewis FA, Axon AT, Tompkins DS, Dixon MF, Quirke P (1993) PCR identification of *Helicobacter pylori* in faeces from gastritis patients. Lancet 341:447

Marchetti M, Arico B, Burroni O, Figura N, Rappuoli R, Ghiara P (1995) Development of a mouse model of *Helicobacter pylori* infection that mimics human disease. Science 267:1655

Marshall BJ (1993) Treatment strategies for *Helicobacter pylori* infection. Gastroenterol Clin North Am 22:183–198

Marshall BJ, Langton SR (1986) Urea hydrolysis in patients with *Campylobacter pylori* infection. Lancet 2:965–966

Marshall BJ, Surveyor I (1988) Carbon-14 urea breath tests for the diagnosis of *Campylobacter pylori*-associated gastritis. J Nucl Med 29:11–16

Marshall BJ, Armstrong JA, McGechie DB, Glancy RJ (1985) Attempts to fulfill Koch's postulates for pyloric Campylobacter. Med J Aust 142:436–439

Marshall BJ, Goodwin CS, Warren JR, Murray R, Blincow ED, Blackbourn SJ, Phillips M, Waters TE, Sanderson CR (1988) Prospective double-blind trial of duodenal ulcer relapse after eradication of *Campylobacter pylori*. Lancet 2:1437–1442

Marshall BJ, Plankey MW, Hoffman SR, Boyd CL, Dye KR, Frierson HF, Guerrant RL, McCallum RW (1991) A 20-minute breath test for *Helicobacter pylori*. Am J Gastroenterol 86:438–445

McCarthy CJ, Collins R, Beattie S, Hamilton H, O'Morain C (1993) Short report: treatment of *Helicobacter pylori*-associated duodenal ulcer with omeprazole plus antibiotics. Alim Pharmacol Ther 7:463–466

McGowan FD, Cover TL, Blaser MJ (1996) *Helicobacter pylori* and gastric acid: biological and therapeutic implications. Gastroenterology 110:926–938

McMichael AJ, McCall MG, Hartshone JM, Woddings TL (1980) Patterns of gastro-intestinal cancer in European migrants to Australia: the role of dietary change. Int J Cancer 25:431–437

McNulty CA, Dent JC (1988) Susceptibility of clinical isolates of *Campylobacter pylori* to twenty one antimicrobial agents. Eur J Clin Microbiol 7:566–569

McQueen S, Hutton DA, Allen A, Garner A (1983) Gastric and duodenal surface mucus gel thickness in the rat: effect of prostaglandins and damaging agents. Am J Physiol 8:388–394

Megraud F (1993) Epidemiology of *Helicobacter pylori* infection. Gastroenterol Clin North Am 22:73–88

Megraud F (1995) Transmission of *Helicobacter pylori*: faecal-oral versus oral-oral. Aliment Pharmacol Ther 9:85–91

Mertz-Nielsen AJH, Frokiare H, Bukhave K, Rask-Madsen J (1996) Gastric bicarbonate secretion and release of prostaglandin E2 are increased in duodenal ulcer patients but not in *Helicobacter pylori* positive healthy subjects. Scand J Gastrenterol 31:38–43

Mitchell HM, Bohane TD, Tobias V, Bullpitt P, Daskalopoulos G, Carrick J, Mitchell JD, Lee A (1993) *Helicobacter pylori* infection in children: potential clues to pathogenesis. J Pediatr Gastroenterol Nutr 16:120–125

Mitchell HM, Li YY, Hu PJ, Liu Q, Chen M, Du GG, Wang ZJ, Lee A, Hazell SJ (1992) Epidemiology of *Helicobacter pylori* in southern China: identification of early childhood as the critical period for acquisition. J Infect Dis 166:149–153

Moayyedi P, Axon ATR (1994) Efficacy of a new one week triple therapy regime in eradicating *Helicobacter pylori*. Gut 35[Suppl]:F248

Mobley HLT, Island MD, Hausinger RP (1995) Molecular biology of microbial ureases. Microbiol Rev 59:451–480

Moonka D, Lichtenstein GR, Levine MS, Rombeau JL, Furth EE, MacDermott (1993) Giant gastric ulcers: an unusual manifestation of Crohn's disease. Am J Gastroenterol 88:297–299

Murphy MS, Eastham EJ, Jimenez M, Nelson R, Jackson RH (1987) Duodenal ulceration: a review of 110 cases. Arch Dis Child 62:544–548

Nagita A, Amemoto K, Yoden A, Aoki S, Sakuguchi M, Ashida K, Mino M (1996) Diurnal variation in intragastric pH in children with and without peptic ulcers. Pediatr Res 40:528–532

Negrini R, Coiesi C, Savio A et al (1994) Molecular mimicr of gastric antigens by *Helicobacter pylori*: a role in the pathogenesis of atrophic gastritis (abstract)? Am J Gastroenterol 89:1329

Newell DG, Rathbone BJ (1989) The serodiagnosis of *Campylobacter pylori* infection. Serodiagn Immunother Infect Dis 3:1–6

Newell DG, Stacey AR (1992) The serology of *Helicobacter pylori* infection. In: Rathbone BJ (ed) *Helicobacter pylori* and gastroduodenal disease, vol 1. Blackwell Scientific, Oxford, pp 64–73

Nguyen AM, Engstrand L, Genta RM, Graham DY, el-Zaatari FA (1993) Detection of *Helicobacter pylori* in dental plaque by reverse transcription polymerase chain reaction. J Clin Microbiol 31: 783–787

NIH Consensus Development Panel on *Helicobacter pylori* in peptic ulcer disease (1994) *Helicobacter pylori* in peptic ulcer disease. JAMA 272:65–69

Oderda G, Vaira D, Dell'Olio D, Holton J, Forni M, Altare N (1990) Serum pepsinogen I and gastrin concentrations in children positive for *Helicobacter pylori*. J Clin Pathol 43:762–765

Oppenheimer EH, Esterly JR (1975) Pathology of cystic fibrosis: review of the literature and comparison of 146 autopsied cases. Perspect Pediatr Pathol 2:241–278

Osato MS, Le HH, Ayoub C, Graham DY (1997) Houseflies as a reservoir for *Helicobacter pylori*. Gastroenterology112:A247

O'Toole PW, Kostrzynska M, Trust TJ (1994) Non-motile mutants of *Helicobacter pylori* and Helicobacter mustelae defective in hook production. Mol Microbiol 14:691–703

Owen RJ, Bickley J, Hurtado A, Fraser A, Pounder RE (1994) Comparison of PCR-based restriction length polymorphism analysis of urease genes with rRNA gene profiling for monitoring *Helicobacter pylori* infections in patients on triple therapy. J Clin Microbiol 32:1203–1210

Parkin DM (1986) Cancer occurrence in developing countries. IARC Sci Publ 75:1–39

Parsonnet J (1995) The incidence of *Helicobacter pylori* infection. Aliment Pharmacol Ther 9:45–51

Parsonnet J, Friedman GD, Vandersteen DP, Chang Y, Vogleman JH, Orentreich N, Sibley RK (1991a) *Helicobacter pylori* infection and the risk of gastric carcinoma. N Engl J Med 325:1127–1131

Parsonnet J, Vandersteen D, Goates J, Sibley RK, Pritikin J, Chang Y (1991b) *Helicobacter pylori* infection in intestinal and diffuse type gastric adenocarcinoma. J Natl Cancer Inst 83:640–643

Parsonnet J, Hansen S, Rodriguez L, Gelb AB, Warnke FA, Jellum E, Orentreich N, Vogleman JH, Friedman GD (1994) *Helicobacter pylori* infection and gastric lymphoma. N Engl J Med 330: 1267–1271

Perkins SE, Fox JG, Walsh JH (1996) Helicobacter mustelae-associated hypergastrinemia in ferrets (Mustelae putorius furo). Am J Vet Res 57:147–150

Peterson WL (1991) *Helicobacter pylori* and peptic ulcer disease. N Engl J Med 324:1043–1048

Prieto G, Polanco I, Larrauri J, Rota L, Lama R, Carrasco S (1992) *Helicobacter pylori* infection in children: clinical, endoscopic, and histologic correlations. J Pediatr Gastroenterol Nutr 14:420–425

Rao S, Royal LE, Conrad HA, Harris V, Ahuja J (1990) Duodenal ulcer in sickle cell disease. J Pediatr Gastroenterol Nutr 10:117–120

Rauws EAJ, Tytgat GNJ (1990) Cure of duodenal ulcer associated with eradication of *Helicobacter pylori*. Lancet 335:1233–1235

Recavarren-Arce S, Leon-Barua R, Cok J, Berendson R, Gilman RH, Ramirez-Ramirez A, Rodriguez C, Spira WM (1991) *Helicobacter pylori* and progressive gastric pathology that predisposes to gastric cancer. Scand J Gastroenterol 18:51–57

Robert ME, Weinstein WM (1993) *Helicobacter pylori*-associated gastric pathology. Gastroenterol Clin North Am 22:59–72

Rosenstein B, Perman JA, Kramer SS (1986) Peptic ulcer disease in cystic fibrosis: an unusual occurrence in black adolescents. Am J Dis Child 140:66–69

Rosenwaike I (1984) Cancer mortality among Puerto Rican-born residents in New York City. Am J Epidemiol 119:177–185

Rosioru C, Glassman MS, Berezin SH, Bostwick HE, Halata M, Schwarz SM (1993) Treatment of *Helicobacter pylori*-associated gastroduodenal disease in children. Clinical evaluation of antisecretory vs. antibacterial therapy. Dig Dis Sci 38:123–128

Rotter JI, Sones JQ, Samloff IM, Richardson CT, Gursky JM, Walsh JH, Rimoin DL (1979) Duodenal ulcer disease associated with elevated serum pepsinogen I: an autosomal inherited disorder. N Engl J Med 300:63–66

Rowland M, Kuman D, O'Connor P, Daly LE, Drumm B (1997) Reinfection with *Helicobacter pylori* in children. Gastroenterology 112:A273

Rubin E, Farber JL (1990) The gastrointestinal tract. In: Rubin E, Farber JL (eds) Essential pathology, vol 1. Lippincott, Philadelphia, pp 352–392

Ruuska T, Vaajalahti P, Arajarvi P, Maki M (1994) Prospective evaluation of upper gastrointestinal mucosal lesions in children with ulcerative colitis and Crohn's disease. J Pediatr Gastroenterol Nutr 19:181–186

Sauerbruch T, Schreiber MA, Schüssler P, Permanetter W (1984) Endoscopy in the diagnosis of gastritis: diagnostic value of endoscopic criteria in relation to histologic diagnosis. Endoscopy 16:101–104

Sbeih F, Abdullah A, Sullivan S, Merenkov Z (1996) Antral nodularity, gastric lymphoid hyperplasia, and *Helicobacter pylori*. J Clin Gastroenterol 22:227–230

Schmitz A, Josenhans C, Suerbaum S (1995) The H pylori flagellar biosynthesis regulatory protein FlbA affects the expression of flagellar components on the transcriptional level and is probably a membrane protein. Gut 37:A245

Seppala K, Farkkila M, Nautinan H et al. (1992) Triple therapy of *Helicobacter pylori* infection in peptic ulcer. A 12 month follow-up study of 93 patients. Scand J Gastroenterol 27:973–976

Serjeant GR, May H, Patrick A, Slifer E (1973) Duodenal ulceration in sickle cell anemia. Trans R Soc Trop Med Hyg 67:59–63

Sherman PM (1994) Peptic ulcer disease in children. Gastroenterol Clin North Am 23:707–725

Silen W (1987) The clinical problem of stress ulcers. Clin Invest Med 10:270–274

Sonnenberg A, Everhart JE (1996) The prevalence of self reported peptic ulcer in the United States. Am J Publ Health 86:200–205

Sonnenberg A (1988) Factors which influence the incidence and the course of peptic ulcer. Scand J Gastroenterol 23:119–140

Sonnenberg A (1995) Temporal trends and geographical variations of peptic ulcer disease. Aliment Pharmacol Ther 2:3–12

Spiro HM (1983) Gastric lymphomas. Clinical gastroenterology. Macmillan, New York, pp 292–297

Staat MA, Kruszon-Moran D, McQuillan GM, Kaslow RA (1996) A population-based serologic survey of Helicobacter. J Infect Dis 174:1120–1123

Steen T, Berstad K, Meling T, and Berstad A (1995) Reproducibility of the ^{14}C urea breath test repeated after 1 week. Am J Gastroenterol 90:2103–2105

Stolte M, Eidt S (1989) Lymphoid follicles in the antral mucosa: immune response to *Campylobacter pylori*. J Clin Pathol 42:1269–1271

Stone JW, Wise R, Donovan IA, Gearty JC (1988) Failure of ciprofloxacin to eradicate *Campylobacter pylori* from the stomach. J Antimicrob Chemother 22:92–93

Talley NJ, Zinsmeister AR, Weaver A, Dimagno EP, Carpener HA, Perez-Perez GI, Blaser MJ (1991) Gastric adenocarcinoma and *Helicobacter pylori* infection. J Natl Cancer Inst 83:1734–1739

Taylor IL (1984) Gastrointestinal hormones in the pathogenesis of peptic ulcer disease. Clin Gastroenterol 13:355–382

Thijs JC, Van Zweet AA, Oey HB (1993) Efficacy and side effects of a triple drug regimen for the eradication of *Helicobacter pylori*. Scand J Gastroenterol 28:934–938

Tomb J-F, White O, Kerlavage AR, Clayton RA, Sutton FF, Fleischman RD, Ketchum KA, Lenk HP et al (1997) The complete genome sequence of the gastric pathogen *Helicobacter pylori*. Nature 338:539–547

Tucci A, Corinaldesi R, Stanghellini V, Paparo GF, Gasperoni S, Biasco G, Varoli O, Ricci-Maccarinin M, Barbara L (1993) One-day therapy for treatment of *Helicobacter pylori* infection. Dig Dis Sci 38:1670–1673

Tummuru MKR, Cover TL, Blaser MJ (1993) Cloning and expression of a high molecular weight major antigen of *Helicobacter pylori*: evidence of linkage to cytotoxin production. Infect Immun 61: 1799–1809

Unge P, Gad A, Gnarpe H, Olsson J (1989) Does omeprazole improve antimicrobial therapy directed towards gastric *Campylobacter pylori* in patients with antral gastritis? A pilot study. Scand J Gastroenterol 167:S49–S54

Veldhuyzen van Zanten SJ, Pollack PT, Best LM, Bezanson GS, Marrie T (1994) Increasing prevalence of *Helicobacter pylori* infection with age: continuous risk of infection in adults rather than cohort effect. J Infect Dis 169:434–437

Villar HV, Wong R, Paz B, Bull D, Neumayer L, Grogan T, Spier C (1991) Immuno-phenotyping in the management of gastric lymphoma. Am J Surg 161:171–175

Wang JT, JC Seu, Lin JT, Wang TH, Wu MS (1993) Direct DNA amplification and restriction pattern analysis of *Helicobacter pylori* in patients with duodenal ulcers and their families. J Infect Dis 169:1544–1548

Wang JD, Zhou DY, Yang HT, Zhang WD, Xu ZM (1994) Using polymerase chain reaction to detect *Helicobacter pylori* in clinical samples and gastric mucosa of some domestic animals (abstract). Am J Gastroenterol 89:1300

Warren JR, Marshall BJ (1983) Unidentified curved bacilli on gastric epithelium in active chronic gastritis. Lancet 1:1273–1275

Watanabe T, Tada M, Nagai H, Sasaki S, Nakao M (1998) *Helicobacter pylori* infection induces gastric cancer in Mongolian gerbils. Gastroenterology 118:642–648

Webb PM, Knight T, Greaves S, Wilson A, Newell DG, Forman D (1994) Relationship between infection with *Helicobacter pylori* and living conditions in childhood: evidence for person to person transmission in early life. Br Med J 308:750–753

Westblom TU, Madan E, Gudipati S, Midkiff BR, Czinn SJ (1992) Diagnosis of *Helicobacter pylori* infection in adult and pediatric patients by using Pyloriset, a rapid latex agglutination test. J Clin Microbiol 30:96–98

Westblom TU, Phadnis S, Yang P, Czinn SJ (1993) Diagnosis of *Helicobacter pylori* infection by means of a polymerase chain reaction assay for gastric juice aspirates. Clin Infect Dis 16:367–371

Whitney AE, Guarner J, Hutwagner L, Gold BD (1998) Histopathological differences between *Helicobacter pylori* gastritis of children and adults. Gastroenterology 114(4):A331

Whitney AEW, Emory TS, Marty AM, O'Shea PA, Newman GW, Otterbeck V, Gold BD (1996) Macrophage infiltration of the gastric mucosa in children with and without *Helicobacter pylori* infection. J Pediatr Gastroenterol Nutr 23:348

Wilhelmsen I, Weberg R, Berstad K, Hausken T, Hundal O, Berstad A (1994) *Helicobacter pylori* eradication with bismuth subcitrate, oxytetracyclines and metronidazole in patients with peptic ulcer disease. Hepatogastroenterology 41:43–47

Wotherspoon AC, Ortiz-Hidalgo C, Falzon MJ, Isaacson PG (1991) *Helicobacter pylori*-associated gastritis and primary B-cell gastric lymphoma. Lancet 338:1175–1176

Wotherspoon AC, Doglioni C, Diss TC, Pan L, Mschini A, De Boni M, Isaacson PG (1993) Regression of primary low-grade B-cell gastric lymphoma of mucosa-associated lymphoid tissue type after eradication of *Helicobacter pylori*. Lancet 342:575–577

Wyatt JI, Primrose J, Dixon MF (1988) Distribution of *Campylobacter pylori* in gastric biopsies. J Pathol 155:350

Wyatt JI, Rathbone BJ (1988) Immune response of the gastric mucosa to *Campylobacter pylori*. Scand J Gastroenterol 23[Suppl 142]:44–49

Wyatt JI (1995) Histopathology of gastroduodenal inflammation: the impact of *Helicobacter pylori*. Histopathology 26:1–15

Xiang Z, Censini S, Bayelli PF, Telford JL, Figura N, Rappoulir A, Covacci A (1995) Analysis of expression of cagA and vacA virulence factors in 43 strains of *Helicobacter pylori* reveals that the clinical isolates can be divided into two major and that cagA is not necessary for expression of the vacuolating toxin. Infect Immun 63:94–98

Yamashiro Y, Shioya T, Ohtsuka Y, Nakata S, Oguchi S, Shimizu T, Sato M (1995) Patterns of 24 h intragastric acidity in duodenal ulcers in children: the importance of monitoring and inhibiting nocturnal activity. Acta Paediatr Jpn 37:557–561

Yeung CK, Fu KH, Yuen KY, Ng WF, Tsang TM, Braniki FJ, Saing H (1990) *Helicobacter pylori* and associated duodenal ulcer. Arch Dis Child 65:1212–1216

Yip R, Limburg PJ, Ahlquist DA, Carpenter JH, O'Neill A, Kruse D, Stitham S, Gold BD et al. (1997) Pervasive occult gastrointestinal bleeding in an Alaska Native Population with prevalent iron deficiency anemia. JAMA 277:1135–1139

Younan R, Pearson J, Allen A, Venables C (1982) Changes in the structure of the mucus gel on the mucosal surface of the stomach in association with peptic ulcer disease. Gastroenterology 82:827–831

Young JL, Percy CL, Asire AJ, Berg JW, Cusan MM, Gloeckler LA, Horn JW, Lourie WI, Pollack ES, Shambaugh EM (1981) Cancer incidence and mortality in the United States, 1973–1977. Natl Cancer Inst Monogr 57:1–187

Yu J, Russell M, Salomen RN, Murphy JC, Palley LS, Fox JG (1995) Effect of *Helicobacter mustelae* infection on ferret gastric epithelial cell proliferation. Carcinogenesis 16:1927–1931

Microbiology of *Helicobacter pylori*

A. Marais, L. Monteiro, and F. Mégraud

1 Introduction

Since the complete genome sequence of *Helicobacter pylori* (strain 26695) was published (Tomb et al. 1997), an important amount of information concerning the microbiology of this organism must be added to already known features (Fig. 1). In fact, a new era in microbiology has dawned, and microbiologists cannot ignore the

Laboratoire de Bactériologie, Université de Bordeaux 2 et Hôpital Pellegrin, 33076 Bordeaux Cedex, France numerous data provided by this extraordinary work. This chapter gives an overview of the microbiology of *H. pylori* and includes new sequence data.

2 Taxonomy

Three phases may be distinguished in the history of the taxonomy; the first two are based on a phenotypic study and the third on a genotypic analysis.

In the seventeenth century, LINNÉ attempted to define taxonomic rules. The principles of this classification consisted of putting together in a same group (or taxon), organisms sharing some phenotypic characteristics. However, this method presents some limits: the characteristic to be considered may be chosen arbitrarily; examination of some other characteristics may lead to another classification; and the failure to detect a given characteristic in only one strain renders its classification difficult. In order to circumvent this drawback, a numerical taxonomy was developed when computer science emerged. This method takes into account a great number of characteristics, to which the same value is given, and a statistical analysis then allows a classification of the organisms. Nevertheless, phenotypic characteristics may be dependent on environmental conditions.

More recently, the genomic taxonomy has been developed. It is based on the comparison of the degree of similarity existing between nucleotide sequences from different strains. Currently, a bacterial species is defined if the level of DNA/DNA hybridization between strains is at least 70% (WAYNE et al. 1987).

The comparison of the 16S rDNA sequences is also a criterion for defining a bacterial species. Two organisms with identical 16S rDNA sequences (i.e., less than

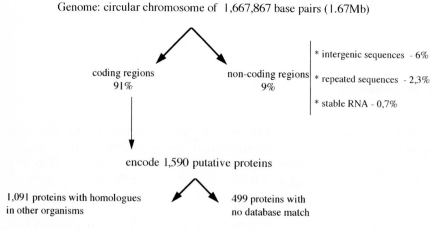

Genome: circular chromosome of 1,667,867 base pairs (1.67Mb)

coding regions 91%

non-coding regions 9%

* intergenic sequences - 6%
* repeated sequences - 2,3%
* stable RNA - 0,7%

encode 1,590 putative proteins

1,091 proteins with homologues in other organisms

499 proteins with no database match

Fig. 1. General features of the *H. pylori* genome (strain 26695)

5–15 differences out of 1500 base pairs sequenced) are assumed to belong to the same species (WOESE 1994). Based on the 16S rDNA sequence and its comparison with that of *Campylobacter* spp, the *Helicobacter* genus was proposed in 1989 and included *Helicobacter mustelae* and *H. pylori* (GOODWIN et al. 1989). Since then, more than ten species have been attributed to this genus (Table 1).

3 Morphology

3.1 Ultrastructure

H. pylori is a curved gram-negative bacillus. The organisms are 3–5μm in length and about 0.5μm in diameter. The ability of *H. pylori* to convert into a coccoidal form has been demonstrated and has suggested different hypotheses concerning the significance of this conversion (Fig. 2).

During infection, most of the bacteria are present in the host gastric mucus as spiral forms (WARREN and MARSHALL 1983; MARSHALL et al. 1984), but coccoidal forms have also been found in the human stomach (CHAN et al. 1994). However, the role of these forms in the pathogenicity is controversial. Studies using animal

Table 1. The genus *Helicobacter*

Species	Host
Gastric *Helicobacter* spp.	
H. pylori	Man
H. bizzozeroni	Dog
H. heilmannii[a]	Cat, dog, pig, monkey, (man)
H. felis	Cat, dog, (man)
H. mustelae	Ferret
H. nemestrinae	Macaque
H. acinonyx	Cheetah
Intestinal *Helicobacter* spp.	
H. cinaedi	Hamster (man)
H. fennelliae	Man
H. muridarum	Mouse
H. bilis	Mouse
H. canis	Dog
H. hepaticus	Mouse
H. pametensis	Seagull
H. cholecystus	Hamster
H. pullorum	Poultry
H. rodentium	Mouse
H. trogontum	Rat
H. wesmaedi	Mouse
H. salomonis	Mouse

[a] Also known as *Gastrospirillum hominis* or *Gastrospirillum suis*.

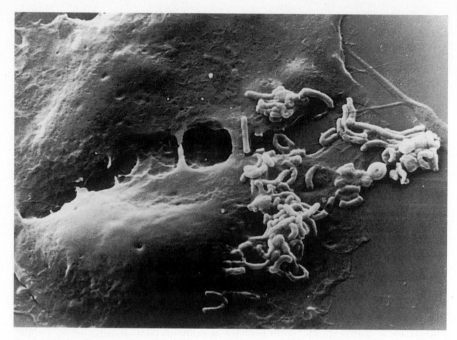

Fig. 2. Adherence of spiral and coccoidal forms of *H. pylori* visualized by scanning electron microscopy

models also gave conflicting results: coccoidal forms seem to be infectious in mice (Cellini et al. 1994a) but not in piglets (Eaton et al. 1995).

Under favorable culture conditions, *H. pylori* maintains its spiral form. Nevertheless, the conversion into a coccoidal form has been observed under unfavorable conditions (West et al. 1990; Mai et al. 1989). A similar phenomenon has been described for the *Campylobacter* genus (Moran and Upton 1986, 1987). The conversion of spiral forms into coccoidal forms can be induced by an increase in oxygen tension (Catrenich and Makin 1991), by alkaline pH (Jones and Curry 1991), an increase in temperature (Shahamat et al. 1993), an extended incubation (Reynolds and Penn 1994), and treating the culture with omeprazole (Cellini et al. 1994b) or antibiotics such as amoxicillin (Berry et al. 1995).

Coccoidal forms are nonculturable, but some studies have suggested that they are viable and even infectious (Cellini et al. 1994b; Cole et al. 1997; Sorberg et al. 1996). In contrast, other studies have shown that coccoidal forms are the morphological manifestation of bacterial cell death (Moran and Upton 1986; Buck et al. 1983). Recently, Kusters et al. (1997) observed that, independently of conditions leading to the conversion into coccoidal forms, the transformation is accompanied by several ultrastructural and antigenic modifications: (a) the amount of RNA and DNA as well as their integrity are significantly decreased in the coccoidal forms; (b) a loss of membrane potential is observed; and (c) inhibition of RNA or protein synthesis by the action of antibiotics does not prevent the transformation into coccoidal forms but leads to an increase in the conversion rate. These observations led the authors to propose that the conversion of *H. pylori* into coccoidal forms is a passive process which does not require protein synthesis, and that the coccoidal form is more likely the morphological manifestation of bacterial cell death rather than a viable metabolizing but nonculturable entity.

Based on the few regulatory networks suggested by the *H. pylori* genome sequence annotation (Tomb et al. 1997), the molecular data support the concept that coccoidal forms are degenerative forms of *H. pylori*. The significance of these coccoidal forms is still under debate, and more experiments concerning the regulation of gene expression will contribute to elucidate this question.

3.2 Motility

The capacity of *H. pylori* to spread through the viscous mucus covering the epithelial cells of the gastric mucosa, is due to the presence of five or six unipolar flagella. These units are essential for *H. pylori* colonization (see "Mechanisms of *Helicobacter pylori* Infection: Bacterial Factors," this volume). The flagellar filaments are composed of two different proteins: the major flagellin is a 53-kDa protein named FlaA, and the minor flagellin, FlaB, is a 54-kDa protein.

A property of these flagella is that the flagellar filament is covered by a double layer of phospholipids. This sheath is thought to protect the flagella from the gastric acidity, which otherwise would depolymerize the flagellar filaments (Suerbaum et al. 1993). In 1997, Jones et al. reported the existence of a flagellar sheath protein identical to the HpaA protein, which was shown to be a N-acetyl neuraminyllactose-binding hemagglutinin (Evans et al. 1993).

The two genes (*flaA* and *flaB*) encoding the proteins FlaA and FlaB were characterized (Leying et al. 1992; Suerbaum et al. 1993). These genes were shown to be expressed from promoters using different sigma factors (sigma 28 and 54). This result suggests that the composition of the flagellar filament might vary in response to changes in environmental conditions. This modulation might confer to the bacteria, motility properties adapted to environmental conditions (Josenhans et al. 1995). Sigma 28- and sigma 54-like promoters have been found upstream of many flagellar genes by Tomb et al. (1997) who suggested a complex transcriptional regulation of the flagellar regulon.

Moreover, orthologues of proteins involved in the control of flagellar gene expression in *Bacillus subtilis* were found to be encoded by *H. pylori* DNA (Tomb et al. 1997), for example, the FlhF protein which is a GTP-binding protein and the FliS protein involved in the negative control of flagellar gene expression.

In addition, Schmitz et al. (1997) have characterized the *flbB* gene which encodes a protein that is similar to InvA, LcrD, and FlbF proteins implicated in the regulation of virulence or motility.

Examination of *H. pylori* genome sequence annotation shows that numerous genes involved in the secretion and assembly of the flagellar structure are present in *H. pylori* DNA including genes involved in hook structure and basal body synthesis. Orthologous proteins responsible for motor rotation and motor switching seem to be encoded by *H. pylori*.

4 Chemotaxis

Despite a well-developed adaptation to its environment, some studies have suggested that *H. pylori* demonstrates chemotactic activity, mediated in particular, through four amino acids (lysine, alanine, glutamine and histidine), and toward urea and bicarbonate (WORKU et al. 1997; YOSHIYAMA et al. 1997).

Moreover, JACKSON et al. (1995) have characterized two genes encoding the major regulators of chemotaxis in bacteria (CheA and CheY). The latter has been shown to belong to a stress-responsive operon (BEIER et al. 1997). Orthologous genes namely *cheV*, *cheF*, and *cheW*, have also been identified (PITTMAN et al. 1997). As additional evidence to this chemotactic activity, genome sequence analysis has also allowed the identification of genes encoding putative receptors/transducers and genes involved in intermediate signal processing.

5 Metabolism

As a microaerophilic bacterium living in an acidic environment, *H. pylori* has developed strategies to survive and grow under such particular conditions. In addition to a brief overview of the *H. pylori* metabolism, we will focus on a few metabolic features that account for this adaptation to a restricted ecological niche.

5.1 Glucose Metabolism

H. pylori seems to be able to metabolize glucose by using both fermentative and oxidative pathways, as shown experimentally (for review, HAZELL and MENDZ 1997) and also by analyzing the whole genome sequence (TOMB et al. 1997). However, glucose is the only source of carbohydrates and the main source for substrate-level phosphorylation.

The importation of glucose into cells is mediated by a permease. No phosphotransferase system nor general glucokinase seems to be encoded by *H. pylori* DNA. This feature could reflect the limited range of carbohydrates used and the adaptation to a restricted niche.

Three pathways are believed to be involved in glucose catabolism: the pentose phosphate pathway, glycolysis, and the primitive Entner-Doudoroff pathway (MENDZ et al. 1994a; CHALK et al. 1994; HOFFMAN et al. 1996; MENDZ and HAZELL

1991). The latter is less energetic than glycolysis but offers the possibility to metabolize aldonic acids. Genes involved in these different pathways have been identified in the *H. pylori* DNA sequence.

5.2 Pyruvate Metabolism and the Krebs Cycle

Pyruvate is the final product of glycolysis and the Entner-Doudoroff pathway. The fate of pyruvate in *H. pylori* has been investigated under anaerobic and aerobic conditions (CHALK et al. 1994; MENDZ et al. 1994b). These studies and the genome sequence annotation provide some outline for the microaerophilic character of *H. pylori*.

For example, the oxidative decarboxylation of pyruvate was shown to be carried out by a pyruvate:flavodoxin oxidoreductase (HUGHES et al. 1995), instead of the aerobic pyruvate dehydrogenase (AceCF), and the strictly anaerobic pyruvate-formate-lyase (Pfl) associated with mixed fermentation, whose corresponding genes seem to be absent from the *H. pylori* genome sequence (TOMB et al. 1997).

Orthologous genes encoding enzymes involved in the Krebs cycle or in fermentative metabolism have been found in *H. pylori* DNA. An interesting finding is the presence of 2-oxoglutarate:acceptor oxidoreductase which catalyzes one of the reactions in the Krebs cycle. Moreover, some studies report the existence of a reductive pathway in the Krebs cycle (MENDZ et al. 1993; HAZELL and MENDZ 1997). What is interesting in this reductive pathway is that fumarate may act as an electron acceptor in anaerobic respiration (see below).

The pyruvate:flavodoxin oxidoreductase from *H. pylori* has been shown to be related to pyruvate ferredoxin oxidoreductases, previously associated with hyperthermophilic organisms (HUGHES et al. 1995). The same observation should be made for the 2-oxoglutarate:acceptor oxidoreductase, based on gene sequence similarities (TOMB et al. 1997).

The putative anaerobic respiration and the characterization of both the pyruvate:flavodoxin oxidoreductase and the 2-oxoglutarate:acceptor oxidoreductase are elements that contribute to the microaerophilic phenotype of *H. pylori* and support the concept of an anaerobic metabolic system in this bacterium, even if oxygen is required for growth.

5.3 Amino Acid Metabolism

The development of a defined medium for the culture of *H. pylori* and the subsequent determination of its amino acid requirement were important steps in understanding *H. pylori* metabolism (REYNOLDS and PENN 1994). In 1995, MENDZ and HAZELL (1995) showed that carbohydrates can be removed from a medium in which amino acids constituted the basic nutrients. When analyzing the genome sequence annotation, a very high correlation was observed with experimental data. Orthologous genes encoding enzymes involved in amino acid biosynthesis or catabolism were identified in *H. pylori* DNA. In summary, when an amino acid is found to be required for growth (REYNOLDS and PENN 1994), the analysis of the molecular data reveals that the biosynthetic pathway for it is not complete. In contrast, dispensable amino acids are thought to be synthesized by the bacterium through conventional pathways.

5.4 Fatty Acid and Phospholipid Metabolism

Degradation of lipids could provide an additional source of carbon and energy. Moreover, phospholipids are a potential source of phosphate. *H. pylori* seems to have the coding capacity for few enzymes involved in the β-oxidation cycle (TOMB et al. 1997). Some studies have reported phospholipase activity in *H. pylori*, involving phospholipase A1, A2, or C (LICHTENBERGER et al. 1990; OTTLECZ et al. 1993; WEITKAMP et al. 1993; BODE et al. 1997). The role of these phospholipases in gastric mucosa alterations is discussed elsewhere in this volume (see "Mechanisms of *Helicobacter pylori* Infection: Bacterial Factors").

Concerning the biosynthesis of fatty acids and phospholipids, few experimental studies have been carried out. Considering the genome sequence, at least 14 genes, encoding enzymes involved in biosynthetic pathway of lipids have been identified in *H. pylori* DNA (TOMB et al. 1997). The finding of a *cfa* orthologous gene from *C. coli* suggests the presence of cyclopropane fatty acids in the *H. pylori* genome, as in many other bacteria. Regarding the phospholipid biosynthetic pathway, genes involved in it have been found in *H. pylori* sequence (TOMB et al. 1997). Moreover, GE and TAYLOR (1997) have identified the phosphatidylserine synthase and the corresponding gene (*pssA*).

5.5 Nucleotide Biosynthesis

Ribonucleotide monophosphates (NMP), from which deoxyribonucleotide monophosphates (dNMP) are derived, may be synthesized de novo from simple precursors or they may be formed via the so-called salvage pathway.

Data provided from experimental studies (MENDZ et al. 1994c,d) and molecular data from the sequence annotation (TOMB et al. 1997) have led to the conclusion that *H. pylori* can synthesize de novo many of the pyrimidine nucleotides and has a limited utilization of the pyrimidine salvage pathways. On the other hand, the purine nucleotides are thought to be synthesized by the purine salvage pathways rather than by the de novo pathways.

5.6 Respiratory Chains

In *H. pylori*, there is some evidence that aerobic and anaerobic respiration occurs. Proton translocation is mediated by NDH-1 dehydrogenase and various cytochromes. The NDH-1 complex is also able to catalyze the reduction in quinones by NADH (SMITH and EDWARDS 1997). Some studies report that the primitive cbb3-type cytochrome oxidase acts as a terminal oxidase in the aerobic respiration in *H. pylori* (NAGATA et al. 1996; ALDERSON et al. 1997). In addition to the NDH-1 complex, four other respiratory electron-generating dehydrogenases have been identified by gene sequence similarities (TOMB et al. 1997): a hydrogenase complex (HydABC), a D-lactate dehydrogenase and two *sn*-glycerol-3-phosphate dehydrogenases (aerobic and anaerobic forms).

In aerobic respiration, oxygen is the terminal respiratory acceptor for electrons. MENDZ and HAZELL (1993) have demonstrated that *H. pylori* contains a fumarate reductase whose existence suggests the possibility of ATP generation via anaerobic respiration, in a similar fashion to other anaerobic or facultative bacteria. Thus, fumarate can serve as an electron acceptor in anaerobic respiration. MARCELLI et al. (1996) have shown that the major isoprenoid quinone is menaquinone-6, which implies that the anaerobic respiratory chain is used more frequently in *H. pylori* than the aerobic respiratory chain (TATUSOV et al. 1996).

6 Nitrogen Sources

Analysis of the genome sequence of *H. pylori* leads to the hypothesis that the bacterium is able to use several substrates as a nitrogen source, including urea, ammonia, and three amino acids (alanine, serine, and glutamine).

Ammonia can be produced by the activity of urease (WILLIAMS et al. 1996) which allows access to urea nitrogen in the form of ammonium ions. *H. pylori* also seems to have the coding capacity for an aliphatic amidase (SKOULOUBRIS et al. 1997; DEREUSE et al. 1997). This enzyme catalyzes the degradation of amides, which supplies a nitrogen source also by ammonia production.

7 Iron Acquisition

As with other bacteria, *H. pylori* requires an iron-scavenging system to provide iron, which is an extremely important element for biological systems. What is very interesting, when analyzing the genome sequence of *H. pylori*, is the complexity of iron acquisition mechanisms and the redundancy of the iron-scavenging systems. One wonders about the relevance and the signification of this feature. Genome sequence analysis suggests the existence of a system for iron uptake analogous to the siderophore-mediated iron uptake *fec* system of *Escherichia coli*.

Components of a periplasmic binding protein-dependent transport system for the uptake of a ferric siderophore seem to be encoded by *H. pylori* DNA. The bacterium should be able to assimilate ferrous iron, since a feo-like system has been found in *H. pylori*. In *E. coli*, the system provides an important contribution to the iron supply under anaerobic conditions (KAMMLER et al. 1993). FRAZIER et al., in 1993, and later EVANS et al. (1995) identified a nonheme cytoplasmic iron-containing ferritin used for storage of iron (Pfr). In addition to this component, *H. pylori* contains NapA, a bacterio-ferritin possibly involved in the storage of residual iron.

Concerning the regulation of the iron uptake, three copies of the *frpB* orthologous gene from *Neisseria meningitidis* have been found in *H. pylori*. The encoded protein is homologous to several TonB-dependent outer membrane receptors of *E. coli* (BEUCHER and SPARLING 1995). The TonB protein is an essential component in iron-siderophore uptake in bacteria. Moreover, the important regulatory protein Fur (ferric uptake regulator) seems to be encoded by *H. pylori*. Consensus sequences for Fur-binding boxes were found upstream of two *fecA* genes, three *frpB* genes and the *fur* gene (TOMB et al. 1997).

8 pH Regulation

H. pylori must have developed physiological strategies to colonize an acidic environment due to the high activity of gastric H^+, K^+ ATPase. In vitro, *H. pylori* cannot survive at pH 3, whereas when urea is adding at a similar concentration as in the stomach, the bacteria are protected (CLYNE et al. 1995). Therefore the urease produced by *H. pylori* allows it to extend its survival into the acidic range of pH. However, MEYER-ROSBERG et al. (1996) have shown that urease decreases the bacteria's survival at alkaline pH (Fig. 3).

Other mechanisms of pH homeostasis have been developed by *H. pylori*. As in other bacteria, *H. pylori* is able to maintain the proton motive force, by adjusting the potential difference across the plasmic membrane to compensate for the changes in pH gradient (SACHS et al. 1996). Its ability to create a positive inside-membrane potential seems more likely to be provided by concentrating cations than by pumping out anions, as suggested by the few mechanisms for anion efflux encoded by *H. pylori* DNA. Three proton-translocating P-type ATPases have been identified in *H. pylori*: ATPase-439, ATPase-948, and ATPase-115 (GE et al. 1995; MELCHERS et al. 1996, 1998).

H^+-coupled ion-transport systems have also been identified in *H. pylori* involving two orthologous proteins of NapA from *Enterococcus hirae* and NhaA from *E. coli* which are Na^+/H^+ antiporters and responsible for controlling the flow of ions into and out of the cell.

The pH of a host microenvironment can be considered as one of the physicochemical signals that then results in the induction or repression of appropriate genes. In this area, McGOWAN et al. (1996, 1997) reported a change in *H. pylori* protein content following a shift in extracellular pH.

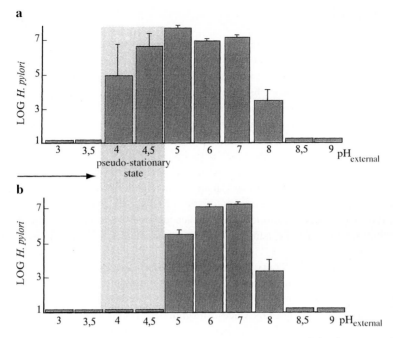

Fig. 3a,b. Comparison of *H. pylori* survival **a** and growth **b** in different pH conditions in presence of urea. (From SACHS et al. 1996)

9 Diversity

H. pylori was cultured in 1982 by WARREN and MARSHALL (1983) from human stomach biopsies of patients with type B gastritis. During the following years this bacterium was shown to be associated with diverse diseases (see "Diagnosis of *Helicobacter pylori* Infection," this volume). The occurrence of one of these diseases can be related to host genetic factors and environmental factors, but might also be dependent on the specific properties of the infectious bacteria. Hence, it is of interest to evaluate the heterogeneity of *H. pylori* populations and to attempt to find a relationship between the bacterial genetic background and a given disease. Numerous studies have shown by diverse typing methods, that there are substantial levels of variation among natural isolates of *H. pylori* and that the degree of diversity seems to exceed that recorded in virtually all bacterial species (Go et al. 1996; VAN DOORN et al. 1997; WOLLE et al. 1997).

Many different mechanisms could contribute to this genetic diversity. One of the most interesting is the point mutation which is the change in only one single base pair. Such a mutation has been shown to be associated with diversity in the *ureC* gene (KANSAU et al. 1996; COURCOUX et al. 1990) and the *iceA* gene (PEEK et al. 1996), for example. The acquisition of exogenous DNA may also have contributed to this diversity as well as multiple genomic rearrangements.

9.1 Cag Locus

The cag locus (Fig. 4) provides an extraordinary illustration of multiple mechanisms by which diversity can occur. First, the *cagA* gene was the first *H. pylori* gene to be described which is not conserved in all strains (Tummuru et al. 1993; Covacci et al. 1993). The molecular characterization of the *cagA* gene, the gene currently used as the marker for the cag locus, provides an example of heterogeneity by variation in the number of intragenic cassettes. The number of DNA repeats accounts for the observed size heterogeneity of the CagA protein (Blaser 1996).

Finally, the cag locus was shown to be most likely acquired by horizontal transfer and integrated into a bacterial housekeeping gene, and then to evolve by chromosomal rearrangements and acquisition of insertion sequence elements (Censini et al. 1996). Several characteristics of this locus such as the presence of short repeated sequences and insertion sequences, its $G + C$ content (35%) which is different than that of the genome (39%), its prevalence with the most virulent strains, and its capacity to encode proteins probably involved in the export of virulence determinants (Tummuru et al. 1995; Tomb et al. 1997), have led to the consideration of this genetic locus as a so-called pathogenicity island (see "Mechanisms of *Helicobacter pylori* Infection: Bacterial Factors," this volume).

The success of foreign DNA acquisition depends on the DNA transfer and on its integration into the *H. pylori* genome by a recombinant event. Despite the natural competence of *H. pylori* (Wang et al. 1993), the efficiency of a foreign DNA successful transfer might be reduced by the presence of numerous restriction and modification systems existing in *H. pylori* (Tomb et al. 1997).

In contrast, recombination events might be responsible for genetic shifts in *H. pylori*. Indeed, the bacterium has the coding capacity for a recombination pathway (RecF), and numerous homologous sequences such as DNA repeats and paralogous genes are present in *H. pylori* DNA.

9.2 *vacA* Gene

The *vacA* gene encodes the vacuolating cytotoxin A which is produced by approximatively 50% of *H. pylori* strains (Cover and Blaser 1992). The role of this cytotoxin in the pathogenicity of *H. pylori* is discussed elsewhere in this volume (see "Mechanisms of *Helicobacter pylori* Infection: Bacterial Factors"). In this section we will consider this gene as an example of diversity.

Atherton et al. (1995) demonstrated the mosaic structure of the *vacA* gene in which both conserved regions and diverse regions exist (Fig. 5). The authors defined two types of midregion sequences (m1 and m2) and three different families of *vacA* signal sequences (s1a, s1b, and s2). More recently two other allelic types were defined in the midregion of the gene: m1-like (m1*) and the hybrid m1*-m2 (Pan et al. 1998) and one in the signal sequence (s1c) (van Doorn et al. 1998). The analysis of the whole genome sequence of *H. pylori* led to the identification of three other genes sharing sequence similarity with the *vacA* gene. The mosaic structure as

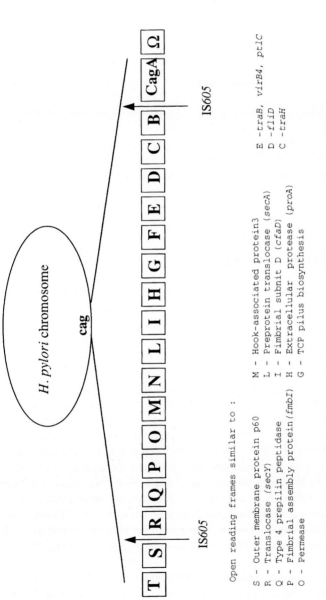

Open reading frames similar to :

S – Outer membrane protein p60   M – Hook-associated protein3   E – *traB, virB4, ptlC*
R – Translocase *(secY)*   L – Preprotein translocase *(secA)*   D – *fliD*
Q – Type 4 prepilin peptidase   I – Fimbrial subnit D *(cfaD)*   C – *traH*
P – Fimbrial assembly protein *(fmbI)* H – Extracellular protease *(proA)*
O – Permease   G – TCP pilus biosynthesis

IS*605*: insertion sequence which can be localized at different sites indicated by the arrows

Fig. 4. The cag pathogenicity island

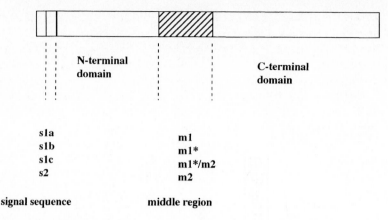

Fig. 5. The *vacA* gene diversity

well as the putative intragenic recombination events between *vacA*-related genes might contribute to the heterogeneity of *H. pylori* strains, by generating new VacA variants. An association between the *vacA* allelic type and the amount of cytotoxin produced has been made.

9.3 Adhesins and Lipopolysaccharide

H. pylori also exhibits some diversity in adhesin expression. Despite the fact that the majority of *H. pylori* is free-living in the gastric mucosa (LEE and MITCHELL 1994), some are found adhering to epithelial cells (HESSEY et al. 1990; LEE et al. 1993). The presence of adhesins in *H. pylori* was proved by the characterization of the adhesins themselves or of a cellular receptor (CLYNE and DRUMM 1997). Their contribution to *H. pylori* colonization is reviewed elsewhere in this volume (see "Mechanisms of *Helicobacter pylori* Infection: Bacterial Factors").

Adhesins also contribute to the observed heterogeneity of *H. pylori* strains. Indeed, three previously identified adhesins, AlpA, AlpB, and BabA (ODENBREIT et al. 1997; LLVER et al. 1998), belong to the large family of outer membrane proteins (OMPs) (TOMB et al. 1997). What is interesting is that all the members of this family (32 in *H. pylori*) contain one highly similar domain at the amino-terminal end and seven homologous domains at the carboxy terminus. Furthermore, 11 of these 32 OMPs share extensive similarities over their entire length. Considering these sequence similarities and the great number of OMP genes encoding surface-exposed proteins, it seems that recombination events could occur and lead to mosaic organization. This structure may be the basis for antigenic variation in *H. pylori*.

In addition to this mosaic structure, OMP genes seem to be submitted to transcriptional regulation which would likewise provide antigenic variation. In this category, eight OMP genes have been found with potential promoter regions containing oligonucleotide repeats (Tomb et al. 1997). The synthesis of functional versus nonfunctional proteins depends on the stretch length (Jonsson et al. 1991; Yogev et al. 1991). Until recently such antigenic variation had not been documented for OMPs. However, another mechanism of phase variation was identified for the BabA adhesin (Llver et al. 1998). There is a duplication or deletion of ten base pairs, which induces the conversion of a silent gene to an expressed gene and vice versa.

With regard to the lipopolysaccharide (LPS) of *H. pylori*, its main characteristic is to contain Lewis^x and Lewis^y antigenic moieties that mimic the Lewis antigens present on parietal cells and in human gastric mucosa (see "Mechanisms of *Helicobacter pylori* Infection: Host Factors," this volume) (Fig. 6).

In addition to the genes necessary to ensure the biosynthesis of lipid A and the core region, the whole genome sequence allowed the identification of two copies of α 1,3 fucosyl transferase genes. The corresponding enzyme is involved in the expression of sialyl-Lewis^x antigens in humans. As in some OMP genes, stretches of repeats have been identified in the promoter region of these genes. Recently, Appelmelk et al. (1998) described phase variation in Lewis and non-Lewis LPS serotypes due to "on/off" switching of these genes.

9.4 Extragenic Elements

Extrachromosomal DNA and transposon elements can also contribute to *H. pylori* diversity.

Approximatively 40% of *H. pylori* strains contain cryptic plasmids (Dunn et al. 1997). Other extragenic elements contribute to the diversity such as insertion sequences or transposons. As mentioned above, *H. pylori* was shown to contain insertion sequence IS605. In the sequenced *H. pylori* strain (26695), two distinct insertion sequences were found: five full-length copies of IS605 and two of a novel IS606, as well as partial copies of both.

Lewis^x

$$\begin{array}{l} \text{Gal } \beta \ 1 - 4 \text{ GlcNAc} \\ \quad | \ \alpha 1,3 \\ \quad \text{Fuc} \end{array}$$

Lewis^y

$$\begin{array}{l} \text{Fuc}\alpha 1 - 2 \text{ Gal}\beta 1 - 4 \text{ GlcNAc} \\ \quad | \ \alpha 1,3 \\ \quad \text{Fuc} \end{array}$$

Fig. 6. Lewis^x and Lewis^y antigen structure. *Gal*, D-Galactose; *GlcNAc*, N-acetyl-D-glucosamine; *Fuc*, L-fucose

These extragenic elements are not widely distributed in the *H. pylori* population and hence could confer different phenotypic characters. Finally, there is evidence that *H. pylori* populations are highly diverse and that this diversity is still increasing. For this reason, it will probably be difficult to predict disease development even when the infectious strain of *H. pylori* is identified and characterized.

10 Conclusion

In summary, *H. pylori* is a bacterium which has developed a great number of specialized systems allowing it to grow and persist in a restricted ecological niche.

The variability of the *H. pylori* genome sequence has confirmed some previous experimental data and has helped to solve some ambiguities, in iron-scavenging systems for example. These molecular data have indeed provided some explanations concerning the limited carbohydrate range used by *H. pylori*. The sequence also provides new insights into the acid tolerance and microaerophilic character of *H. pylori*, as we have tried to show in this chapter.

Interestingly, molecular data provided by the whole-genome sequencing as well as recent studies (APPELMELK et al. 1998; LLVER et al. 1998) have shown that this organism has developed mechanisms which induce antigenic variation within a population. In the future, experiments concerning such antigenic variation will no doubt provide insight into its biological significance, and in particular into its contribution to evade the host immune response.

Nevertheless, the availability of the complete genome sequence of *H. pylori* is not an ending itself but the starting point for further experiments. One of the principal genome-oriented experimental approaches would involve the inactivation of genes, followed by evaluation of the effects of gene disruption in biochemical and biological test systems as well as in animal models.

There is no doubt that *H. pylori* research will benefit from the sequence data, in particular pathogenesis, vaccine and therapeutic developments.

References

Alderson J, Clayton CL, Kelly DJ (1997) Investigations into the aerobic respiratory chain of *Helicobacter pylori*. Gut 41 [Suppl 1]:A7

Appelmelk BJ, Shiberu B, Trinks C, Tapsi N, Zheng PY, Verboom T, Maaskant J, Hokke CH, Schiphorst WE, Blanchard D, Simoons-Smit IM, Van den Eijnden DH, Vandenbroucke-Grauls CM (1998) Phase variation in *Helicobacter pylori* lipopolysaccharide. Infect Immun 66:70–76

Atherton JC, Cao P, Peek RM, Tummuru MKR, Blaser MJ, Cover TL (1995) Mosaicism in vacuolating cytotoxin alleles of *Helicobacter pylori*. Association of specific *vacA* types with cytotoxin production and peptic ulceration. J Biol Chem 270:17771–17777

Beier D, Spohn G, Rappuoli R, Scarlato V (1997) Identification and characterization of an operon of *Helicobacter pylori* that is involved in motility and stress adaptation. J Bacteriol 179:4676–4683

Berry V, Jennings K, Woodnutt G (1995) Bactericidal and morphological effects of amoxicillin on *Helicobacter pylori*. Antimicrob Agents Chemother 39:1859–1861

Beucher M, Sparling PF (1995) Cloning, sequencing and characterization of the gene encoding FrpB, a major iron-regulated outer membrane protein of *Neisseria gonorrhoeae*. J Bacteriol 177:2041–2049

Blaser MJ (1996) Genetic bases for heterogeneity of *Helicobacter pylori*. In: Hunt RH, Tytgat GNJ (eds) *Helicobacter pylori*-Basic mechanisms to clinical cure. Kluwer, Dordrecht, pp 33–39

Bode G, Song Q, Barth R, Adler G (1997) Phospholipase C activity of *Helicobacter pylori* is not associated with the prevalence of the *cagA* gene. Gut 41 [Suppl 1]:A14

Buck GE, Parshall KA, Davis CP (1983) Electron microscopy of coccoid form of *Campylobacter jejuni*. J Clin Microbiol 18:420–421

Catrenich CE, Makin KM (1991) Characterization of the morphologic conversion of *Helicobacter pylori* from bacillary to coccoid forms. Scand J Gastroenterol 26 [Suppl 181]:58–64

Cellini L, Allocati N, Angelucci D, Iezzi T, Di Campli E, Marzio L, Dainelli B (1994a) Coccoid *Helicobacter pylori* not culturable in vitro reverts in mice. Microbiol Immunol 38:843–850

Cellini L, Allocati N, Di Campli E, Dainelli B (1994b) *Helicobacter pylori*: a fickle germ. Microbiol Immunol 38:25–30

Censini S, Lange C, Xiang ZY, Crabtree JE, Ghiara P, Borodovsky M, Rappuoli R, Covacci A (1996) Cag, a pathogenicity island of *Helicobacter pylori*, encodes type I-specific and disease-associated virulence factors. Proc Natl Acad Sci USA 93:14648–14653

Chalk PA, Roberts AD, Blows WM (1994) Metabolism of pyruvate and glucose by intact cells of *Helicobacter pylori* studied by C-13 NMR spectroscopy. Microbiology UK 140:2085–2092

Chan WY, Hui PK, Leung K, Chow J Kwok F, Ng CS (1994) Coccoid forms of *Helicobacter pylori* in human stomach. Am J Clin Pathol 102:503–507

Clyne M, Drumm B (1997) Adherence of *Helicobacter pylori* to gastric mucosa. Can J Gastroenterol 11:243–248

Clyne M, Labigne A, Drumm B (1995) *Helicobacter pylori* requires an acidic environment to survive in presence of urea. Infect Immun 63:1669–1673

Cole SP, Cirillo D, Kagnoff MF, Guiney DG, Eckmann L (1997) Coccoid and spiral *Helicobacter pylori* differ in their abilities to adhere to gastric epithelial cells and induce interleukin-8 secretion. Infect Immun 65:843–846

Courcoux P, Freland C, Piemond Y, Fauchère JL, Labigne A (1990) Polymerase chain reaction and direct DNA sequencing as a method for distinguishing between different strains of *Helicobacter pylori*. Rev Esp Enferm Dig 78:29

Covacci A, Censini S, Bugnoli M, Petracca R, Burroni D, Macchia G, Massone A, Papini E, Xiang Z, Figura N, Rappuoli R (1993) Molecular characterization of the 128 kDa immunodominant antigen of *Helicobacter pylori* associated with cytotoxicity and duodenal ulcer. Proc Natl Acad Sci USA 90:5791–5795

Cover TL, Blaser MJ (1992) Purification and characterization of the vacuolating toxin from *Helicobacter pylori*. J Biol Chem 267:10570–10575

De Reuse H, Skouloubris S, Labigne A (1997) Identification of an aliphatic amidase in *H. pylori*. 9th International Workshop on Campylobacter, Helicobacter, and related organisms, Cape Town, South Africa, p 59

van Doorn LJ, Figueiredo C, Carneiro F, Sanna R, Pena S, Midolo P, Blaser MJ (1997) Worldwide heterogeneity of the *Helicobacter pylori vacA* gene. Gut 41 [Suppl 1]:A34

van Doorn LJ, Figueiredo CG, Schneeberger P, de Boer W, Quint W (1998) Peptic ulcer disease is related to the *vacA*, *cagA* and *iceA* status of *Helicobacter pylori*. Proceedings in Second Annual Winter *H. pylori* Workshop, 27–28 Feb 1998, Phoenix, Arizona, USA

Dunn BE, Cohen H, Blaser MJ (1997) *Helicobacter pylori*. Clin Microbiol Rev 10:720–741

Eaton KA, Catrenich CE, Makin KM, Krakowkas S (1995) Virulence of coccoid and bacillary forms of *Helicobacter pylori* in gnotobiotic piglets. J Infect Dis 171:459–462

Evans DG, Karjalainen RK, Evans DJR, Graham DY, Lee CH (1993) Cloning, nucleotide sequence, and expression of a gene encoding an adhesin subunit protein of *Helicobacter pylori*. J Bacteriol 175:674–683

Evans DJ Jr, Evans DG, Lampert HC, Nakano H (1995) Identification of four new prokaryotic bacterioferritins, from *Helicobacter pylori*, *Anabaena variabilis*, *Bacillus subtilis*, and *Treponema pallidum*, by analysis sequence. Gene 153:123–127

Frazier BA, Pgeifer JD, Russell DG, Flak P, Olsen AN, Hammar M, Westblom TU, Normark ST (1993) Paracrystalline inclusions of a novel ferritin containing non-heme iron, produced by the human gastric pathogen *Helicobacter pylori*: evidence for a third class of ferritins. J Bacteriol 175:966–972

Ge Z, Taylor DE (1997) The *Helicobacter pylori* gene encoding phosphatidylserine synthase: sequence, expression, and insertional mutagenesis. J Bacteriol 179:4970–4976

Ge Z, Hiratsuka K, Taylor DE (1995) Nucleotide sequence and mutational analysis indicate that two *Helicobacter pylori* genes encode a P-type ATPase and a cation-binding protein associated with copper transport. Mol Microbiol 15:97–106

Go MF, Kapur V, Graham DY, Musser JM (1996) Population genetic analysis of *Helicobacter pylori* by multilocus enzyme electrophoresis: extensive allelic diversity and recombinational population structure. J Bacteriol 178:3934–3938

Goodwin CS, Armstrong JA, Chilvers T, Peters M, Collins MD, Sly L, Mc Connell W, Harper WES (1989) Transfer of *Campylobacter pylori* and *Campylobacter mustelae* to *Helicobacter* gen nov as *Helicobacter pylori* comb nov and *Helicobacter mustelae* comb nov respectively. Int J Syst Bacteriol 39:397–405

Hazell SL, Mendz GL (1997) How *Helicobacter pylori* works: an overview of the metabolism of *Helicobacter pylori*. Helicobacter 2:1–12

Hessey SJ, Spencer J, Wyatt JI, Sobala G, Rathbone BJ, Axon ATR, Dixon MF (1990) Bacterial adhesion and disease activity in Helicobacter associated chronic gastritis. Gut 31:134–138

Hoffman PS, Goodwin A, Johnsen J, Magu K, Veldhuyzen VanZanten SOV (1996) Metabolic activities of metronidazole-sensitive and -resistant strains of *Helicobacter pylori* – repression of isocitrate lyase activity correlate with resistance. J Bacteriol 178:4822–4829

Hughes NJ, Chalk PA, Clayton CL, Kelly DJ (1995) Identification of carboxylation enzymes and characterization of a novel four-subunit pyruvate:flavodoxin oxidoreductase from *Helicobacter pylori*. J Bacteriol 177:3953–3959

Jackson CJ, Kelly DJ, Clayton CL (1995) The cloning and characterization of chemotaxis genes in *Helicobacter pylori*. Gut 37:A71

Jones DM, Curry A (1991) The genesis of coccal forms of Helicobacter. In: Malfertheiner P, Ditschuneit H (eds) Gastritis and peptic ulcer. Springer, Berlin, pp 29–27

Jones AC, Logan RP, Foynes S, Cockayne A, Wren BW, Penn CW (1997) A flagellar sheath protein of *Helicobacter pylori* is identical to HpaA, a putative N-acetylneuraminyllactose-binding hemagglutinin, but is not an adhesin for AGS cells. J Bacteriol 179:5643–5647

Josenhans C, Labigne A, Suerbaum S (1995) Reporter gene analyses show that expression of both *H. pylori* flagellins is dependent on the growth phase. Gut 37:A246

Jonsson AB, Nyberg G, Norwark S (1991) Phase variation of gonococcal pili by frameshift mutation in *pilC*, a novel gene for pilus assembly. EMBO J 10:477–488

Kammler M, Schon C, Hantke K (1993) Characterization of the ferrous iron uptake system of *Escherichia coli*. J Bacteriol 175:6212–6219

Kansau I, Raymond J, Bingen E (1996) Genotyping of *Helicobacter pylori* isolates by sequencing of PCR products and comparison with the RAPD techniques. Res Microbiol 147:661–669

Kursters JG, Gerrits MM, van Strijp JAG, Vandenbroucke-Grauls MJE (1997) Coccoid forms of *Helicobacter pylori* are the morphologic manifestation of cell death. Infect Immun 65:3672–3679

Lee A, Mitchell H (1994) Basic bacteriology of *H. pylori*: *H. pylori* colonization factors. In: Hunt RH, Tytgat GNT (eds) *Helicobacter pylori*-basic mechanisms to clinical cure. Kluwer, Dordrecht, pp 59–72

Lee A, Fox J, Hazell S (1993) Pathogenicity of *Helicobacter pylori*: a perspective. Infect Immun 61:1601–1610

Leying H, Suerbaum S, Geis G, Haas R (1992) Cloning and genetic characterization of a *Helicobacter pylori* flagellin gene. Mol Microbiol 6:2863–2874

Lichtenberger LM, Hazell SL, Romero JJ, Graham DY (1990) *Helicobacter pylori* hydrolysis of artificial phospholipid monolayers: insight into a potential mechanism of mucosal injury. Gastroenterology 98:A78

Llver D, Arnqvist A, Ögren J, Frick IM, Kersulyte D, Incecik ET, Berg DE, Covacci A, Engstrand L, Borén T (1998) *Helicobacter pylori* adhesin binding fucosylated histo-blood group antigens revealed by retagging. Science 279:373–377

Mai U, Geis G Leying H, Ruhl G, Operkuch W (1989) Dimorphism of *Campylobacter pylori*. In: Mégraud F, Lamouliatte H (eds) Gastroduodenal pathology and *Campylobacter pylori*. Elsevier Science, Amsterdam, pp 29–33

Marcelli SW, Chang HJ, Chapman T, Chalk PA, Miles RJ, Poole RK (1996) The respiratory chain of *Helicobacter pylori*: identification of cytochromes and the effects of oxygen on cytochrome and menaquinone levels. FEMS Microbiol Lett 138:59–64

Marshall BJ, Royce H, Annear DI, Goodwin CS, Pearman JW, Warren JR, Armstrong JA (1984) Original isolation of *Campylobacter pyloridis* from human gastric mucosa. Microbiol Lett 25:83–88

McGowan CC, Cover TL, Blaser MJ (1996) *Helicobacter pylori* and gastric acid: biological and therapeutic implications. Gastroenterology 110:926–938

McGowan CC, Necheva AS, Cover TL, Blaser MJ (1997) Acid-induced expression of oxidative stress protein homologs in *Helicobacter pylori*. Gut 41 [Suppl 1]:A18

Melchers K, Weitzenegger T, Buhmann A, Steinhilber W, Sachs G, Schäfer K (1996) Cloning and membrane topology of a P type ATPase from *Helicobacter pylori*. J Biol Chem 271:446–457

Melchers K, Herrman L, Mauch F, Bayle D, Heuermann D, Weitzenegger T, Schuhmacher A, Sachs G, Haas R, Bode G, Bensch KW, Schäfer KP (1998) Properties and function of the P type ions pumps cloned from *Helicobacter pylori*. Acta Physiol Scand (in press)

Mendz GL, Hazell SL (1991) Evidence for a pentose phosphate pathway in *Helicobacter pylori*. FEMS Microbiol Lett 84:331–336

Mendz GL, Hazell SL (1993) Fumarate catabolism in *Helicobacter pylori*. Biochem Mol Biol Int 31:325–332

Mendz GL, Hazell SL (1995) Aminoacid utilization by *Helicobacter pylori*. Int J Biochem Cell Biol 27:1085–1093

Mendz GL, Hazell SL, Burns BP (1993) Glucose utilization and lactate production by *Helicobacter pylori*. J Gen Microbiol 139:3023–3028

Mendz GL, Hazell SL, Burns BP (1994a) The Entner-Doudoroff pathway in *Helicobacter pylori*. Arch Biochem Biophys 312:349–356

Mendz GL, Hazell SL, Vangorkam L (1994b) Pyruvate metabolism in *Helicobacter pylori*. Arch Microbiol 162:187–192

Mendz GL, Jimenez BM, Hazell SL, Gero AM, O'Sullivan WJ (1994c) Salvage synthesis of pyrimidine nucleotides by *Helicobacter pylori*. J Appl Bacteriol 77:1–8

Mendz GL, Jimenez BM, Hazell SL, Gero AM, O'Sullivan WJ (1994d) Salvage synthesis of purine nucleotides by *Helicobacter pylori*. J Appl Bacteriol 77:674–681

Meyer-Rosberg K, Scott DR, Rex D, Melchers K, Sachs G (1996) The effect of environmental pH on the proton motive force of *Helicobacter pylori*. Gastroenterology 111:886–900

Moran AP, Upton ME (1986) A comparative study of the rod and coccoid forms of *Campylobacter jejuni* ATCC 29428. J Appl Bacteriol 60:103–110

Moran AP, Upton ME (1987) Factors affecting production of coccoid forms by *Campylobacter jejuni* on solid media during incubation. J Appl Bacteriol 62:527–537

Nagata K, Tsukita S, Tamura T, Sone N (1996) A cb- type cytochrome-c oxidase terminates the respiratory chain in *Helicobacter pylori*. Microbiology 142:1757–1763

Odenbreit S, Till M, Hofreuter D, Haas R (1997) Outer membrane proteins AlpA and AlpB are involved in *H. pylori* binding to epithelial cells. Gut 41 [Suppl 1]:A107

Ottlecz A, Romero JJ, Hazell SL, Graham DY, Lichtenberger LM (1993) Phospholipase activity of *Helicobacter pylori* and its inhibition by bismuth salts. Biochem Biophys Res Commun 38:2071–2080

Pan ZJ, van der Ende A, Su WW, Roorda P, Raudonikiene A, Xiao SD, Dankert J, Tytgat GNJ, Berg DE (1998) High prevalence of vacuolating cytotoxin production and unusual distribution of vacA alleles in *Helicobacter pylori* from China. In: Hunt RH, Tytgat GNJ (eds) *Helicobacter pylori*-Basic mechanisms to clinical cure 1998. Kluwer, Dordrecht (in press)

Peek RM, Thompson SA, Atherton JC, Blaser MJ, Miller GG (1996) Expression of *iceA*, a novel ulcer-associated *Helicobacter pylori* gene, is induced by contact with gastric epithelial cells and is associated with enhanced mucosal IL-8. Gut 39 [Suppl 2]:A71

Pittman MS, Jackson CJ, Kelly DJ, Clayton CL (1997) Novel chemotaxis like genes in *Helicobacter pylori*: characterization of CheY and CheF, a homologue of the myxobacterial FRZE protein. Gut 41 [Suppl 1]:A15

Reynolds DJ, Penn CW (1994) Characteristics of *Helicobacter pylori* growth in a defined medium and determination of its aminoacid requirement. Microbiology 140:2649–2656

Sachs G, Meyer-Rosberg K, Scott DR, Melchers K (1996) Acid, protons and *Helicobacter pylori*. Yale J Biol Med 69:301–316

Schmitz A, Josenhans C, Sauerbaum S (1997) Cloning and characterization of the *flbA* gene, which codes for a membrane protein involved in coordinated expression of flagellar genes. J Bacteriol 179:987–997

Shahamat M, Mai U, Paszko-Kolva C, Kessel M, Colwell RR (1993) Use of autoradiography to assess viability of *Helicobacter pylori* in water. Appl Environm Microbiol 59:1231–1235

Skouloubris S, Labigne A, De Reuse H (1997) The aliphatic amidase: another way to produce ammonia in *H. pylori*. Gut 41 [Suppl 1]:A14

Smith MA, Edwards DI (1997) Oxygen scavenging, NADH oxidase and metronidazole resistance in *Helicobacter pylori*. J Antimicrob Chemother 39:347–353

Sorberg M, Nilsson M, Hanberger H, Nilson LE (1996) Morphologic conversion of *Helicobacter pylori* from bacillary to coccoid form. Eur J Clin Microbiol Dis 15:216–219

Suerbaum S, Josenhans C, Labigne A (1993) Cloning and genetic characterization of the *Helicobacter pylori* and *Helicobacter mustelae flaB* flagellin genes and construction of *H. pylori flaA-* and *flaB-* negative mutants by electroporation-mediated allelic exchange. J Bacteriol 175:3278–3288

Tatusov RL, Mushegian AR, Bork P, Brown NP, Hayes WS, Borodovsky M, Rudd KE, Koonin EV (1996) Metabolism and evolution of *Haemophilus influenzae* deduced from a whole-genome comparison with *Escherichia coli*. Curr Biol 6:279–291

Tomb JF, White O, Kerlavage AR, Clayton RA, Sutton GG, Fleischmann RD, Ketchum KA, Klenk HP, Gill S, Dougherty BA, Nelson K, Quackenbuch J, Zhou L, Kirkness EF, Peterson S, Loftus B, Richardson D, Dodson R, Khalk HG, Glodek A, McKenney K, Fitzgerald LM, Lee M, Adams MD, Hickey EK, Berg DE, Gocayne ID, Fujii C, Bowman C, Watthey L, Wallin E, Hayes WS, Borodovsky M, Karp PD, Smith HO, Fraser CM, Venter JC (1997) The complete genome sequence of the gastric pathogen *Helicobacter pylori*. Nature 388:539–547

Tummuru MKR, Cover TL, Blaser MJ (1993) Cloning and expression of a high-molecular-mass major antigen of *Helicobacter pylori*: evidence of linkage to cytotoxin production. Infect Immun 61: 1799–1809

Tummuru MKR, Sharma SA, Blaser MJ (1995) *Helicobacter pylori picB*, a homolog of the *Bordetella pertussis* toxin secretion protein, is required for induction of IL-8 in gastric epithelial cells. Mol Microbiol 18:867–876

Wang Y, Roos KP, Taylor DE (1993) Transformation of *Helicobacter pylori* by chromosomal metronidazole resistance and by a plasmid with a selectable chloramphenicol resistance marker. J Gen Microbiol 139:2485–2493

Warren JR, Marshall BJ (1983) Unidentified curved bacilli on gastric epithelium in active gastritis. Lancet i:1273–1275

Wayne LG, Brenner DJ, Colwell RR, Grimont PAD, Kaudler O, Krichevsky MI, Moore LH, Moore WEC, Murray RGE, Stacklebrant E, Starr MR, Trüjer HG (1987) Report of the AdHoc Committee on Reconciliation of Approaches to Bacterial Systematics. Int J Syst Bacteriol 37:463–464

Weitkamp HJH, Pérez-Pérez GI, Bode G, Malfertheiner P, Blaser MJ (1993) Identification and characterization of *Helicobacter pylori* phospholipase C activity. Int J Med Microbiol Virol Parasitol Infect Dis 280:11–27

West AP, Millar MR, Tompkins DS (1990) Survival of *Helicobacter pylori* in water and saline. J Clin Pathol 43:609

Williams CL, Preston T, Hossack M, Slater C, Mc Coll K (1996) *Helicobacter pylori* utilizes urea for amino acid synthesis. FEMS Immunol Med Microbiol 13:87–94

Woese CR (1994) There must be a prokaryote somewhere: microbiology's search for itself. Microbiol Rev 58:1–9

Wolle K, Leodolter A, Malfertheiner P, König W (1997) Genomic diversity of urease gene among *Helicobacter pylori* strains isolated from one geographical area. Gut 41 [Suppl 1]:A40

Worku M, Sidebotham RL, Wren BW, Karim QN (1997) Chemotaxis of *H. pylori* in presence of human plasma. Gut 41 [Suppl 1]:A25

Yogev D, Rosengarten R, Watson-McKown, Wise K (1991) Molecular basis of Mycoplasma surface antigenic variation: a novel set of divergent genes undergo spontaneous mutation of periodic coding regions and 5′ regulatory sequences. EMBO J 10:4069–4079

Yoshiyama H, Nakamura H, Mizote T, Nakazawa T (1997) Chemotaxis of *Helicobacter pylori* in a viscous environment is urease dependent. Gut 41 [Suppl 1]:A23

Animal Models of *Helicobacter* Gastritis

K.A. Eaton

1 Introduction

Development of animal models of *Helicobacter* gastritis has been a priority since MARSHALL and WARREN first identified the association between gastritis, peptic ulcer, and infection with *Helicobacter pylori* (MARSHALL and WARREN 1984). In

Department of Veterinary Biosciences, Ohio State University, 1925 Coffey Rd., Columbus, OH 43210, USA the approximately 10 years since the introduction of the first animal model (the germ-free piglet; KRAKOWKA et al. 1987; LAMBERT et al. 1987), a bewildering array of new animal models has been introduced, involving host species as disparate as monkeys and mice, and bacterial species isolated from primates, carnivores, and pigs as well as humans. Investigators have used different methods to induce *Helicobacter*-associated disease in animals, and have examined aspects of *Helicobacter*-associated disease ranging from mechanisms of bacterial colonization and induction of gastritis to carcinogenic potential. The result is a large body of sometimes conflicting information regarding animal models, their uses, and their relevance to the pathogenesis of human disease associated with *H. pylori*.

When evaluating animal models of *H. pylori*, several factors must be acknowledged. First, it must be remembered that human disease associated with *H. pylori* encompasses a wide range of pathological changes from asymptomatic chronic gastritis (MARSHALL and WARREN 1984) to gastric cancer (PARSONNET et al. 1991, 1994). It is likely that both host and bacterial factors contribute to this variability, and thus it is to be expected that marked variability in responsiveness is found in animal models as well. Second, it must be understood that there is currently little standardization in the field of animal models of *H. pylori*. Different laboratories use different host strains or species, different bacterial strains or species, and different methodologies. This variation is expected because the study of animal models is still young, and details of standardization are yet to be established. Still, such variability presents a challenge when animal models are to be compared with each other or to human disease. Third, the histological evaluation of animal models is poorly standardized, confusing, and often misleading. It is the purpose of this review to discuss the currently available models in light of these considerations, and to present a strategy whereby nonpathologists may critically evaluate published data as well as compare findings between models and between laboratories. First, currently available animal models will be described. Second, published findings based on these models will be briefly reviewed. Finally, the histological evaluation of animal models will be reviewed, and suggestions for standardization proposed.

2 The Gastric *Helicobacter* spp.

Since the first report of the culture of *H. pylori* (then *Campylobacter pyloridis*) in 1984 (MARSHALL and WARREN 1984), more than 20 *Helicobacter* spp. have been described (BRONSDON et al. 1991; BURNENS et al. 1993; DEWHIRST et al. 1994; EATON et al. 1993; FOX et al. 1989, 1995, 1996a,b; FRANKLIN et al. 1996; HANNINEN et al. 1996; LEE et al. 1992; MENDES et al. 1996; PASTER et al. 1991; STANLEY et al. 1993; TRIVETTMOORE et al. 1997). *Helicobacter* spp. have been

isolated from all parts of the gastrointestinal tract and liver, culturable and unculturable species have been identified, and numerous schemes have been used to
classify these organisms. It is beyond the scope of this review to describe all of
these organisms and classification schemes. However, to properly evaluate animal
models of gastric *Helicobacter* at least a cursory discussion of the bacterial species
used is essential.

Taxonomically, *Helicobacter* spp. have been most commonly categorized based
on genetic methods, usually rRNA gene sequencing (DEWHIRST et al. 1994; DRAZEK
et al. 1994; ECKLOFF et al. 1994; FRANKLIN et al. 1996; HOOK-NIKANNE et al. 1991;
LEE et al. 1992; SLY et al. 1993). This method has several advantages. It is available
to many laboratories, reproducible, and applicable to both culturable and unculturable species. Classification based on rRNA homology is consistent and closely
parallels both biochemical methods of classification and DNA hybridization, and
thus this method has become the most widely used means of taxonomic classification of *Helicobacter* spp. That said, rRNA gene sequence homology suffers from
the characteristic defect inherent in all classification schemes based on DNA sequence data: the relevance of these classifications to functional, biological characteristics of the organisms in question is not always apparent. Fortunately, in the
case of *Helicobacter* spp., genetic classification does appear to be correlated with
biological differences between the strains most of the time. However, in order to
evaluate the pathological relationships between bacteria and host, phenotypic
characteristics of the bacteria are more likely to be biologically relevant. Thus, for
the purposes of this review, gastric *Helicobacter* spp. are discussed in groups based
on phenotypic characteristics.

Gastric *Helicobacter* spp. fall into roughly two groups based on differences in
morphology, host range, and pattern of colonization within the stomach. The first
group, the *Helicobacter pylori*-like organisms includes *H. pylori* (GOODWIN et al.
1989), *H. acinonyx* (EATON et al. 1993), *H. nemestrinae* (BRONSDON et al. 1991),
and *H. mustelae* (FOX et al. 1989). These organisms are characterized morpho-
logically by small size (approximately 5μm in length), one or two loose spirals,
and most commonly a single unipolar tuft of flagella (Fig. 1A). *H. pylori*-like
bacteria colonize the gastric mucus, surface epithelium and pits, but do not
penetrate far into the gastric glands. This group of *Helicobacter* spp. tends to be
host-specific. With few exceptions (see below), *H. pylori* is only found in the
human host, and *H. acinonyx*, *H. nemestrinae*, and *H. mustelae* have only been
described in their natural hosts (cheetahs, monkeys, ferrets, and mink). Indeed,
experimental colonization of aberrant hosts by this group of *Helicobacter* spp. is
difficult. Under some experimental conditions, some strains of *H. pylori* have been
shown to colonize some animal species (FOX et al. 1995; KARITA et al. 1991;
KRAKOWKA et al. 1987; MARCHETTI et al. 1995; LEE et al. 1997; see below), but
such colonization is bacterial strain-specific, and sometimes requires complex
manipulation and results in low colonization rates. Naturally occurring *H. pylori*
infection in nonhumans is sporadic and usually involves laboratory animal colonies with close contact with human workers and often without the normal
endogenous *Helicobacter* species (HANDT et al. 1994, 1995). Even in nonhuman

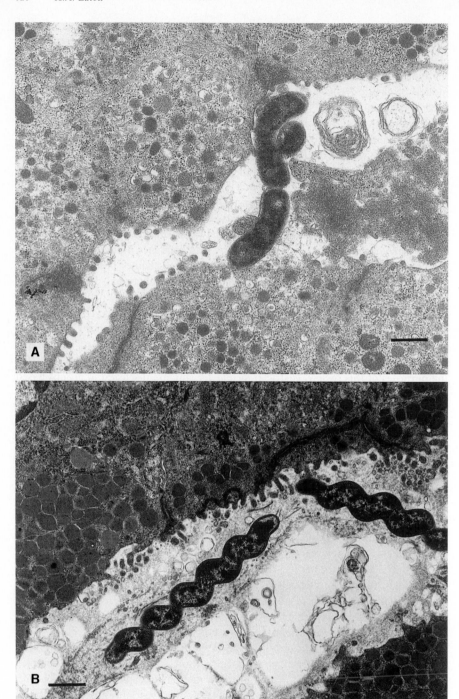

Fig. 1. A Electron micrograph of *H. pylori* in the stomach of a gnotobiotic piglet. Note the small size and gently curved morphology. *Bar*, 0.76μm. **B** Electron micrograph of *Gastrospirillum/H. heilmannii* in the stomach of a mouse. Bacteria are longer than *H. pylori* and more tightly coiled (compare **A**). *Bar*, 1.0μm

primates, *H. pylori* of monkey origin is more infectious for monkeys than *H. pylori* of human origin (EULER et al. 1990).

The second group of *Helicobacter* spp., the *H. felis*-like organisms, are represented by *H.* felis (PASTER et al. 1991), *Gastrospirillum/H. heilmannii* (McNULTY et al. 1989; MENDES et al. 1990; SOLNICK et al. 1993), and *H. bizzozeronii* (HANNINEN et al. 1996). These organisms are longer than *H. pylori* (approximately 10 μm) with more coils, and are sometimes tightly coiled or contain periplasmic fibrils which encircle the organism under the outer membrane (Fig. 1B). They tend to have bipolar tufts of flagella. In contrast to *H. pylori*-like bacteria, *H. felis*-like bacteria are able to colonize deep in the gastric fundic glands and sometimes are found actually within gastric parietal cell canaliculi as well as in the pits and gastric mucus (EATON et al. 1996a). In addition, *H. felis*-like bacteria appear to have a much wider host range than *H. pylori*-like organisms. Experimentally, *H. felis* easily colonizes species as disparate as cats, mice, and ferrets (Fox et al. 1991a; LEE et al. 1990; PASTER et al. 1991), and colonization rates are often high. Nonculturable organisms of the *H. felis* group isolated from baboons, humans, cats, and cheetahs readily colonize mice (DICK et al. 1989; EATON et al. 1993; MOURA et al. 1993). Furthermore, many carnivore and omnivore species support endogenous *Gastrospirillum/H. heilmannii*-like organisms (CURRY et al. 1989; EATON et al. 1993; HENRY et al. 1987; HERMANNS et al. 1995; LEE et al. 1988; MENDES et al. 1990). While these organisms are most often not culturable, and their identity cannot be firmly established, their widespread distribution in nature suggests that they easily colonize many different mammalian species.

A word about the genus and species designations of these organisms is in order. Culturable species, such as *H. pylori* and *H. felis*, can be easily identified and named. However, many of the *H. felis* group of organisms have not been cultured. These organisms were originally called *Gastrospirillum*, *Gastrospirillum hominis* or *Gastrospirillum suis*, and rRNA gene sequences from two of these, *Gastrospirillum* 1 and 2, have been determined and used to definitively classify these organisms as *Helicobacter* spp. (McNULTY et al. 1989; MENDES et al. 1990; SOLNICK et al. 1993). PCR amplification of rRNA sequences from tissue has also been used to propose the name *H. heilmannii* for these unculturable organisms (SOLNICK et al. 1993). However, because many of them remain uncultured, definitive taxonomic classification is not possible. For the purposes of this review, these unculturable organisms of the *H. felis* group will be referred to as *Gastrospirillum/H. heilmannii*.

3 The Animal Models

The following discussion will list the animal models described as of this writing, and will briefly describe them in terms of the host and bacterial species, method of production, bacteriological and histological findings reported, and most frequent use. Details of the individual models and studies using these models to investigate pathogenesis of disease will be described in later sections. The models are divided according to bacterial species used (*H. pylori*-type vs *H. felis*-type). They are summarized in Table 1.

3.1 Animal Models Using *H. pylori*-Type Bacteria

3.1.1 Gnotobiotic Piglets

Germ-free piglets are susceptible to colonization by *H. pylori* of human origin (EATON et al. 1989; KRAKOWKA et al. 1987). Piglets are derived by Caesarian section and housed in germ-free sterile isolators. Between 3 days and 3 weeks of age, piglets are challenged with a single dose of broth-cultured human *H. pylori*. They are susceptible to many different human-derived strains, and to doses as low as 10^2 organisms (unpublished observations). All challenged piglets become infected, and colonization ranges from 10^5 to 10^8cfu/g gastric mucosa depending on bacterial strain and individual piglet (EATON and KRAKOWKA 1992, 1996; EATON et al. 1989, 1996b). Bacterial strains can be piglet-adapted to increase their colonization efficiency (AKOPYANTS et al. 1995). Piglets remain infected for the duration of the study (up to 90 days) and after removal to conventional housing (EATON et al. 1990).

Colonization results in chronic gastritis characterized by lymphocytes, plasma cells, and mucosal and submucosal lymphoid follicles in the glandular gastric mucosa (EATON and KRAKOWKA 1992, 1996; EATON et al. 1989, 1990; KRAKOWKA et al. 1987). Neutrophils (polymorphonuclear leukocytes, PMNs) may be present early in infection or in piglets rendered immune by parenteral vaccination with bacterial antigen prior to challenge (EATON and KRAKOWKA 1992). Gastric ulcers have been reported in infected piglets (KRAKOWKA et al. 1995).

The piglet model has been most useful for studies of putative bacterial colonization factors, such as urease, flagellin, and VacA cytotoxin (see below; EATON 1992, 1994, 1997; EATON et al. 1989, 1991, 1995, 1996b). In addition, piglets have been used for vaccination studies (EATON and KRAKOWKA 1992), and for evaluation of the host immune response (KRAKOWKA et al. 1996). Similar models include germ-free neonatal puppies (RADIN et al. 1990) and barrier-raised, colostrum deprived piglets (ENGSTRAND et al. 1990), both of which are susceptible to *H. pylori* of human origin. The puppy model has been used to demonstrate the occurrence of oral-oral transmission of *Helicobacter* spp. (RADIN et al. 1990).

3.1.2 Nonhuman Primates

Many different species of monkeys have been used to study gastric *Helicobacter* spp., but the macaque species are most commonly used (BASKERVILLE and NEWELL 1988; BRONSDON and SCHOENKNECHT 1988; DRAZEK et al. 1994; DUBOIS et al. 1994,

Table 1. Commonly used animal models of *Helicobacter*-associated gastritis

Host species	Bacterial species	Lesions	Uses	References
Models using *H. pylori*-type bacteria: Germ-free piglet	*H. pylori*, human origin	Lymphoplasmacytic and follicular gastritis Inconsistent neutrophilic inflammation Inconsistent gastric ulceration	Bacterial colonization factors Host immune response Host-bacterial interactions Bacterial interactions in vivo Therapy Vaccination	AKOPYANTS et al. 1995; EATON et al. 1989, 1990, 1991, 1995; EATON 1992, 1994, 1996b, 1997; EATON and KRAKOWKA 1992, 1996; EATON et al. 1990; KRAKOWKA et al. 1987; KRAKOWKA et al. 1996; LAMBERT et al. 1987
Ferret	*H. mustelae*	Lymphocytic and plasmacytic gastritis Inconsistent epithelial necrosis and gastric ulcers Inconsistent gland atrophy	Bacterial colonization factors Host physiological response Epidemiology and transmission Carcinogenesis Therapy Vaccination	ALDER et al. 1996; ANDRUTIS et al. 1995, 1997; CUENCA et al. 1996; CZINN and NEDRUD 1991; Fox et al. 1988, 1990, 1991a,b, 1992, 1993a,b; GOTTFRIED et al. 1990; OTTO et al. 1990; TOMPKINS et al. 1988; YU et al. 1995
Cat	*H. pylori*, feline origin and human origin, *H. acinonyx*	Lymphofollicular gastritis	–	EATON et al. 1993; Fox et al. 1995
Nonhuman primate	*H. pylori*, monkey origin and human origin	Lymphoplasmacytic superficial gastritis Inconsistent neutrophilic inflammation	Epidemiology and transmission Host physiological response Therapy Vaccination	BASKERVILLE and NEWELL 1988; BRONSDON and SCHOENKNECHT 1988; DRAZEK et al. 1994;

Table 1. (Cont.)

Host species	Bacterial species	Lesions	Uses	References
Mouse	*H. pylori*, human origin	Variable dependent on mouse strain Lymphocytic gastritis Variable neutrophilic inflammation Variable follicular gastritis	Bacterial colonization factors Therapy Vaccination	DUBOIS et al. 1991, 1994, 1995, 1996; EULER et al. 1990; HAZELL et al. 1992; SHUTO et al. 1993; STADTLANDER et al. 1996; TAKAHASHI et al. 1993 CANTORNA and BALISH 1990; EHLERS et al. 1988; GHIARA et al. 1995; KARITA et al. 1991, 1993, 1994; LEE et al. 1997; MARCHETTI et al.1995; McCOLM et al. 1995a,b; TELFORD et al. 1994; TSUDA et al. 1994
Models using *H. felis*-type bacteria				
Mouse	*H. felis*, various *Gastrospirillum*/ *H. heilmannii* isolates	Variable, dependent on mouse strain Lymphoplasmacytic and follicular gastritis Variable neutrophilic inflammation, sometimes with gland abscesses Polypoid or diffuse epithelial proliferation and mucus metaplasia Variable gland atrophy	Host immune response Carcinogenesis studies Therapy Vaccination	BLANCHARD et al. 1995a,b; BROMANDER et al. 1996; CHEN et al. 1993; CORTHESYTHEULAZ et al. 1995; CZINN et al. 1993; DANON et al. 1995; DICK et al. 1989; DOIDGE et al. 1994; EATON et al. 1993, 1995; FERRERO et al. 1994, 1995; FOX et al. 1993a, 1996b; LEE and CHEN 1994; LEE et al. 1990, 1995; MICHETTI et al. 1994; MOHAMMADI et al.

Others	Variable host and bacteria species, mostly naturally occurring models	Lymphoid follicles characteristic of all host/bacterial species Lymphocytic and plasmacytic gastritis variable among species and individuals	Role of the host in inflammation	1996a,b, 1997; PAPPO et al. 1995; RADCLIFF et al. 1996a,b; SAKAGAMI et al. 1996; TAKAHASHI et al. 1996; WANG et al. 1996 CURRY et al. 1989; DICK et al. 1989; EATON et al. 1993, 1996; HANNINEN et al. 1996; HENRY et al. 1987; HERMANNS et al. 1995; LEE et al. 1988; MENDES et al. 1990; OTTO et al. 1994

1996; EULER et al. 1990; HAZELL et al. 1992; SHUTO et al. 1993; TAKAHASHI et al. 1993). These animals often carry naturally occurring gastric bacteria of both the *H. pylori*-type (*H. nemestrinae* and *H. pylori*), and the *H. felis* type (*Gastrospirillum/H. heilmannii*). Natural infection is associated with chronic superficial gastritis, most severe in the antrum. Neutrophils and endoscopically identified erosions have been described, but ulcers or histologically identified erosions have not. Experimentally, uninfected rhesus monkeys are susceptible to *H. pylori* of human or monkey origin, although strains from monkeys colonize better than human strains (DUBOIS et al. 1996; EULER et al. 1990). Experimental inoculation with 10^8–10^9cfu of *H. pylori* results in mild-moderate chronic gastritis which resolves after clearance of infection either naturally or as a result of antibiotic therapy.

Nonhuman primates have been used to investigate the epidemiology and transmission of gastric *Helicobacter* spp. (DUBOIS et al. 1995), the role of *Helicobacter* spp. in hypochlorhydria (DUBOIS et al. 1991; TAKAHASHI et al. 1993), the role of bacterial strain in virulence (DUBOIS et al. 1996), and vaccination protocols (STADTLANDER et al. 1996).

3.1.3 Domestic Cats

Normal domestic cats are almost universally colonized with endogenous *H. felis*-type bacteria (see below), and do not harbor gastric bacteria of the *H. pylori* type (DICK et al. 1989; DICK and LEE 1991; ELZAATARI et al. 1997; HERMANNS et al. 1995; LEE et al. 1988). However, some specific pathogen free colonies of laboratory cats have been described which do not harbor *H. felis-like* bacteria (EATON et al. 1993; HANDT et al. 1994, 1995). These cats are susceptible to bacteria of the *H. pylori*-type (*H. acinonyx* and *H. pylori*), either by natural or experimental infection. Inoculation of approximately 10^9cfu of *H. acinonyx* (EATON et al. 1993) or *H. pylori* (Fox et al. 1995) results in persistent colonization with *H. acinonyx* for up to 11 months and with *H. pylori* for up to 7 months. Colonization by either bacterial species results in chronic lymphofollicular gastritis in the gastric antrum characterized primarily by large mucosal lymphoid follicles.

3.1.4 Ferrets

Ferrets and mink are naturally colonized with *H. mustelae*, an *H. pylori*-like organism (Fox et al. 1988, 1990, 1991a; GOTTFRIED et al. 1990; TOMPKINS et al. 1988). In ferrets, naturally occurring infection with *H. mustelae* results in chronic gastritis characterized by primarily lymphocytic and plasmacytic inflammation in the gastric fundus and antrum (Fox et al. 1988, 1990, 1991a; GOTTFRIED et al. 1990). Inflammation is most severe and widespread in the proximal antrum, and epithelial necrosis, gland atrophy and gastric ulcers have been described. Ferrets can be treated with triple therapy (tetracycline or amoxicillin, metronidazole, and bismuth) to clear infection, and inflammatory lesions resolve after successful eradication (Fox et al. 1991a; OTTO et al. 1990). Gastritis due to *H. mustelae* does not appear to be universal in ferrets. Infected colonies of ferrets have been described in which gastritis was not present. Host factors which may contribute to these differences have not been explored (TOMPKINS et al. 1988).

Almost universal colonization of ferret colonies originally hindered evaluation of this model, but *H. mustelae*-free ferrets have been developed, permitting use of this model to examine the pathogenesis of *Helicobacter*-associated disease (Fox et al. 1991a). Antibiotic treatment of dams throughout parturition and nursing has resulted in the development of *H. mustelae*-negative offspring (Fox et al. 1991a) which have been used to investigate the lesions caused by *H. mustelae* as well as the roles of putative bacterial colonization factors (ANDRUTIS et al. 1995, 1997). *H. mustelae*-infected ferrets have been used to investigate the effect of gastric *Helicobacter* on gastric pH (Fox et al. 1991b) and gastric epithelial proliferation (YU et al. 1995), the epidemiology and transmission of gastric *Helicobacter* spp. (Fox et al. 1992, 1993b), and treatment (ALDER et al. 1996; OTTO et al. 1990) and vaccination (CUENCA et al. 1996; CZINN and NEDRUD 1991) protocols. In addition, ferrets have been used to evaluate the role of gastric *Helicobacter* in gastric carcinogenesis associated with cocarcinogenic agents (Fox et al. 1993). Of 10 infected ferrets given a single oral dose of 50–100mg of MNNG, 9 developed gastric carcinoma, compared to 0/5 infected but untreated ferrets. This demonstrates that MNNG is carcinogenic in *H. mustelae*-infected ferrets but the effect of MNNG in uninfected ferrets has not yet been determined.

3.1.5 Mice

Early reports suggested that mice either were not susceptible to colonization by *H. pylori*, or that colonization was sporadic, low, and not associated with gastritis (CANTORNA and BALISH 1990; EHLERS et al. 1988; KARITA et al. 1991; MARCHETTI et al. 1995; McCOLM et al. 1995a). However, recently it has been shown that some strains of human *H. pylori* can be adapted to colonization of mice (LEE et al. 1997). Particularly in C57BL/6 mice, one mouse-adapted strain reaches a high level of colonization (10^7–10^8cfu/g gastric mucosa) and is associated with lymphoplasmacytic and follicular gastritis, sometimes with neutrophils. Colonization and gastritis are mouse-strain dependent (see *H. felis* models, below). Mouse models have been used to evaluate bacterial colonization factors (GHIARA et al. 1995; TELFORD et al. 1994; TSUDA et al. 1994), treatment protocols (KARITA et al. 1993; McCOLM et al. 1995b), and the interaction of *H. pylori* with normal flora (KARITA et al. 1994). Recently mouse *H. pylori* models have also been used in vaccination studies (see "Host Response and Vaccine Development to *Helicobacter pylori* Infection," this volume).

3.1.6 Other Rodents

Although only described in abstract form to date, it is likely that rats are susceptible to mouse-adapted strains of *H. pylori* (BLANCHARD et al. 1996). Mongolian gerbils have been reported to be susceptible to strains of *H. pylori* as well (MATSUMOTO et al. 1997; YOKOTA et al. 1991) (also see note added in proof).

3.2 Animal Models Using *H. felis*-Type Bacteria

3.2.1 Mice

Mice appear to be susceptible to all *H. felis* type bacteria evaluated including *H. felis* and various isolates of *Gastrospirillum/H. heilmannii* (DICK et al. 1989; EATON et al. 1993, 1995; LEE et al. 1990). Challenge with one to three doses of broth cultured bacteria or gastric homogenate containing bacteria results in 100% colonization with large numbers of bacteria and attendant lymphoplasmacytic, follicular, and sometimes neutrophilic gastritis, ranging from minimal to severe, depending on the mouse strain (MOHAMMADI et al. 1996b; SAKAGAMI et al. 1996). Gastritis in mice colonized with *H. felis*-type bacteria is more severe than gastritis due to *H. pylori* (LEE et al. 1997).

Mice colonized with *H. felis* have been most often used for evaluation of vaccination and treatment protocols (BLANCHARD et al. 1995a; CHEN et al. 1993; CORTHESYTHEULAZ et al. 1995; CZINN et al. 1993; DOIDGE et al. 1994; FERRERO et al. 1994, 1995; LEE and CHEN 1994; LEE et al. 1995; MICHETTI et al. 1994; PAPPO et al. 1995; RADCLIFF et al. 1996a; see "Host Response and Vaccine Development to *Helicobacter pylori* Infection this volume). However, the *H. felis*-mouse model also offers potential for pathogenesis studies because of the intense inflammation associated with infection, the availability of mouse strains, mutants, and immunological reagents, and because of the observation that strains of mice differ in their responsiveness to the same strain of *Helicobacter* (see below). To date, mice colonized with *H. felis*-type bacteria have been used to investigate normal immune responses (BLANCHARD et al. 1995b; Fox et al. 1993a; MOHAMMADI et al. 1996a), the role of interleukins in interleukin (IL) 6 and IL4 knockout mice (BROMANDER et al. 1996; RADCLIFF et al. 1996b), the role of T cells in gastritis and protective immunity (MOHAMMADI 1997), the role of p53 in epithelial proliferation (Fox et al. 1996b), and the role of gastric acid in epithelial proliferation and distribution of bacteria in the stomach (DANON et al. 1995).

In addition to gastric inflammation, mice colonized with *H. felis*-like bacteria develop marked gastric epithelial proliferation often with epithelial metaplasia (EATON et al. 1993, 1995; Fox et al. 1996b). This epithelial proliferation has been used to investigate the potential ulcerogenic and carcinogenic effects of gastric *Helicobacter*. It has been shown, for example, that gastric proliferative lesions due to *Gastrospirillum/H. heilmannii* increase susceptibility of mice to ulcerogenesis (EATON et al. 1995), demonstrating that gastric *Helicobacter* can act as a cofactor for epithelial damage. Carcinogenesis studies in mice have been less successful in demonstrating a role for *Helicobacter* in cancer. To date, neoplastic transformation of proliferative lesions has not been described in mice, even when animals are treated with the carcinogenic agents MNU (WANG et al. 1996) or MNNG (TAKAHASHI et al. 1996) (see note added in proof).

3.2.2 Other Models

In nature, cats, dogs, pigs, wild carnivores, and many species of nonhuman primates are almost universally colonized by gastric bacteria of the *H. felis* group (Curry et al. 1989; Dick et al. 1989; Eaton et al. 1993, 1996; Hanninen et al. 1996; Henry et al. 1987; Hermanns et al. 1995; Lee et al. 1988; Mendes et al. 1990; Otto et al. 1994). Because of the high prevalence of naturally occurring colonization, evaluation of the role of these organisms in gastric disease is difficult. Studies implicating *H. felis*-like organisms in gastric disease in both dogs and cats have suffered from the lack of "normal" uninfected controls, hindering definitive interpretation of the significance of the bacteria in disease (Eaton et al. 1996; Hermanns et al. 1995; Otto et al. 1994). Experimental colonization of natural and aberrant hosts has been useful in demonstrating the role of the host in disease due to gastric *Helicobacter* spp, however. For example, gastric *Helicobacter* spp which cause severe disease in naturally infected cheetahs and experimentally infected mice result in minimal disease in experimentally infected cats, indicating that host factors have at least some role in determining disease severity (Eaton et al. 1993). In general, however, experimental manipulation of these models which use outbred hosts, undefined normal flora, and naturally occurring *Helicobacter* infection are unwieldy and difficult to adequately control.

4 What Can We Learn from Animal Models?

Studies of disease due to gastric *Helicobacter* spp. in animal models fall into roughly three categories: bacterial colonization factors, treatment and vaccination studies, and pathogenesis of disease. Of these, animal models have been most intensely used to study bacterial colonization factors and treatment and vaccination protocols. Studies which involve pathogenesis of disease (including host and bacterial factors which contribute to disease) have been limited by variability in host responsiveness to gastric *Helicobacter* spp., mentioned above, and by weaknesses in histological evaluation of models, discussed below. The three types of studies are discussed and their results summarized below.

4.1 Bacterial Colonization Factors

Bacterial factors which contribute to disease can be divided into *colonization factors*, which promote survival of bacteria in the host but do not necessarily contribute directly to disease, and *virulence factors*, which contribute to disease in the host. (For additional details on this subject see "Mechanisms of *Helicobacter pylori* Infection: Bacterial Factors," this volume) It is in the study of bacterial colonization factors that animal models have been most useful. Inoculum dose and extent of resultant colonization (both cfu/g and number of animals colonized) are relatively easily quantified in most animal models, allowing straightforward evaluation of differential colonization by different bacterial strains. Recent successes in genetic engineering of bacteria, leading to bacterial "knockout" mutants with deletional or insertional mutations in putative colonization factors of interest has led to several studies which demonstrate the role of these colonization factors. Studies in piglets, ferrets, and mice have demonstrated unequivocally that bacterial urease is essential for colonization by *H. pylori* (ANDRUTIS et al. 1995; EATON et al. 1991; TSUDA et al. 1994). Studies in piglets and ferrets have shown that expression of both flagellins A and B is also necessary for colonization, but that bacteria that express Fla A, but not Fla B may colonize, although at a lower efficiency than wild-type bacteria (ANDRUTIS et al. 1997; EATON et al. 1996b). Studies in piglets have demonstrated that, in contrast to urease and flagellin, bacterial cytotoxin (VacA) is not needed for bacterial colonization (EATON et al. 1997).

In addition to simple yes/no experiments in which the role of specified colonization factors is determined, animal models have been useful in evaluating the mechanisms by which colonization is promoted by colonization factors. In piglets, it has been shown that while urease is essential for colonization, it may not be solely because urease protects against gastric acid (EATON and KRAKOWKA 1994). Although in vitro urease allows *H. pylori* to survive low pH more effectively (PEREZ et al. 1992), elimination of gastric acid in vivo does not permit colonization by urease-negative *H. pylori*, suggesting that urease must fulfill some other function in colonization. Furthermore, it has been shown that colonization dependance on flagella is not an all-or-none phenomenon. In ferrets, *H. mustelae* Fla A is more important for colonization than is Fla B, suggesting that these flagellins have differing roles in promoting colonization (ANDRUTIS et al. 1995). In addition, it is likely that variation of expression of flagellin may determine virulence of some strains. In germ-free piglets, piglet-passage and adaptation of *H. pylori* is accompanied by continually increased expression of flaA by bacteria, suggesting that flagellin expression may be one mechanism whereby *H. pylori* adapts to its host (MANKOSKI and EATON 1997). Increased understanding of the genetics of *H. pylori*, identification of putative colonization factors, and the published sequence of the *H. pylori* genome (TOMB et al. 1997) will greatly facilitate the study of colonization factors in vivo and eventual understanding of the factors which allow bacterial colonization. Such understanding could promote use of selected factors as therapeutic or vaccine targets. Already, urease is under development as a vaccine target (FERRERO et al. 1994; MICHETTI et al. 1994; PAPPO et al. 1995). Other colonization factors may also prove useful in treating or preventing *H. pylori* colonization in the human host.

4.2 Vaccine and Treatment Studies

Mouse models, primarily models which use *H. felis* have been the most commonly used for treatment and vaccination studies. *H. felis* has a similar antibiotic sensitivity level to *H. pylori*, and mice infected with this organisms have been used as a screening model for drug efficacy studies (DICK and LEE 1991; HOOK-NIKANNE et al. 1996; SMITH et al. 1997). Germ-free piglets infected with *H. pylori*, mice infected with *H. pylori*, and ferrets infected with *H. mustelae* have also been used to screen potential therapies (ALDER et al. 1996; KARITA et al. 1993; OTTO et al. 1990; KRAKOWKA et al. 1998). In piglets, patterns of antibiotic susceptibility are similar to those in humans and incomplete clearance by antibiotic therapy results in recrudescence of the organism occurs as it does in humans. This suggests that simple treat and culture studies may not always be sufficient to demonstrate complete efficacy (KRAKOWKA et al. 1998).

Animal models have proven useful in evaluating vaccine efficacy for both prevention and cure of gastric *Helicobacter* spp. The earliest studies in germ-free piglets infected with *H. pylori* suggested that parenteral vaccination is ineffective against subsequent infection with *H. pylori*, and that such vaccination might even intensify host immune response to bacterial challenge (EATON and KRAKOWKA 1992). More recently it has been shown that oral vaccination of mice can both protect some strains of mice against *H. felis* challenge, and cure established infection (BLANCHARD et al. 1995a; CHEN et al. 1992; CORTHESYTHEULAZ et al. 1995; CZINN et al. 1993; DOIDGE et al. 1994; FERRERO et al. 1994, 1995; LEE and CHEN 1994; LEE et al. 1995; MICHETTI et al. 1994; PAPPO et al. 1995; RADCLIFF et al. 1996a). Either prior to challenge or following challenge with live bacteria, mice are immunized orally with *H. felis* or *H. pylori* antigens mixed with cholera toxin, an oral adjuvant. This model has been used to demonstrate protective efficacy of such bacterial antigens as urease (FERRERO et al. 1994; LEE et al. 1995; MICHETTI et al. 1994; PAPPO et al. 1995) and heat shock protein (FERRERO et al. 1995). Its advantages include ease of use, relatively low cost, the potential for use of large numbers of animals, and its effectiveness in preventing and curing infection. Its disadvantage, however, is that it is not directly applicable to nonrodent mammalian species because of the toxicity of cholera toxin in these species. Attempts to circumvent this difficulty using the less toxic *E. coli* labile toxin or low doses of cholera toxin have so far shown only partial efficacy in oral vaccination of piglets, cats, ferrets, and primates (Eaton, unpublished observations; BATCHELDER et al. 1996; CUENCA et al. 1996; DUBOIS et al. 1996; LEE et al. 1996; STADTLANDER et al. 1996). In all studies, colonization density was diminished in vaccinated animals, but most animals were not protected from challenge or cured of infection. Ongoing studies evaluating different adjuvants, antigens, and vaccine protocols may prove more successful (for additional details, "Host Response and Vaccine Development to *Helicobacter pylori* Infection," this volume).

4.3 Pathogenesis of Disease due to *H. pylori*

Investigations into the mechanisms whereby *H. pylori* causes disease include the carcinogenesis studies in ferrets and mice, described above, and studies which investigate the host and bacterial factors which lead to gastritis and gastric damage. Largely because of studies in animals it has become increasingly clear that differences in disease severity associated with gastric *Helicobacter* spp. are attributable to both host and bacterial factors. The role of the host is demonstrated by the fact that different hosts colonized by the same bacteria develop very different manifestations of disease. In an early study, cats and mice colonized with the same *Helicobacter* spp. from cheetahs demonstrated marked differences in the severity and character of gastritis (EATON et al. 1993). Mice developed severe gastritis with gastric epithelial proliferation and ulcers, similar to the original lesion in cheetahs. In contrast, cats showed only mild, lymphofollicular gastritis. Strains or populations of animals may also differ in response to gastric *Helicobacter* spp. For example, some *H. mustelae*-infected ferret colonies fail to develop gastritis (TOMPKINS et al. 1988). The critical role of the host in determining severity of gastritis due to gastric *Helicobacter* spp. is most clearly demonstrated in mice. Strains of mice vary greatly in their response to the same strain of *H. felis* (MOHAMMADI et al. 1996b; SAKAGAMI et al. 1996). Responder strains, such as C57Bl/6 mice, develop severe gastritis, while nonresponder strains (e.g., BALB/c) develop only mild or moderate gastritis. Comparison between strains of mice infected with the same bacterial strains and immunological manipulation of these mouse models will likely result in important information regarding the host immune factors which contribute to differences in host responses and ultimately in differences between humans infected with *H. pylori*. (For additional details on host responses see chapter by BLANCHARD et al. this volume.) Understanding these differences could allow physicians to predict which infected individuals will respond with severe disease, thus allowing treatment of only those individuals at risk for disease. Such understanding could also lead to therapies designed to ameliorate the host response in those individuals in whom treatment is unsuccessful.

In contrast to the role of the host, the role of bacterial factors has been more difficult to demonstrate in animal models. Epidemiological studies clearly show associations between severe manifestations of disease (such as peptic ulcer, neutrophilic gastritis, and cancer) and bacterial virulence factors such as those expressed in the *cag*-pathogenicity island (PAI; CRABTREE and FARMERY 1995) as well as certain genotypes of vacA (ATHERTON et al. 1995). In vitro cell culture models support the suggestion that cag-PAI proteins are associated with induction of IL8 and thus neutrophils which presumably lead to severe disease in the host (CENSINI et al. 1996; HUANG et al. 1995; TUMMURU et al. 1995). However, animal model studies have been less definitive. In piglets, different strains of *H. pylori* appear to lead to differences in severity of inflammation, but the specific bacterial factors responsible for these differences have not yet been identified (EATON and KRAKOWKA 1996). Similarly, in mice, *H. felis*-type bacteria lead to more severe disease than does *H. pylori*, but the pathogenesis of these differences are not known (LEE et al. 1997; SAKAGAMI et al. 1996). Studies with bacterial mutants in piglets, have shown that vacA does not lead to more severe disease in piglets, but cag-PAI proteins have not yet been examined (EATON et al. 1997). Similar studies in mice designed to determine the role of VacA are hindered by the lack of epithelial changes in *H. pylori*-infected mice (GHIARA et al. 1995; TELFORD et al. 1994). In general, the natural variability in host response to the same bacterial strain to some degree hinders evaluation of bacterial virulence factors in vivo. In pigs (EATON and KRAKOWKA 1992; EATON et al. 1990), mice (EATON et al. 1993, 1995), dogs (EATON et al. 1996), and probably most other species, severity of gastritis in individual hosts varies markedly in response to the same bacterial strain. Thus, evaluation of large numbers of animals is necessary to determine if differences are due to normal host variation or to the bacterial strain used.

Taken together, pathogenesis studies in animals suggest that both host and bacterial factors do contribute to disease severity, but the specific factors involved remain unknown. Animal models are likely to prove useful in elucidating some of these factors. However, standardization and improved interpretation of animals models is essential if pathogenesis studies are to be useful in dissecting the mechanisms of disease due to *H. pylori*. First, the variability of individual host response to gastric *Helicobacter* spp. greatly hinders direct evaluation of bacterial virulence factors in vivo in any host species. Thus development of quantifiable markers of severe disease is necessary. Second, as discussed below, histological interpretation of animal models as currently practiced is fraught with inconsistencies and confusion. Since pathogenesis studies require reliable histological evaluation, such studies must be standardized.

5 Histological Interpretation of Animal Models

Studies of the mechanisms by which gastric *Helicobacter* spp. induce lesions in the host are necessarily dependent on histological evaluation of those lesions. While inflammatory cells and cytokines can be quantified by molecular and immunological methods, the actual effects of bacterial infection on host tissues must be evaluated by microscopic examination of tissue. Most studies of pathogenesis therefore use histological description and interpretation as part of their evaluation of disease. Unfortunately, as currently practiced, histological evaluation of animal models of *H. pylori* suffers from sufficient inconsistencies as to render many studies uninterpretable, or at least not comparable between laboratories. Problems associated with histological evaluation fall into two categories: (a) use of different terminology by different investigators and (b) investigators who are inexperienced or untrained in *Helicobacter* pathology. The following discussion provides examples of these and makes suggestions for improvement.

5.1 Terminology of *Helicobacter*-Induced Lesions in Animals

Lesions associated with gastric *Helicobacter* in animals include gastritis (inflammation of the gastric mucosa), epithelial damage (including epithelial necrosis, erosion, and ulceration), epithelial atrophy, and proliferation (both neoplastic and nonneoplastic) of epithelial and lymphoid tissue. Other lesions have been described, but these are the most common. The following discussion addresses each of these terms, their varying definitions, and suggestions for standardization.

5.2 Gastritis

Gastritis may include a variety of cell types (lymphocytes, plasma cells, neutrophils, macrophages, mast cells, and others), variable numbers of cells, and variable patterns or distributions of cells. Often, shorthand terms such as chronic gastritis (meaning gastritis consisting mostly of lymphocytes and plasma cells), chronic active gastritis (chronic gastritis which includes neutrophils), or lymphofollicular gastritis (chronic gastritis which includes lymphoid follicles) are used. While these terms may be useful in a clinical situation in which the clinician and pathologist both use the same definitions of the words, they are less useful in experimental studies which require precise descriptions. Terms such as "chronic active gastritis," for example, give no information as to the actual types of cells present (lymphocytes, plasma cells, and macrophages, for example), the relative numbers of cells (mononuclear cells vs granulocytes), the pattern of distribution (widespread, multifocal, superficial or deep), or the presence of related changes (gland abscesses, mucosal or submucosal lymphoid follicles). Furthermore, such terms do not indicate the intensity of the inflammatory infiltrate. Similarly, "chronic gastritis" may not distinguish diffuse, superficial lymphoplasmacytic gastritis from gastritis which extends throughout the mucosa (Fig. 2), follicular gastritis, or even from hyperplasia of gastric mucosa-associated lymphoid tissue (Fig. 3). All four lesions illustrated in Figs. 2 and 3 could legitimately be described as "chronic gastritis," but the character of the inflammation and pathogenetic implications vary widely according to the different morphological appearances. Finally, the pattern of infiltration of neutrophils ("chronic active gastritis") may differ resulting in differing pathogenetic implications (Fig. 4).

5.3 Ulceration and Erosion

Epithelial ulceration is defined as a defect in the epithelium which extends through the muscularis mucosae (CRAWFORD 1994). Epithelial erosion is a defect which is less deep. Currently, in the description of animal models of *Helicobacter* gastritis, definitions differ as to what constitutes a true ulcer (breaching of the basement membrane vs the muscularis mucosae, for example), and often definitions are not clearly stated. Sometimes the words "ulcer" or "erosion" are used to refer to the macroscopic (endoscopic) appearance of a lesion, and histological correlates are not described at all, hindering interpretation. Equally important, differences in the morphology of epithelial defects (e.g., acute or chronic, inflamed or not) are rarely described even though they may be pathogenically important. For example, in piglets infected with *H. pylori*, epithelial damage ranges from vacuolation and necrosis of single epithelial cells (EATON et al. 1997) to acute gastric ulcers char-

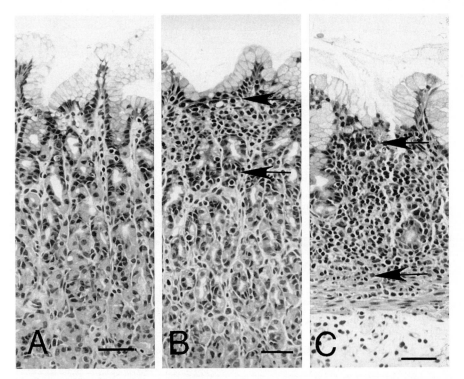

Fig. 2A–C. Hematoxylin and eosin stained sections of gastric mucosa from gnotobiotic piglets. **A** Normal gastric mucosa from an uninfected piglet. Most lamina propria nuclei are those of stromal cells (fibroblasts). **B** Mild superficial gastritis characterized by infiltrates of lymphocytes, plasma cells, and macrophages in the superficial lamina propria (*between arrows*) in a piglet infected with *H. pylori*. **C** Severe transmural gastritis characterized by intense infiltration of lymphocytes, macrophages, and plasma cells throughout the lamina propria (*between arrows*) in a piglet infected with *H. pylori*. *Bars*, 73μm

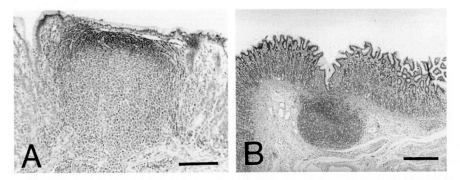

Fig. 3A,B. Hematoxylin and eosin stained sections of gastric mucosa from gnotobiotic piglets infected with *H. pylori*. **A** Well-developed mucosal lymphoid follicle characteristic of follicular gastritis. *Bar*, 105μm. **B** Submucosal lymphoid follicle (mucosa-associated lymphoid tissue), indicative of local immune stimulation and often accompanied by gastritis. *Bar*, 370μm

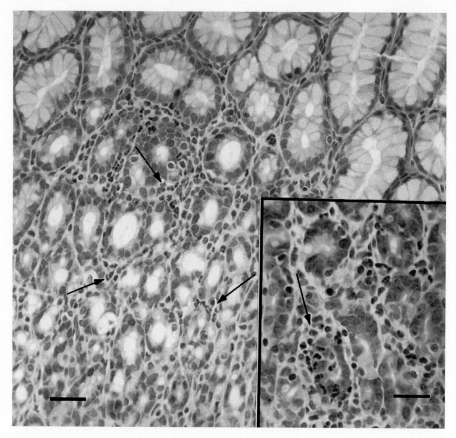

Fig. 4. Hematoxylin and eosin stained sections of gastric mucosa a gnotobiotic piglet infected with *H. pylori*. Gastritis is characterized by scattered neutrophils in the lamina propria (*arrows*). These cells are most likely in transit between the vasculature and the lumen. *Bar*, 48μm. *Inset*, in this piglet neutrophils cluster around individual gastric glands and are associated with destruction of epithelial cells (*arrow*). *Bar*, 28μm. The presence of inflamed glands (*inset*) as opposed to diffuse neutrophilic infiltration may have pathogenetic significance and should be reported

acterized by necrosis of the epithelium which extends to the muscularis mucosae and is accompanied by marked inflammatory cell debris (KRAKOWKA et al. 1995). These lesions are most suggestive of a response to a surface epithelial insult. In contrast, erosions and ulcers associated with *H. heilmannii* infection in BALB/c mice are characterized by acute coagulation necrosis of epithelium with only minimal inflammation, most reminiscent of stress ulcers, likely of vascular pathogenesis (see below; EATON et al. 1995). For proper interpretation, of pathogenetic significance complete description of such lesions is necessary to allow adequate evaluation. In many cases, not only are histological lesions not adequately interpreted, but they are not examined. For example, in some studies, erosions are identified based on macroscopic findings alone, and histopathology is not described, precluding definitive interpretation (TAKAHASHI et al. 1993). Finally, it should be noted that although gastric ulcers and erosions have been described in a number of different animal models, peptic ulcer disease, characterized by chronic persistent ulcers of the duodenal bulb as seen in *H. pylori* infected persons, has not been described in any animal model.

5.4 Atrophy

Atrophic gastritis is an important lesion in human patients with *H. pylori*, and it has been suggested that atrophy represents a precursor to gastric carcinoma (Co-RREA 1992). For that reason, diagnosis of atrophy has become important in animal model development. Atrophy is defined as loss of tissue. Unfortunately, because such loss or absence can be due to a number of causes, many different lesions are identified as atrophy. Figure 5 illustrates epithelial atrophy due to displacement of glands by inflammatory infiltrate. The glands which were present are no longer there, and thus this lesions fits the technical definition of atrophy. However, in this case the loss of tissue is clearly secondary to the massive inflammatory infiltrate. Thus, identification of this lesion as atrophy may be somewhat misleading. Gastritis with displacement of glands would be a better diagnosis.

A second lesion which is sometimes identified as atrophy is illustrated in Fig. 6. In this case, the glands are present, but the gastric parietal and chief cells have

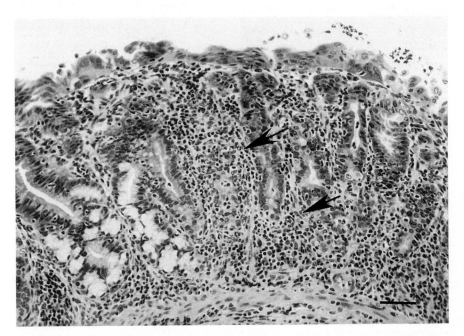

Fig. 5. Hematoxylin and eosin stained section of gastric mucosa from a mouse infected with *Gastrospirillum/H. heilmannii*. Massive inflammatory infiltrate displaces gastric glands (*arrows*). *Bar*, 53μm

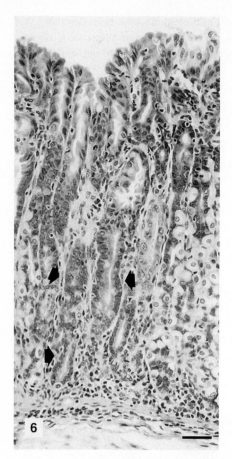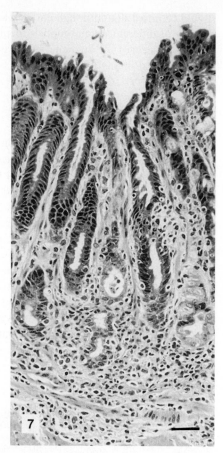

Fig. 6. Hematoxylin and eosin stained section of gastric mucosa from a mouse infected with *Gastrospirillum/H. heilmannii*. Normal fundic glands surround a metaplastic gland (*arrows*) in which parietal and chief cells have been replaced by mucus cells. *Bar*, 30μm

Fig. 7. Hematoxylin and eosin stained section of gastric mucosa from a mouse infected with *Gastrospirillum/H. heilmannii*. Gastric glands are sparse, and separated by connective tissue stroma and a few inflammatory cells. *Bar*, 47μm

disappeared and been replaced with mucus cells. This is a common lesion in mice infected with *H. felis*-type bacteria. The lesion technically meets the definition of atrophy (of parietal cells rather than entire glands, in this case), but because the gland is still present a less misleading description of this lesion is metaplasia, or change, of one gland type (fundic, containing many parietal and chief cells) to another (cardiac, with mostly mucus cells). This type of metaplasia must be distinguished from intestinal metaplasia, a preneoplastic lesions in human stomachs (CORREA 1992).

Finally, Fig. 7 illustrates another form of atrophy. In this case, entire glands are missing and are replaced primarily with fibrous connective tissue stroma. Inflammatory cells are present, but do not obscure the lesion as in Fig. 5. This is likely "true" atrophy, in which damage to glands has lead to their eventually disappearance without replacement by glandular tissue or inflammation (APPELMAN 1994; DIXON et al. 1996). This lesion is occasionally seen in mice infected with *H. felis*-type bacteria, and may be analogous to the atrophic gastritis described in *H. pylori* infected persons.

It is worth noting that the confusion surrounding the definition of atrophy in animal models is also reflected in human medicine. At least one study has shown that concordance between diagnoses of different pathologists is good with respect to gastritis, but poor with respect to atrophy (EL-ZIMAITY et al. 1996). This is likely due to varying definitions of atrophy (APPELMAN 1994; EL-ZIMAITY et al. 1996). Attempts by pathologists to adhere to stringent criteria appear to improve concordance (ANDREW et al. 1994).

5.5 Neoplasia

Because *H. pylori* has been associated with both gastric carcinoma (PARSONNET et al. 1991) and gastric mucosa-associated lymphoid tissue lymphoma (PARSONNET et al. 1994), there is a great deal of interest in gastric cellular proliferation in animal models. Proliferative lesions of both epithelium and lymphoid tissue are most common in mice (EATON et al. 1993, 1995; ENNO et al. 1995; Fox et al. 1996b). In mice of all strains chronic infection with bacteria of the *H. felis* group causes focal polypoid proliferations of gastric mucosa with loss of parietal cells, hyperplasia and disorganization of mucus neck cells, and often accompanied by lymphocytic or follicular inflammation. Lymphoid proliferation, often extending throughout the lamina propria, submucosa, and sometimes extending into the muscularis, is also common in these animals. Unfortunately, definitive diagnosis of neoplasia as opposed to hyperplasia in these lesions is difficult and subjective.

Neoplasia is a functional condition, rather than a morphological one. A neoplastic cell is one that is no longer under growth control. Because this change is functional, it cannot be easily identified by morphological methods. Only functional evaluation (eg, evidence of metastasis, growth in culture, evidence of clonality) can definitively identify a lesion as neoplastic.

The *Helicobacter*-associated proliferative changes described in animals to date have all been either benign, or not clearly malignant based on functional criteria. In the case of epithelial proliferations it may be possible to devise morphological criteria for recognition of neoplastic change once sufficient numbers of animals with tumors have been examined. However, because of the unique characteristics of lymphoid proliferative lesions, it is likely to be difficult if not impossible to distinguish them on the basis of morphology. In order to diagnose lymphoma with certainty, functional criteria will be necessary.

5.6 Standardization of Terminology

As illustrated by the foregoing discussion, standardization of terminology used to described animal models of *Helicobacter* gastritis is necessary to allow comparison between studies. In all cases descriptions of gastritis should include the types of inflammatory cells present, associated lesions, and some at least semiquantitative estimate of their relative prominence and distribution. Lymphoid follicles should be described as mucosal (indicating inflammation), or submucosal (indicating immune stimulation of the mucosa-associated lymphoid tissue). In addition, indications of severity, pattern (diffuse vs follicular) and distribution of inflammation (multifocal vs. widespread) should be included. Cells may be counted or semiquantified, but the quantification scheme should be clearly described. For description of epithelial damage, the terms ulcer and erosion should be defined and used appropriately. In all cases the presence of epithelial defects should be confirmed by histological examination, and the morphological appearance of the defects (depth, chronicity, associated changes such as inflammation or epithelial response) should be described and illustrated. Other lesions should be defined and described fully. Atrophy must be defined, preferably as loss of glands with replacement by fibrosis (DIXON et al. 1996), and criteria for diagnosis of malignancy must be clearly stated. Finally, photomicrographs should be included which illustrate the salient features of the lesions described as closely as possible. The publication of photographs which are inadequate to illustrate the lesions described (MARCHETTI et al. 1995; TELFORD et al. 1994) should be discouraged.

In addition to standardization of terminology, care must be taken to distinguish between artefactual or postmortem autolytic changes in tissue and those changes which represent true *Helicobacter* related pathologies. These two classes of changes can often be distinguished from each other by a careful examination of the surrounding tissue to discern the context of the changes. For example acute necrosis of epithelium may not by itself be distinguishable from postmortem autolysis, but dilation of adjacent glands with flattening of the epithelium and/or presence of inflammatory cells and/or proliferative cellular responses would be consistent with *Helicobacter* associated pathology whereas absence of any adjacent tissue changes would be more consistent with postmortem autolysis.

5.7 Species Differences

A final issue is animal species and strain variations in interpretation of gastric lesions. One example of this is the presence of lymphoepithelial lesions (clusters of neoplastic lymphocytes within gastric epithelia) which may represent low grade B cell mucosa-associated lymphoma tissue lymphomas in humans (ISAACSON 1994) or mice (ENNO et al. 1997) but are much more likely to be of T cell origin in dogs (FRENCH et al. 1996; STEINBERG 1995). Another example involves the diagnosis and interpretation of neutrophilic gastritis in mice. It has been known for some time that mice respond easily with neutrophilic gastric inflamation and that this response can be mouse strain dependent (MARLEY et al. 1994). In BALB/c mice neutrophilic infiltrates in specific pathogen free mice are generally mild and do not interfere with interpretation in *Helicobacter*-infected animals (EATON et al. 1993). However, in C57BL/6 mice high background neutrophilic inflammation of unknown etiology may occur in animals with no known *Helicobacter* infections. While the causes of this inflammation are unknown, housing conditions and the background "normal" bacterial flora may contribute. It is important, however, to recognize that animal species and strain differences do exist when evaluating *Helicobacter* associated gastric lesions in animal models.

6 Conclusions

Several excellent animal models of *H. pylori* gastritis are currently available. Different host and bacterial species offer models with varying characteristics which present opportunities to study different aspects of disease. To date, animal models have been instrumental in promoting our understanding of aspects of *H. pylori*-related disease as disparate as bacterial colonization factors, therapeutic strategies, and host and bacterial interactions. Use of these models continues to hold promise for furthering our understanding of these and other aspects of *Helicobacter*-associated gastric disease. Standardization of methods for evaluating animal models of disease will be increasingly important as we seek to compare models, and to use animal model studies effectively to further our understanding of the pathogenesis of human disease.

Note added in proof. The study of animal models of *H. pylori* has advanced rapidly. Since submission of this review, a number of important developments have been published, including the colonization of rats by *H. pylori* of human origin (LI et al. 1998), the use of interleukin-deficient "knockout" mice for determination of the role of host response in helicobacter-associated gastritis (BERG et al. 1998), and the description of gastric ulceration and cancer in Mongolian gerbils infected with *H. pylori* of human origin (SUGIYAMA et al. 1998; WATANABE et al. 1998). New models should be interpreted in light of the histologic considerations described in this review, particularly with respect to the large variation in interpretation of histologic lesions related to carcinogenesis.

References

Akopyants NS, Eaton KA, Berg DE (1995) Adaptive mutation and co-colonization during *Helicobacter pylori* infection of gnotobiotic piglets. Infect Immun 63:116–121
Alder JD, Ewing PJ, Mitten MJ, Oleksijew A, Tanaka SK (1996) Relevance of the ferret model of *Helicobacter*-induced gastritis to evaluation of antibacterial therapies. Am J Gastroenterol 91:2347–2354

148   K.A. Eaton

Andrew A, Wyatt JI, Dixon MF (1994) Observer variation in the assessment of chronic gastritis ac-
cording to the Sydney system. Histopathology 25:317–322
Andrutis KA, Fox JG, Schauer DB, Marini RP, Li XT, Yan LL, Josenhans C, Suerbaum S (1997)
Infection of the ferret stomach by isogenic flagellar mutant strains of Helicobacter mustelae. Infect
Immun 65:1962–1966
Andrutis KA, Fox JG, Schauer DB, Marini RP, Murphy JC, Yan LL, Solnick JV (1995) Inability of an
isogenic urease-negative mutant strain of Helicobacter mustelae to colonize the ferret stomach. Infect
Immun 63:3722–3725
Appelman HD (1994) Gastritis: terminology, etiology, and clinicopathologic correlations: another biased
view. Hum Pathol 25:1006–1019
Atherton JC, Cao P, Peek RM, Tummuru MKR, Blaser MJ, Cover TL (1995) Mosaicism in vacuolating
cytotoxin alleles of Helicobacter pylori-association of specific vacA types with cytotoxin production
and peptic ulceration. J Biol Chem 270:17771–17777
Baskerville A, Newell DG (1988) Naturally occurring chronic gastritis and C. pylori infection in the
rhesus monkey: a potential model for gastritis in man. Gut 29:465–472
Batchelder M, Fox JG, Monath T, Yan L, Attardo L, Georgakopoulos K, Li X, Marini R, Shen Z,
Pappo J, Lee C (1996) Oral vaccination with recombinant urease reduces gastric Helicobacter pylori
colonization in the cat. Gastroenterology 110:A58
Berg DJ, Lynch NA, Lynch RG, Lauricella DM (1998) Rapid development of severe hyperplastic gas-
tritis with gastric epithelial dedifferentiation in Helicobacter felis-infected IL-10(−/−) mice. American
Journal of Pathology 152:1377–1386
Blanchard TG, Czinn SJ, Maurer R, Thomas WD, Soman G, Nedrud JG (1995a) Urease-specific
monoclonal antibodies prevent Helicobacter felis infection in mice. Infect Immun 63:1394–1399
Blanchard TG, Czinn SJ, Nedrud JG, Redline RW (1995b) Helicobacter-associated gastritis in SCID
mice. Infect Immun 63:1113–1115
Blanchard TG, Nedrud JG, Czinn SJ (1996) Development of a rat model of H. pylori infection and
disease to study the role of H. pylori in gastric cancer incidence. Gut 39 [Suppl 2]:A76
Bromander AK, Ekman L, Kopf M, Nedrud JG, Lycke NY (1996) IL-6-deficient mice exhibit normal
mucosal IgA responses to local immunizations and Helicobacter felis infection. J Immunol 156:4290–
4297
Bronsdon MA, Goodwin CS, Sly LI, Chilvers T, Schoenknecht FD (1991) Helicobacter nemestrinae sp.
nov., a spiral bacterium found in the stomach of a pigtailed macaque (Macaca nemestrina). Int J Syst
Bact 41:148–153
Bronsdon MA, Schoenknecht FD (1988) Campylobacter pylori isolated from the stomach of the monkey,
Macaca nemestrina. J Clin Microbiol 26:1725–1728
Burnens AP, Stanley J, Schaad UB, Nicolet J (1993) Novel Campylobacter-like organism resembling
Helicobacter fennelliae isolated from a boy with gastroenteritis and from dogs. J Clin Microbiol
31:1916–1917
Cantorna MT, Balish E (1990) Inability of human clinical strains of Helicobacter pylori to colonize the
alimentary tract of germfree rodents. Can J Microbiol 36:237–241
Censini S, Lange C, Xiang Z, Crabtree JE, Ghiara P, Borodovsky M, Rappuoli R, Covacci A (1996) cag,
a pathogenicity island of Helicobacter pylori, encodes type-I specific and disease-associated virulence
factors. Proc Natl Acad Sci USA 93:14648–14654
Chen M, Lee A, Hazell S, Hu P, Li Y (1993) Immunisation against gastric infection with Helicobacter
species: first step in the prophylaxis of gastric cancer? Zentrabl Bakteriol 280:155
Correa P (1992) Human gastric carcinogenesis: a multistep and multifactorial process. Cancer Res
52:6735–6740
Corthesytheulaz I, Porta N, Glauser M, Saraga E, Vaney AC, Haas R, Kraehenbuhl JP, Blum AL,
Michetti P (1995) Oral immunization with Helicobacter pylori urease B subunit as a treatment against
Helicobacter infection in mice. Gastroenterology 109:115–121
Crabtree JE, Farmery SM (1995) Helicobacter pylori and gastric mucosal cytokines: evidence that CagA-
positive strains are more virulent. Lab Invest 73:742–745
Crawford JM (1994) The gastrointestinal tract. In: Cotran RS, Kumar V, Robbins SL (eds) Robbins
pathologic basis of disease. Saunders, Philadelphia
Cuenca R, Blanchard TG, Czinn SJ, Nedrud JG, Monath TP, Lee CK, Redline RW (1996) Therapeutic
immunization against Helicobacter mustelae in naturally infected ferrets. Gastroenterology 110: 1770–
1775
Curry A, Jones DM, Skelton-Stroud P (1989) Novel ultrastructural findings in a helical bacterium found
in the baboon (papio anubis) stomach. J Gen Microbiol 135:2223–2231

Czinn SJ, Cai A, Nedrud JG (1993) Protection of germ-free mice from infection by *Helicobacter* felis after active oral or passive IgA immunization. Vaccine 11:637–642

Czinn SJ, Nedrud JG (1991) Oral immunization against *Helicobacter pylori*. Infect Immun 59:2359–2363

Danon SD, O'Rourke JL, Moss ND, Lee A (1995) The importance of local acid production in the distribution of *Helicobacter felis* in the mouse stomach. Gastroenterology 108:1386–1395

Dewhirst FE, Seymour C, Fraser GJ, Paster BJ, Fox JG (1994) Phylogeny of *Helicobacter* isolates from bird and swine feces and description of *Helicobacter pametensis* sp. nov. Int J Syst Bact 44:553–560

Dick E, Lee A, Watson G, O'Rourke J (1989) Use of the mouse for the isolation and investigation of stomach-associated, spiral-helical shaped bacteria from man and other animals. J Med Microbiol 29:55–62

Dick HE, Lee A (1991) Use of a mouse model to examine anti-*Helicobacter pylori* agents. Scand J Gastroenterol 26:909–915

Dixon MF, Genta RM, Yardley JH, Correa P, Batts KP, Dahms BB, Filipe MI, Haggitt RC, Haot J, Hui PK, Lechago J, Lewin K, Offerhaus JA, Price AB, Riddell RH, Sipponen P, Solcia E, Watanabe H (1996) Classification and grading of gastritis – The updated Sydney System. Am J Surg Pathol 20:1161–1181

Doidge C, Crust I, Lee A, Buck F, Hazell S, Manne U (1994) Therapeutic immunisation against *Helicobacter* infection. Lancet 343:914–915

Drazek ES, Dubois A, Holmes RK (1994) Characterization and Presumptive Identification of *Helicobacter pylori* Isolates from Rhesus Monkeys. J Clin Microbiol 32:1799–1804

Dubois A, Berg DE, Incecik ET, Fiala N, Hemanackah LM, Perezperez GI, Blaser MJ (1996) Transient and persistent experimental infection of nonhuman primates with *Helicobacter pylori*: Implications for human disease. Infect Immun 64:2885–2891

Dubois A, Fiala N, Heman AL, Drazek ES, Tarnawski A, Fishbein WN, Perez PG, Blaser MJ (1994) Natural gastric infection with *Helicobacter pylori* in monkeys: a model for spiral bacteria infection in humans. Gastroenterology 106:1405–1417

Dubois A, Fiala N, Weichbrod RH, Ward GS, Nix M, Mehlman PT, Taub DM, Perezperez GI, Blaser MJ (1995) Seroepizootiology of *Helicobacter pylori* gastric infection in nonhuman primates housed in social environments. J Clin Microbiol 33:1492–1495

Dubois A, Lee C, Fiala N, Kleanthougs H, Monath T (1996) Immunization against natural *Helicobacter pylori* infection in rhesus monkeys. Proceedings of the IXth European *Helicobacter pylori* Study Group International Conference, Copenhagen, Denmark

Dubois A, Tarnawski A, Newell DG, Fiala N, Dabros W, Stachura J, Krivan H, Heman AL (1991) Gastric injury and invasion of parietal cells by spiral bacteria in rhesus monkeys. Are gastritis and hyperchlorhydria infectious diseases? Gastroenterology 100:884–891

Eaton KA, Brooks CL, Morgan DR, Krakowka S (1991) Essential role of urease in pathogenesis of gastritis induced by *Helicobacter pylori* in gnotobiotic piglets. Infect Immun 59:2470–2475

Eaton KA, Catrenich CE, Makin KM, Krakowka S (1995) Virulence of coccoid and bacillary forms of *Helicobacter pylori* in gnotobiotic piglets. J Infect Dis 171:459–462

Eaton KA, Cover TL, Tummuru MKR, Blaser M, Krakowka S (1997) The role of vacuolating cytotoxin in gastritis due to *Helicobacter pylori* in gnotobiotic piglets. Infect Immun 65:3462–3464

Eaton KA, Dewhirst FE, Paster BJ, Tzellas N, Coleman BE, Paola J, Sherding R (1996) Prevalence and varieties of Helicobacter species in dogs from random sources and pet dogs: animal and public health implications. J Clin Microbiol 34:3165–3170

Eaton KA, Dewhirst FE, Radin MJ, Fox JG, Paster BJ, Krakowka S, Morgan DR (1993) *Helicobacter acinonyx* sp. nov., isolated from cheetahs with gastritis. Int J Syst Bacteriol 43:99–106

Eaton KA, Krakowka S (1992) Chronic active gastritis due to *Helicobacter pylori* in immunized gnotobiotic piglets. Gastroenterology 103:1580–1586

Eaton KA, Krakowka S (1994) Effect of gastric pH on urease-dependent colonization of gnotobiotic piglets by *Helicobacter pylori*. Infect Immun 62:3604–3607

Eaton KA, Krakowka S (1996) H pylori strain differences and their role in early, transient neutrophilic inflammation in gnotobiotic piglets. Gastroenterology 108:A100

Eaton KA, Morgan DR, Krakowka S (1989) *Campylobacter pylori* virulence factors in gnotobiotic piglets. Infect Immun 57:1119–1125

Eaton KA, Morgan DR, Krakowka S (1990) Persistence of *Helicobacter pylori* in conventionalized piglets. J Infect Dis 161:1299–1301

Eaton KA, Radin MJ, Krakowka S (1993) Animal models of bacterial gastritis: the role of host, bacterial species and duration of infection on severity of gastritis. Zentalbl Bakteriol 280:28–37

Eaton KA, Radin MJ, Krakowka S (1995) An animal model of gastric ulcer due to bacterial gastritis in mice. Vet Pathol 32:489–497

Eaton KA, Radin MJ, Kramer L, Wack R, Sherding R, Krakowka S, Fox JG, Morgan DR (1993) Epizootic gastritis associated with gastric spiral bacilli in cheetahs (*Acinonyx jubatus*). Vet Pathol 30:55–63

Eaton KA, Ringler SS, Krakowka S (1996a) Isolation of pure populations of Helicobacter heilmannii-like bacteria. In: Newell DG, Ketley JM, Feldman RA (eds) Campylobacters, helicobacters, and related organisms. Plenum, New York

Eaton KA, Suerbaum S, Josenhans C, Krakowka S (1996b) Colonization of gnotobiotic piglets by *Helicobacter pylori* deficient in two flagellin genes. Infect Immun 64:2445–2448

Eckloff BW, Podzorski RP, Kline BC, Cockerill F3 (1994) A comparison of 16 S ribosomal DNA sequences from five isolates of *Helicobacter pylori*. Int J Syst Bacteriol 44:320–323

Ehlers S, Warrelmann M, Hahn H (1988) In search of an animal model for experimental *Campylobacter pylori* infection: administration of *Campylobacter pylori* to rodents. Zentralbl Bakteriol 268:341–346

El-Zimaity HMT, Graham DY, Alassi MT, Malaty H, Karttunen TJ, Graham DP, Huberman RM, Genta RM (1996) Interobserver variation in the histopathological assessment of *Helicobacter pylori* gastritis. Hum Pathol 27:35–41

Elzaatari FAK, Woo JS, Badr A, Osato MS, Serna H, Lichtenberger LM, Genta RM, Graham DY (1997) Failure to isolate *Helicobacter pylori* from stray cats indicates that H. pylori in cats may be an anthroponosis – an animal infection with a human pathogen. J Med Microbiol 46:372–376

Engstrand L, Gustavsson S, Jorgensen A, Schwan A, Scheynius A (1990) Inoculation of barrier-born pigs with *Helicobacter pylori*: a useful animal model for gastritis type B. Infect Immun 58:1763–1768

Enno A, O'Rourke JL, Howlett CR, Jack A, Dixon MF, Lee A (1995) MALToma-like lesions in the murine gastric mucosa after long-term infection with *Helicobacter felis*: a mouse model of *Helicobacter pylori*-induced gastric lymphoma. Am J Pathol 147:217–222

Euler AR, Zurenko GE, Moe JB, Ulrich RG, Yagi Y (1990) Evaluation of two monkey species (Macaca mulatta and Macaca fascicularis) as possible models for human *Helicobacter pylori* disease. J Clin Microbiol 28:2285–2290

Ferrero RL, Thiberge J, Huerre M, Labigne A (1994) Recombinant antigens prepared from the urease subunits of helicobacter spp: evidence of protection in a mouse model of gastric infection. Infect Immun 62:4981–4989

Ferrero RL, Thiberge JM, Kansau I, Wuscher N, Huerre M, Labigne A (1995) The GroES homolog of *Helicobacter pylori* confers protective immunity against mucosal infection in mice. Proc Natl Acad Sci USA 92:6499–6503

Fox JG, Batchelder M, Marini R, Yan L, Handt L, Li X, Shames B, Hayward A, Campbell J, Murphy JC (1995) *Helicobacter pylori*-induced gastritis in the domestic cat. Infect Immun 63:2674–2681

Fox JG, Blanco M, Murphy JC, Taylor NS, Lee A, Kabok Z, Pappo J (1993a) Local and systemic immune responses in murine *Helicobacter felis* active chronic gastritis. Infect Immun 61:2309–2315

Fox JG, Blanco MC, Yan L, Shames B, Polidoro D, Dewhirst FE, Paster BJ (1993b) Role of gastric pH in isolation of Helicobacter mustelae from the feces of ferrets. Gastroenterology 104:86–92

Fox JG, Cabot EB, Taylor NS, Laraway R (1988) Gastric colonization by *Campylobacter pylori* subsp. mustelae in ferrets. Infect Immun 56:2994–6

Fox JG, Chilvers T, Goodwin CS, Taylor NS, Edmonds P, Sly LI, Brenner DJ (1989) *Campylobacter mustelae*, a new species resulting from the elevation of *Campylobacter pylori* subsp. mustelae to species status. Int J Syst Bacteriol 39:301–303

Fox JG, Correa P, Taylor NS, Lee A, Otto G, Murphy JC, Rose R (1990) *Helicobacter mustelae*-associated gastritis in ferrets. An animal model of *Helicobacter pylori* gastritis in humans. Gastroenterology 99:352–361

Fox JG, Drolet R, Higgins R, Messier R, Yan L, Coleman BE, Paster BJ, Dewhirst FE (1996a) *Helicobacter canis* isolated from a dog liver with multifocal necrotizing hepatitis. J Clin Microbiol 34:2479–2482

Fox JG, Li XT, Cahill RJ, Andrutis K, Rustgi AK, Odze R, Wang TC (1996b) Hypertrophic gastropathy in *Helicobacter felis* – infected wild-type C57BL/6 mice and p53 hemizygous transgenic mice. Gastroenterology 110:155–166

Fox JG, Otto G, Murphy JC, Taylor NS, Lee A (1991a) Gastric colonization of the ferret with *Helicobacter* species: natural and experimental infections. Rev Inf Dis 13 (supplement 8) S671–S680

Fox JG, Otto G, Taylor NS, Rosenblad W, Murphy JC (1991b) *Helicobacter mustelae*-induced gastritis and elevated gastric pH in the ferret (Mustela putorius furo). Infect Immun 59:1875–1880

Fox JG, Paster BJ, Dewhirst FE, Taylor NS, Yan LL, Macuch PJ, Chmura LM (1992) *Helicobacter mustelae* isolation from feces of ferrets: evidence to support fecal-oral transmission of a gastric Helicobacter. Infect Immun 60:606–611

Fox JG, Wishnok JS, Murphy JC, Tannenbaum SR, Correa P (1993) MNNG-induced gastric carcinoma in ferrets infected with *Helicobacter mustelae*. Carcinogenesis 14:1957–1961

Fox JG, Yan L, Shames B, Campbell J, Murphy JC, Li X (1996) Persistent hepatitis and enterocolitis in germfree mice infected with *Helicobacter hepaticus*. Infect Immun 64:3673–3681

Fox JG, Yan LL, Dewhirst FE, Paster BJ, Shames B, Murphy JC, Hayward A, Belcher JC, Mendes EN (1995) *Helicobacter bilis* sp nov, a novel *Helicobacter* species isolated from bile, livers, and intestines of aged, inbred mice. J Clin Microbiol 33:445–454

Franklin CL, Beckwith CS, Livingston RS, Riley LK, Gibson SV, Beschwilliford CL, Hook RR (1996) Isolation of a novel *Helicobacter* species, *Helicobacter cholecystus* sp nov, from the gallbladders of Syrian hamsters with cholangiofibrosis and centrilobular pancreatitis. J Clin Microbiol 34:2952–2958

French RA, E SS, Valli VEO (1996) Primary epitheliotropic alimentary T-cell lymphoma with hepatic involvement in a dog. Vet Pathol 33:349–352

Ghiara P, Marchetti M, Blaser MJ, Tummuru MKR, Cover TL, Segal ED, Tompkins LS, Rappuoli R (1995) Role of the *Helicobacter pylori* virulence factors vacuolating cytotoxin, CagA, and urease in a mouse model of disease. Infect Immun 63:4154–4160

Goodwin CS, Armstrong JA, Chilvers T, Peters M, Collins MD, Sly L, McConnell S, Harper WES (1989) Transfer of *Campylobacter pylori* and campylobacter mustelae to Helicobacter gen. nov. as *Helicobacter pylori* comb. nov. and *Helicobacter mustelae* comb. nov. respectively. Int J Syst Bacteriol 39:397–405

Gottfried MR, Washington K, Harrell LJ (1990) *Helicobacter pylori*-like microorganisms and chronic active gastritis in ferrets. Am J Gastroenterol 85:813–818

Handt LK, Fox JG, Dewhirst FE, Fraser GJ, Paster BJ, Yan LL, Rozmiarek H, Rufo R, Stalis IH (1994) *Helicobacter pylori* isolated from the domestic cat: public health implications. Infect Immun 62:2367–2374

Handt LK, Fox JG, Stalis IH, Rufo R, Lee G, Linn J, Li XT, Kleanthous H (1995) Characterization of feline *Helicobacter pylori* strains and associated gastritis in a colony of domestic cats. J Clin Microbiol 33:2280–2289

Hanninen ML, Happonen I, Saari S, Jalava K (1996) Culture and characteristics of *Helicobacter bizzozeronii*, a new canine gastric *Helicobacter* sp. Int J Syst Bacteriol 46:160–166

Hazell SL, Eichberg JW, Lee DR, Alpert L, Evans DG, Evans DJ, Graham DY (1992) Selection of the chimpanzee over the baboon as a model for *Helicobacter pylori* infection. Gastroenterology 103:848–854

Henry GA, Long PH, Burns JL, Charbonneau DL (1987) Gastric spirillosis in beagles. Am J Vet Res 48:831–836

Hermanns W, Kregel K, Breuer W, Lechner J (1995) *Helicobacter*-like organisms: Histopathological examination of gastric biopsies from dogs and cats. J Comp Pathol 112:307–318

Hook-Nikanne J, Aho P, Karkkainen P, Kosunen TU, Salaspuro M (1996) The Helicobacter felis mouse model in assessing anti-Helicobacter therapies and gastric mucosal prostaglandin E(2) levels. Scand J Gastroenterol 31:334–338

Hook-Nikanne J, Solin M, Kosunen TU, Kaartinen M (1991) Comparison of partial 16 S rRNA sequences of different *Helicobacter pylori* strains, Helicobacter mustelae, and a Gastric Campylobacter-like Organism (GCLO). Syst App Microbiol 14:270–274

Huang JZ, Otoole PW, Doig P, Trust TJ (1995) Stimulation of interleukin-8 production in epithelial cell lines by *Helicobacter pylori*. Infect Immun 63:1732–1738

Isaacson PG (1994) Gastrointestinal lymphoma. Hum Pathol 25:1020–1029

Karita M, Kouchiyama T, Okita K, Nakazawa T (1991) New small animal model for human gastric *Helicobacter pylori* infection: success in both nude and euthymic mice. Am J Gastroenterol 86:1596–1603

Karita M, Li Q, Cantero D, Okita K (1994) Establishment of a small animal model for human *Helicobacter pylori* infection using germ-free mouse. Am J Gastroenterol 89:208–213

Karita M, Li Q, Okita K (1993) Evaluation of new therapy for eradication of H. pylori infection in nude mouse model. Am J Gastroenterol 88:1366–1372

Krakowka S, Eaton KA, Leonk RD (1998) Antimicrobial therapies for *Helicobacter pylori* infection in gnotobiotic piglets. Antimicrob Agents. Chemother 42:1549–1554

Krakowka S, Eaton KA, Rings DM (1995) Occurrence of gastric ulcers in gnotobiotic piglets colonized by *Helicobacter pylori*. Infect Immun 63:2352–2355

Krakowka S, Morgan DR, Kraft WG, Leunk RD (1987) Establishment of gastric Campylobacter pylori infection in the neonatal gnotobiotic piglet. Infect Immun 55:2789–2796

Krakowka S, Ringler SS, Eaton KA, Green WB, Leunk R (1996) Manifestations of the local gastric immune response in gnotobiotic piglets infected with *Helicobacter pylori*. Vet Immunol Immunopathol 52:159–173

Lambert JR, Borromeo M, Pinkard KJ, Turner H, Chapman CB, Smith ML (1987) Colonization of gnotobiotic piglets with Campylobacter Pyloridis – an animal model? J Infect Dis 155

Lee A, Chen MH (1994) Successful immunization against gastric infection with Helicobacter species: use of a cholera toxin B-subunit-whole-cell vaccine. Infect Immun 62:3594–3597

Lee A, Fox JG, Otto G, Murphy J (1990) A small animal model of human *Helicobacter pylori* active chronic gastritis. Gastroenterology 99:1315–1323

Lee A, Hazell SL, O'Rourke J, Kouprach S (1988) Isolation of a spiral-shaped bacterium from the cat stomach. Infect Immun 56:2843–2850

Lee A, O'Rourke J, Deungria MC, Robertson B, Daskalopoulos G, Dixon MF (1997) A standardized mouse model of *Helicobacter pylori* infection: Introducing the Sydney strain. Gastroenterology 112:1386–1397

Lee A, Phillips MW, O'Rourke JL, Paster BJ, Dewhirst FE, Fraser GJ, Fox JG, Sly LI, Romaniuk PJ, Trust TJ et al (1992) Helicobacter muridarum sp. nov., a microaerophilic helical bacterium with a novel ultrastructure isolated from the intestinal mucosa of rodents. Int J Syst Bacteriol 42:27–36

Lee CK, Soike K, Tibbitts T, Georgakopoulos K, Bakios J, Blanchard J, Hill J, Pappo J, Kleanthous H, Monath TP (1996) Urease immunization protects against reinfection by *Helicobacter pylori* in rhesus monkeys. Proceedings of the IXth European *Helicobacter pylori* Study Group International Conference, Copenhagen, Denmark

Lee CK, Weltzin R, Thomas WD, Kleanthous H, Ermak TH, Soman G, Hill JE, Ackerman SK, Monath TP (1995) Oral immunization with recombinant *Helicobacter pylori* urease induces secretory IgA antibodies and protects mice from challenge with Helicobacter felis. J Infect Dis 172:161–172

Li H, Kalies I, Mellgard B, Helander HF (1998) A rat model of chronic *Helicobacter pylori* infection – Studies of epithelial cell turnover and gastric ulcer healing. Scandinavian Journal of Gastroenterology 33:370–378

Mankoski RE, Eaton KA (1998) FlaA mRNA transcription level correlates with *Helicobacter pylori* colonizing efficiency in gnotobiotic piglets. J Med Microbiol, in press

Marchetti M, Arico B, Burroni D, Figura N, Rappuoli R, Ghiara P (1995) Development of a mouse model of *Helicobacter pylori* infection that mimics human disease. Science 267:1655–1658

Marley SB, Hadley CL, Wakelin D (1994) Effect of genetic variation on induced neutrophilia in mice. Infect Immun 62:4304–4309

Marshall BJ, Warren JR (1984) Unidentified curved bacilli in the stomach of patients with gastritis and peptic ulceration. Lancet 1:1311–1315

Matsumoto S, Washizuka Y, Matsumoto Y, Tawara S, Ikeda F, Yokota Y, Karita M (1997) Induction of ulceration and severe gastritis in Mongolian gerbil by *Helicobacter pylori* infection. J Med Microbiol 46:391–397

McColm AA, Bagshaw J, O'Malley C, McLaren A (1995a) Development of a mouse model of gastric colonisation with *Helicobacter pylori*. Gut 37:A50

McColm AA, Bagshaw J, Wallis J, McLaren A (1995b) Screening of anti-Helicobacter therapies in mice colonised with H. pylori. Gut 37:A92

McNulty CA, Dent JC, Curry A, Uff JS, Ford GA, Gear MW, Wilkinson SP (1989) New spiral bacterium in gastric mucosa. J Clin Pathol 42:585–591

Mendes EN, Queiroz DM, Rocha GA, Moura SB, Leite VH, Fonseca ME (1990) Ultrastructure of a spiral micro-organism from pig gastric mucosa ("Gastrospirillum suis"). J Med Microbiol 33:61–66

Mendes EN, Queiroz DMM, Dewhirst FE, Paster BJ, Moura SB, Fox JG (1996) Helicobacter trogontum sp nov, isolated from the rat intestine. Int J Syst Bacteriol 46:916–921

Michetti P, Corthesytheulaz I, Davin C, Haas R, Vaney AC, Heitz M, Bille J, Kraehenbuhl JP, Saraga E, Blum AL (1994) Immunization of BALB/c mice against Helicobacter felis infection with *Helicobacter pylori* urease. Gastroenterology 107:1002–1011

Mohammadi M, Czinn S, Redline R, Nedrud J (1996a) Helicobacter-specific cell-mediated immune responses display a predominant Th1 phenotype and promote a delayed-type hypersensitivity response in the stomachs of mice. J Immunol 156:4729–4738

Mohammadi M, Redline R, Nedrud J, Czinn S (1996b) Role of the host in pathogenesis of Helicobacter-associated gastritis: H felis infection of inbred and congenic mouse strains. Infect Immun 64:238–245

Mohammadi M, Nedrud J, Redline R, Lycke N, Czinn S (1997) Murine CD4 T cell responses to Helicobacter infection: TH1 cells enhance gastritis and TH2 cells reduce bacterial load. Gastroenterology 113:1848

Moura SB, Queiroz DM, Mendes EN, Nogueira AM, Rocha GA (1993) The inflammatory response of the gastric mucosa of mice experimentally infected with "Gastrospirillum suis." J Med Microbiol 39:64–68

Otto G, Fox JG, Wu PY, Taylor NS (1990) Eradication of Helicobacter mustelae from the ferret stomach: an animal model of Helicobacter (Campylobacter) pylori chemotherapy. Antimicrob Agents Chemother 34:1232–1236

Otto G, Hazell SH, Fox JG, Howlett CR, Murphy JC, O'Rourke JL, Lee A (1994) Animal and public health implications of gastric colonization of cats by Helicobacter-like organisms. J Clin Microbiol 32:1043–1049

Pappo J, Thomas WD, Kabok Z, Taylor NS, Murphy NS, Fox JG (1995) Effect of oral immunization with recombinant urease on murine Helicobacter felis gastritis. Infect Immun 63:1246–1252

Parsonnet J, Hansen S, Rodriguez L, Gelb AB, Warnke RA, Jellum E, Orentreich N, Vogelman JH, Friedman GD (1994) *Helicobacter pylori* infection and gastric lymphoma. N Engl J Med 330: 1267–1271

Parsonnet J, Vandersteen D, Goates J, Sibley RK, Pritikin J, Chang Y (1991) *Helicobacter pylori* infection in intestinal- and diffuse-type gastric adenocarcinomas. J Nat Cancer Inst 83:640–643

Paster BJ, Lee A, Fox JG, Dewhirst FE, Tordoff LA, Fraser GJ, O'Rourke JL, Taylor NS, Ferrero R (1991) Phylogeny of Helicobacter felis sp. nov., *Helicobacter mustelae*, and related bacteria. Int J Syst Bacteriol 41:31–38

Perez PG, Olivares AZ, Cover TL, Blaser MJ (1992) Characteristics of *Helicobacter pylori* variants selected for urease deficiency. Infect Immun 60:3658–3663

Radcliff FJ, Chen MH, Lee A (1996a) Protective immunization against Helicobacter stimulates long term immunity. Vaccine 14:780–784

Radcliff FJ, Ramsay AJ, AL (1996b) Failure of immunisation against Helicobacter infection in IL-4 deficient mice: evidence of a TH2 immune response as the basis for protective immunity. Gastroenterology 108

Radin MJ, Eaton KA, Krakowka S, Morgan DR, Lee A, Otto G, Fox J (1990) *Helicobacter pylori* gastric infection in gnotobiotic beagle dogs. Infect Immun 58:2606–2612

Sakagami T, Dixon M, O'Rourke J, Howlett R, Alderuccio F, Vella J, Shimoyama T, Lee A (1996) Atrophic gastric changes in both Helicobacter felis and *Helicobacter pylori* infected mice are host dependent and separate from antral gastritis. Gut 39:639–648

Shuto R, Fujioka T, Kubota T, Nasu M (1993) Experimental gastritis induced by *Helicobacter pylori* in Japanese monkeys. Infect Immun 61:933–939

Sly LI, Bronsdon MA, Bowman JP, Holmes A, Stackebrandt E (1993) The phylogenetic position of Helicobacter nemestrinae. Int J Syst Bacteriol 43:386–387

Smith JG, Kong L, Abruzzo GK, Gill CJ, Flattery AM, Scott PM, Silver L, Kropp H, Bartizal K (1997) Evaluation of experimental therapeutics in a new mouse model of Helicobacter felis utilizing 16 S rRNA polymerase chain reaction for detection. Scand J Gastroenterol 32:297–302

Solnick JV, O'Rourke J, Lee A, Paster BJ, Dewhirst FE, Tompkins LS (1993) An uncultured gastric spiral organism is a newly identified Helicobacter in humans. J Infect Dis 168:379–385

Stadtlander CTKH, Gangemi JD, Khanolkar SS, Kitsos CM, Farris HE, Fulton LK, Hill JE, Huntington FK, Lee CK, Monath TP (1996) Immunogenicity and safety of recombinant *Helicobacter pylori* urease in a nonhuman primate. Dig Dis Sci 41:1853–1862

Stanley J, Linton D, Burnens AP, Dewhirst FE, Owen RJ, Porter A, On SL, Costas M (1993) Helicobacter canis sp. nov., a new species from dogs: an integrated study of phenotype and genotype. J Gen Microbiol 139:2495–2504

Steinberg H, Dubeilzig RR, Thomson J, Dzata G (1995) Primary gastrointestinal lymphosarcoma with epitheliotropism in three Shar-Pei and one Boxer dog. Vet Pathol 32:423–436

Sugiyama A, Maruta F, Ikeno T, Ishida K, Kawasaki S, Katsuyama T, Shimizu N, Tatematsu M (1998) *Helicobacter pylori* infection enhances N-methyl-N-nitrosourea-induced stomach carcinogenesis in the Mongolian gerbil. Cancer Res 58:2067–2069

Takahashi S, Igarashi H, Ishiyama N, Nakano M, Ozaki M, Ito M, Masubuchi N, Saito S, Aoyagi T, Yamagishi I et al (1993) Serial change of gastric mucosa after challenging with *Helicobacter pylori* in the cynomolgus monkey. Int J Med Microbiol Parasitol Infect Dis 280:51–57

Takahashi S, Itoh T, Yanagawa Y, Shingaki M, Masubuchi N, Ninomiya H, Hoshiya S, Saito S (1996) A
    Helicobacter heilmannii-like organism accelerates mitosis in mouse gastric epithelial cells induced by
    N-methyl-N'-nitro-N-nitrosoguanidine (MNNG) in vivo. Gastroenterology 108:A973
Telford JL, Ghiara P, Dell'Orco M, Comanducci M, Burroni D, Bugnoli M, Tecce MF, Censini S,
    Covacci A, Xiang Z (1994) Gene structure of the *Helicobacter pylori* cytotoxin and evidence of its key
    role in gastric disease. J Exp Med 179:1653–1658
Tompkins DS, Wyatt JI, Rathbone BJ, West AP (1988) The characterization and pathological signifi-
    cance of gastric Campylobacter-like organisms in the ferret: a model for chronic gastritis? Epid Infect
    101:269–278
Tomb JF, White O, Kerlavage AR, Clayton RA, Sutton GG, Fleischmann RD, Ketchum KA, Dlenk
    HP, Gill S, Dougherty BA, Nelson K, Quackenbush J, Zhou L, Kirkness EF, Peterson S, Loftus B,
    Richardson D, Dodson R, Khalak HG, Glodek A, McKenney K, Fitzgerald LM, Lee N, Adams
    MD, Venter JC et al (1997) The complete genome sequence of the gastric pathogen *Helicobacter
    pylori*. Nature 388:539
Trivettmoore NL, Rawlinson WD, Yuen M, Gilbert GL (1997) Helicobacter westmeadii sp. nov, a new
    species isolated from blood cultures of two AIDS patients. J Clin Microbiol 35:1144–1150
Tsuda M, Karita M, Morshed MG, Okita K, Nakazawa T (1994) A urease-negative mutant of
    Helicobacter pylori constructed by allelic exchange mutagenesis lacks the ability to colonize the nude
    mouse stomach. Infect Immun 62:3586–3589
Tummuru MKR, Sharma SA, Blaser MJ (1995) *Helicobacter pylori* picB, a homologue of the Bordetella
    pertussis toxin secretion protein, is required for induction of IL-8 in gastric epithelial cells. Molec
    Microbiol 18:867–876
Wang TC, Andrutis K, Li X, Cahill R, Rustgi AK, Fox JG (1996) Cooperation of *Helicobacter felis*
    infections with nitrosamines and genetic factors in inducing gastric proliferation in mice. Gastroen-
    terology 108:A218
Watanabe T, Tada M, Nagai H, Sasaki S, Nakao M (1998) *Helicobacter pylori* infection induces gastric
    cancer in Mongolian gerbils. Gastroenterology 115:642–648
Yokota K, Kurebayashi Y, Takayama Y, Hayashi S, Isogai H, Isogai E, Imai K, Yabana T, Yachi A,
    Oguma K (1991) Colonization of *Helicobacter pylori* in the gastric mucosa of Mongolian gerbils.
    Microbiol Immunol 35:475–480
Yu J, Russell RM, Salomon RN, Murphy JC, Palley LS, Fox JG (1995) Effect of *Helicobacter mustelae*
    infection on ferret gastric epithelial cell proliferation. Carcinogenesis 16:1927–1931

Mechanisms of *Helicobacter pylori* Infection: Bacterial Factors

D.J. McGee and H.L.T. Mobley

University of Maryland, Department of Microbiology and Immunology, 655 W Baltimore Street, Howard Hall, Baltimore, MD 21201, USA

1 Introduction

The pathogenesis of *Helicobacter pylori* can be described in three steps: (a) gain of entry and colonization of the unique niche of the human gastric mucosa; (b) avoidance, subversion, or exploitation of the nonspecific and specific human immune system; and (c) multiplication, tissue damage, and transmission to a new susceptible host or spread to adjacent tissue (FALKOW 1991, 1997) (Fig. 1). A virulence factor is a gene product involved in one or more of these steps. To properly assess whether a particular gene is involved in virulence, the candidate gene must be cloned, disrupted in *H. pylori* and be shown to have reduced virulence in an appropriate animal model. This is best determined by testing the interaction of *H. pylori* with human gastric epithelial cells or phagocytic cells or by assessment of infection in *H. pylori* animal models. Finally, "molecular Koch's postulates" (FALKOW 1988) can be completed by cloning the wild-type gene into a shuttle plasmid, which should then complement the *H. pylori* chromosomal defect, resulting in recovery of virulence.

The problem with this approach in *H. pylori* is that shuttle plasmids have only recently been constructed (LEE et al. 1997; H. Kleanthous, personal communication) and these reagents are not yet widely available. Another problem is that animal models currently available, including cat, gnotobiotic piglet, nude mice, transgenic mice and other mice (KRAKOWKA et al. 1987, 1995; EATON et al. 1989; MARCHETTI et al. 1995; DRAZEK et al. 1994; FALK et al. 1995; KARITA et al. 1991; TSUDA et al. 1994; Fox et al. 1995), are not conducive to studying large numbers of *H. pylori* virulence factors. Limited by resources and small numbers of animals per experiment, investigators have used tissue culture lines, including Kato III, ST42, AGS, and Int-407, which may not be representative of the in vivo environment of the gastric mucosa. Use of freshly isolated human primary gastric epithelial cells has been achieved (CLYNE and DRUMM 1993; SMOOT et al. 1993), but has been only rarely used to study virulence factors of *H. pylori* (SMOOT et al. 1996; HARRIS et al. 1996). Finally, freshly isolated human neutrophils and monocytes for *H. pylori* studies have been used and should perhaps be more widely used to study large numbers of potential virulence factors.

H. pylori has adapted itself to survive in the normally hostile, extremely acidic environment of the human stomach. Thus it does not have to compete with other bacterial species in this unique environmental niche, and to be successful *H. pylori* needs only to overcome host innate and acquired immune defense mechanisms. For example, the acid-sensitive *H. pylori* must survive the acidic environment of the stomach and not be washed away into the intestines by peristalsis. Upon encountering the gastric mucosa, *H. pylori* apparently swims through the gastric mucus, propelled by its polar flagella, and adheres to gastric epithelial cells. This is achieved via *H. pylori* adhesins interacting with host cell receptors. During the adhesion process, *H. pylori* has a predilection for intercellular junctions of gastric epithelial cells (DICK 1990; NOACH et al. 1994; BODE et al. 1988). Entrance of *H. pylori* into gastric epithelial cells (NOACH et al. 1994; BODE et al. 1988) or into gastric epithelial cell lines (CRABTREE et al. 1994) is rare and does not appear to be a

A

Adherence Factors

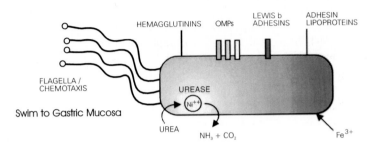

HEMAGGLUTININS   OMPs   LEWIS b ADHESINS   ADHESIN LIPOPROTEINS

FLAGELLA / CHEMOTAXIS

UREASE

Ni^{++}

Swim to Gastric Mucosa

UREA

$NH_3 + CO_2$

Fe^{3+}

Transient Acid Neutralization

Iron Acquisition
Fur
Siderophores
Iron Transporters
Lactoferrin-binding Protein(s)

B

Avoid Peristalsis   Host Mimicry   Phase and Antigenic Variation

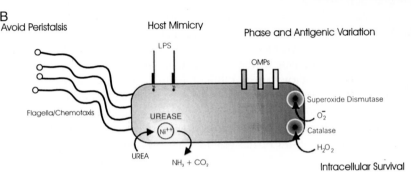

LPS

OMPs

Flagella/Chemotaxis

UREASE

Ni^{++}

Superoxide Dismutase

O_2^-

Catalase

H_2O_2

UREA

$NH_3 + CO_2$

Intracellular Survival

Increase in Gastric pH

Antigenic Shedding

C

Gastric Epithelial Cell Damage   Autoantibodies to Lewis x and Lewis y

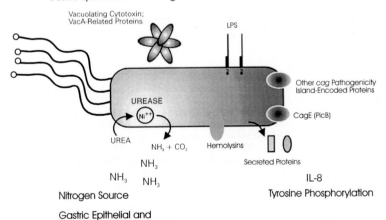

Vacuolating Cytotoxin;
VacA-Related Proteins

LPS

Other cag Pathogenicity Island-Encoded Proteins

UREASE

Ni^{++}

CagE (PicB)

UREA

$NH_3 + CO_2$ Hemolysins

NH_3

Secreted Proteins

NH_3 NH_3

Nitrogen Source

IL-8
Tyrosine Phosphorylation

Gastric Epithelial and
Phagocytic Cell Damage

feature of its pathogenesis. *H. pylori* also induces gastric epithelial cell microvilli damage, weakening of tight junctions, degeneration of the actin cytoskeleton, formation of adherence pedestals, and depletion of mucus granules and mucus in a manner similar to enteropathogenic *Escherichia coli* (SMOOT et al. 1993; BODE et al. 1988; NOACH et al. 1994; SEGAL et al. 1996). Tyrosine phosphorylation of host proteins may occur during intimate attachment (SEGAL et al. 1996, 1997; AIHARA et al. 1997).

During the adhesion of *H. pylori* to gastric epithelial cells, an intense inflammatory response is generated due to unidentified *H. pylori* virulence factors. The cytokine interleukin (IL)-8, a chemotactic factor for human neutrophils, is secreted by gastric epithelial cells. This leads to infiltration of neutrophils and monocytes into the gastric mucosa, causing inflammation and mucosal damage (BODE et al. 1988; GOODWIN et al. 1986; MAI et al. 1991). As *H. pylori* adheres to and is phagocytosed by neutrophils and monocytes, *H. pylori* must survive this onslaught of phagocytic cells and their intracellular reactive oxygen intermediates. It is thought that chronic inflammation leads to further tissue damage that manifests itself as a duodenal or gastric ulcer and predisposes patients to developing gastric adenocarcinoma (BODE et al. 1988; GOODWIN et al. 1986; MAI et al. 1991). This damage may help the organism to be transmitted to a new host via fecal-oral or oral-oral routes.

The recent sequencing of the entire genome of *H. pylori* strain 26695 (TOMB et al. 1997; http://www.tigr.org/tdb/mdb/hpdb/hpdb.html) represents an outstanding new resource that provides researchers with the opportunity of targeting specific putative virulence genes that have strong orthologs (sequence homology not experimentally confirmed) with known virulence factors from other bacteria. We will highlight features of the genome that may be relevant for pathogenesis studies.

2 Urease: Required for Virulence

In the study of bacterial pathogenesis, a successful infection requires that the bacterium colonizes the host, avoids host defense, and damages host tissues (Fig. 1).

Fig. 1A–C. Roles of *H. pylori* virulence factors in various stages of infection and disease. **A** Colonization. Urease and flagella are required for colonization of the gastric mucosa by neutralizing acid and by allowing *H. pylori* to swim to the gastric mucosa, respectively. Adherence factors and proteins involved in iron acquisition may also play a role in colonization. **B** Avoidance of host defense. Urease is required to avoid host defenses by increasing gastric pH and, through antigenic shedding, by binding to secretory immunoglobulins. Flagella are required for avoidance of peristalsis. LPS, outer membrane proteins (*OMPs*), catalase, and superoxide dismutase may also be involved in avoidance of host defenses by host mimicry, phase and antigenic variation, and survival from phagocytic cells. **C** Multiplication and damage to host. Urease and vacuolating cytotoxin cause significant damage to host cells. Urease-generated ammonia also serves as a nitrogen source. LPS may give rise to antibodies that cross-react with host glycoconjugates. Proteins within the *cag* pathogenicity island are necessary for IL-8 induction by gastric epithelial cells and for tyrosine phosphorylation of host proteins. Other bacterial molecules involved in this process could be hemolysins and other secreted proteins. IL-8 recruits phagocytic cells to the site of infection. Cytokines released by the phagocytic cells may lead to additional damage to host tissues

Arguments can be made for urease to be placed in all three categories, and therefore urease may be considered central to the pathogenesis of gastritis and peptic ulcer disease caused by *H. pylori*. *H. pylori* produces copious amounts of urease, which hydrolyzes gastric urea to ammonia (OWEN et al. 1985). Urease is a nickel-containing high molecular weight enzyme composed of UreA and UreB subunits and accounts for 5–10% of the total cellular protein of *H. pylori* (HU and MOBLEY 1990; CLAYTON et al. 1990; LABIGNE et al. 1991; DUNN et al. 1990; EVANS et al. 1991; BAUERFEIND et al. 1997 reviewed by MOBLEY et al. 1995).

2.1 Colonization of the Host

H. pylori is not acidophilic and is sensitive to low pH (BAUERFEIND et al. 1997), unless urea is present (MARSHALL et al. 1988). Upon initial encounter with the stomach, *H. pylori* may be only transiently exposed to an acidic environment. Urease, through hydrolysis of urea to ammonia, serves to protect the bacterium by locally neutralizing the acid in its microenvironment. The ammonia can neutralize gastric acid and provide the bacterium time to safely traverse the mucus layer and colonize the surface of the epithelium. While this mechanism may come into play, it clearly does not represent the whole story on the role of urease as evidenced by a number of animal infection studies.

2.1.1 Urease-Negative Mutants in Animal Models of *Helicobacter* Infection

The role of *H. pylori* urease in colonization has been assessed by testing the virulence of a urease-negative mutant of an *H. pylori* strain, generated by mutagenesis with nitrosoguanidine, in the gnotobiotic piglet model of gastritis (EATON et al. 1991). The mutant, which retained only 0.4% of the urease activity of the parent strain was unable to colonize any of ten orally challenged piglets as assessed at 3 or 21 days after challenge and no pathology was observed in these piglets. In contrast, the parent strain successfully colonized all seven piglets and elicited gastritis. Since complementation techniques are only recently available, it was not possible to determine whether additional defects were present in the nitrosoguanidine-mutated *H. pylori* strain assayed in the piglet. Additional insight, however, was gained in subsequent experiments (EATON and KRAKOWKA 1994) in which an isogenic urease-negative mutant (*ureG*::Km) was used for challenge. Piglets, treated or not with the proton pump inhibitor omeprazole to prevent acid secretion, were challenged with parent and mutant strain. The parent strain colonized normally in numbers ranging from a mean $\log_{10}$ CFU of 4.4–6.9. This urease-negative mutant was unable to colonize the gastric mucosa at normal physiological pH and was recovered only in low numbers (mean $\log_{10}$ CFU < 2) from omeprazole-treated, achlorhydric piglets. The results confirmed that urease enzymatic activity and not simply the inactive apourease protein is essential for colonization. The low capacity to colonize achlorhydric omeprazole-treated piglets suggests that an active urease may also have additional roles necessary for colonization beyond raising gastric pH. Other urease-negative mutants of *H. pylori* also fail to colonize the gastric mucosa of nude mice (Tsuda et al. 1994) and *Cynomolgus* monkeys (Takahashi et al. 1993).

The neutralization of acid appears to be most critical at the time the inoculum is introduced into the gastric mucosa. During the development of acute gastritis, patients can become achlorhydric, demonstrating that acid neutralization does occur. However, after the establishment of chronic gastritis, essentially normal gastric acid output is observed (McColm et al. 1993). Ferrets with established *H. mustelae* infections were administered flurofamide, a powerful urease inhibitor. Urease activity was inhibited, yet under these conditions, colonization persisted, suggesting that high levels of urease activity are not as critical during this phase of infection (McColm et al. 1993). Production of the enzyme, however, still must be essential since isolation of spontaneous urease-negative mutants from fresh gastric biopsies has not been documented in the literature.

2.1.2 Urea as a Nitrogen Source

For survival, it may not be sufficient for the bacterium to use urease simply to neutralize acid. The enzyme also provides a nitrogen source for protein synthesis. The recent description of the gene for glutamine synthetase (*glnA*; Garner et al. 1998) supports the concept that urea-derived ammonium ions can be added to glutamate to make glutamine, which, in turn, can be directly incorporated into protein or converted into other amino acids. This is supported by the finding that urea nitrogen, following incubation with *H. pylori*, ultimately appears in protein (Hazell and Mendz 1993). Therefore, a key role for the urease may be a nutritional one and in the absence of an active enzyme, the organism may starve for nitrogen. Furthermore, it has been suggested that *H. pylori* has a urea cycle (Mendz and Hazell 1996), which may allow very tight control over nitrogen metabolism. An enzyme activity involved in urea production, arginase, has been observed in *H. pylori*. Interestingly, elevated levels of host arginase activity have been observed in gastric cancers (Wu et al. 1996), although at present this is only a correlation.

2.2 Avoidance of Host Defense: Antigenic Shedding of Urease

There is evidence that urease makes its way to the cell surface of *H. pylori* in both stationary phase cultures (Dunn et al. 1990; Evans et al. 1991) and in vivo (Dunn et al. 1997). The enzyme is not covalently attached to the cell as it can be eluted from the surface in vitro under conditions of low ionic strength (Dunn et al. 1990). Since free urease has been localized within gastric tissues by immunohisto-chemical staining (Mai et al. 1992), it is certainly feasible that the protein is shed from the surface in a continuous fashion. This may serve as a means of avoidance of host defense. Secretory immunoglobulin that specifically recognizes and binds to urease could be rendered useless by losing the association of the immune complex with the bacterium as the urease is turned over from the surface. The mechanism of urease shedding is unclear, but may involve autolysis of some portion of the population (PHADNIS et al. 1996; DUNN et al. 1997) or an active transport process (VANET and LABIGNE 1998).

2.3 Damage to Host Tissues

2.3.1 Direct Toxicity to the Host

In addition to the survival benefit of expressing urease, there is evidence that ammonium hydroxide, generated by urea hydrolysis, contributes significantly to histological damage (SMOOT et al. 1990; BARER et al. 1988; XU et al. 1990). It should be emphasized that ammonium ion per se is not toxic but rather damage results from the hydroxide ion generated by the equilibration of ammonia with water. It has also been postulated that ammonia produced by urea hydrolysis has an additional effect: it may interfere with normal hydrogen ion back diffusion across gastric mucosa, resulting in cytotoxicity to the underlying epithelium (HAZELL and LEE 1986).

2.3.2 Damage to the Host Induced by the Immune Response

Urease activity may also be responsible for damage to the gastric epithelium via its interaction with the immune system. *H. pylori* whole cells can stimulate an oxidative burst in human neutrophils (NIELSEN and ANDERSON 1992). The urease enzyme itself can cause activation of monocytes and polymorphonuclear leukocytes and recruitment of inflammatory response cells, resulting in indirect damage to the gastric epithelium. Water extracts of *H. pylori*, known to contain urease in high concentration can activate monocytes by an LPS-independent pathway (MAI et al. 1991). In vitro stimulation of human monocytes led to secretion of inflammatory cytokines and reactive oxygen intermediates, all of which may be involved in mediating the inflammatory response in the gastric epithelium. Further investigation has shown that sonicates of *H. pylori* strains could prime and also cause direct activation of the oxidative burst in human neutrophils and monocytes (NIELSEN and ANDERSON 1992). Both properties were present in two separate molecular weight size ranges, which did not preclude the UreA subunit of urease. In contrast, it was reported that purified urease could not stimulate natural killer cell activity of isolated granular lymphocytes directly, unlike complete cells of *H. pylori* (TARKKANEN et al. 1993). This finding suggests that such damage caused by urease is by its interaction with cells responsible for cellular inflammatory signaling, rather than with the cytotoxic cells themselves.

There is also evidence of urease or urease-containing fractions from *H. pylori* acting as chemotactic factors for leukocyctes, causing further local inflammation (CRAIG et al. 1992; MAI et al. 1992). Such chemotactic activity for human monocytes and neutrophils was present in purified urease samples, and could be inhibited by specific antibody to the UreB urease subunit. Further, a twenty amino acid peptide based on the amino terminus of the UreB subunit protein also exhibited similar levels of chemotaxis in a microchamber test system. Immunocytochemical staining showed urease closely associated with the crypt cells in the lamina propria of patients with duodenal ulcers. It is postulated that urease is absorbed into the mucosa where it attracts leukocytes and causes mucosal inflammation.

Thus, urease, by a variety of mechanisms, may be at least partly responsible for the initial recruitment of monocytes and neutrophils, and further activation and stimulation of the immune system to produce the local inflammatory lesion associated with *H. pylori* infection.

3 Motility: Required for Virulence

Since *H. pylori* is not an acidophile, the organism must move away from the acidic gastric environment to the more pH neutral environment of the gastric epithelium. The organism also needs to move through the viscous gastric mucous layer so that *H. pylori* can encounter the gastric epithelial cell surface. This movement is accomplished through the production of flagella and a chemotactic response, which involves over 40 genes (TOMB et al. 1997). The presence of a chemotactic response suggests an elaborate motility response to environmental conditions in vivo (JACKSON et al. 1995). *H. pylori* cells have four to six unipolar flagella which are surrounded by a membranous sheath (GEIS et al. 1989; SUERBAUM 1995). Flagella are the subcellular structures involved in motility and are composed of flagellin subunits encoded by the *flaA* and *flaB* genes (KOSTRZYNSKA et al. 1991; LEYING et al. 1992; SUERBAUM et al. 1993); as in other motile bacteria, other genes are required for flagellar production (SCHMITZ et al. 1997; O'TOOLE et al. 1994). The *flaA* and *flaB* genes are transcribed by separate sigma factors (28 and 54, respectively) and are regulated under different environmental conditions (JOSENHANS et al. 1995a,b; SCHMITZ et al. 1997).

Motility has been confirmed as a virulence factor for *H. pylori*. Mutants of *H. pylori* that are nonmotile (*flaA⁻* and *flaB⁻*) are unable to colonize and survive in the gnotobiotic piglet (EATON et al. 1989, 1992, 1996), despite still being able to stimulate an IL-8 response (HUANG et al. 1995). It is feasible that any gene disrupted in *H. pylori* that is required for full motility in the wild-type strain, will result in attenuation.

The flagella of *H. pylori* may also serve other functions, such as adhesion, since the membranous sheath surrounding the flagella is composed of LPS and protein (GEIS et al. 1993; LUKE et al. 1995). This, however, has not been directly demonstrated.

4 Adhesins

4.1 Introduction

Since the gastric epithelium and mucus are in continual turnover, and peristalsis ensures constant movement of food and cell debris, *H. pylori* must have evolved mechanisms to keep itself stationed specifically in the gastric mucosal environment. Thus it is postulated that *H. pylori* adhesion factors would represent critical virulence determinants, as has been demonstrated for numerous bacterial species (Leninger et al. 1991; Altmeyer et al. 1993; Pepe and Miller 1993).

H. pylori adheres to human gastric epithelial cells and phagocytic cells via adhesins interacting with host cell receptors. This is an area of very active research. Unfortunately, there is no consensus on which adhesins are most important in vivo, or even whether adhesin(s) and receptor(s) for the *H. pylori*-epithelial cell interactions are similar to the *H. pylori*-phagocytic cell interactions. Several problems with identifying adhesion factors of *H. pylori* are strain adhesion differences, use of nongastric and nonphagocytic cells for experimental studies, presence of more than one adhesion factor in *H. pylori*, autolysis of *H. pylori*, variable expression of adhesion factors in broth versus agar conditions, and possibly variable expression in the coccoid versus bacillary forms of *H. pylori*. With this in mind, we briefly summarize studies on putative adhesins of *H. pylori*.

4.2 Hemagglutination

To investigate the interaction of *H. pylori* with human cells, hemagglutinating activity of *H. pylori* of various species of red blood cells has been extensively studied. Based on studies from numerous laboratories (Evans et al. 1988; Huang et al. 1988; Armstrong et al. 1991; Emödy et al. 1988; Nakazawa et al. 1989; Robinson et al. 1990; Lelwala-Guruge et al. 1992), *H. pylori* exhibits a broad spectrum of hemagglutination. This activity depends on the *H. pylori* strains used, how long they have been passaged in vitro, how the strains are grown, and the species of red blood cells used in the hemagglutination study. Hemagglutinin binding to human red blood cells is mediated by a sialic acid-dependent (either α2,3- or α2,6-specific) interaction for strong hemagglutinating strains and through a sialic acid-independent interaction for weak hemagglutinating strains.

In vivo, *H. pylori* probably does not interact with human red blood cells. Thus, the physiological role(s) of the hemagglutinins needs to be addressed more closely using gastric epithelial cells and human neutrophils and monocytes. Strong hemagglutinating *H. pylori* strains appear to also resist phagocytosis by and have poor adhesion to human neutrophils and monocytes, in contrast with weak hemagglutinating strains (Chmiela et al. 1994, 1995b; Andersen et al. 1993). These results suggest a correlation between possessing sialic acid-dependent lectins and protection from phagocytic killing. However, these studies need to be repeated using freshly isolated patient isolates and mutants bearing isogenic gene disruptions in candidate genes, such as the gene encoding the putative sialic acid lectin, *hpaA*, to address what genes are responsible for adhesion and whether they contribute to the virulence of *H. pylori*.

4.3 Sialic Acid Lectins

So far, the only putative sialic acid lectin discovered in *H. pylori* is HpaA [HP0410]. The gene encoding HpaA, *hpaA*, has been cloned, sequenced and expressed in *E. coli* (EVANS et al. 1993). The purified protein (~29kDa) binds to sialoconjugates mainly in an α2,3-specific manner and can be detected on Western Blots with antiserum directed against HpaA (EVANS et al. 1988, 1993). Antibodies against the putative sialic acid-binding motif, KRTIQK, inhibit *H. pylori* sialic acid-dependent hemagglutination and demonstrate that the protein is surface-exposed, and is functional (EVANS et al. 1993). However, in *E. coli* expressing HpaA, no hemagglutination is observed, suggesting that additional genes are necessary for transport, assembly, or regulation of hemagglutination expression in *H. pylori*. Additionally, HpaA has been shown to be a lipoprotein in *E. coli* expressing *hpaA*, rather than the expected outer membrane location (O'TOOLE et al. 1995). HpaA has also been observed as a component of the flagellar sheath (LUKE et al. 1995; JONES et al. 1997). An isogenic *hpaA* mutant of *H. pylori* still retains sialic acid-dependent hemagglutination activity, and adheres normally to five human gastric carcinoma cell lines and to fixed human gastric tissues (O'TOOLE et al. 1995; JONES et al. 1997), suggesting that other sialic acid lectins exist and that adherence to epithelial cells is multifactorial. Although these latter studies questioned the relevance of HpaA in *H. pylori* virulence, experiments using human neutrophils, monocytes, primary human gastric epithelial cells, and gnotobiotic piglets have not been reported with the *hpaA* mutant. Interestingly, the genome sequence of *H. pylori* has an additional HpaA ortholog (HP0492, 30% identical to HpaA at the amino acid level), which may explain some of the findings obtained with the *hpaA* mutant.

4.4 Lewis b Binding Adhesins

Several reports have indicated that stationary phase *H. pylori* can bind to fucosylated glycoconjugates containing Lewis b structures (FALK et al. 1993; BOREN et al. 1993). Indeed, *H. pylori* was able to bind to the gastric mucosa in transgenic mice expressing the human α1,3/4 fucosyltransferase gene, in contrast with normal mice (FALK et al. 1995). The *H. pylori* adhesin responsible for this interaction is thought to be an outer membrane protein(s) (TOMB et al. 1997; ILVER et al. 1996). Two problems with these studies are that not all *H. pylori* strains bind Lewis b antigens, and Lewis b antigens are widely distributed on epithelial cell types to which *H. pylori* does not interact. Thus, strain heterogeneity may play a role in determining bacterium-host cell interactions. Furthermore, *H. pylori* may not enter stationary phase of growth in vivo.

Another interesting feature is that all *H. pylori* strains examined to date (n = 49) synthesize a neuraminidase and 20% of strains produce fucosidase (DWARAKANATH et al. 1995), which may cleave host cell sialic acid or fucose residues, respectively, from glycoconjugates. This could result in unmasking of other sugar moieties to which putative *H. pylori* adhesins could bind. However, there is no ortholog of either enzyme in the sequenced genome of *H. pylori* strain 26695, suggesting that either presence of these enzymes is artifactual, or that *H. pylori* contains nonhomologous genes.

4.5 Other Adhesins

Other putative adhesins from *H. pylori* include: (a) the 63kDa exoenzyme S-like protein that interacts with host phosphatidylethanolamine in gastric cell membranes (LINGWOOD et al. 1992, 1993); (b) a 25kDa *H. pylori* outer membrane protein, which binds laminin in an $\alpha 2,3$ sialic acid-dependent manner and requires presence of *H. pylori* lipopolysaccharide (MORAN et al. 1995; VALKONEN et al. 1994, 1997). *H. pylori* is also known to interact in vitro with type IV collagen, vitronectin, plasminogen, heparan sulfate, and mucin (CHMIELA et al. 1995a; RINGNÉR et al. 1994; TRUST et al. 1991; DOIG et al. 1992; PIOTROWSKI et al. 1991; TZOUVELEKIS et al. 1991; HIRNO et al. 1995). Thus *H. pylori* appears to be a very sticky bacterium that has evolved numerous adhesins to bind to host cell surfaces. The real challenge is to dissect these adhesive factors and determine which are important in vivo.

5 Iron-Regulated Proteins

Bacteria require iron for incorporation into heme groups in cytochromes. Without the ability to obtain iron from a relatively iron-free environment, most bacteria would die or stop growing. To overcome iron-limitation, bacteria have developed two systems: secreted siderophore production and surface-bound iron-binding proteins such as lactoferrin binding protein (reviewed by CORNELISSEN and SPARLING 1994; NEILANDS et al. 1995). *H. pylori* possess both systems, which contribute to the ability of the organism to assimilate iron that is sequestered by host cell proteins such as lactoferrin.

Lactoferrin-Binding Protein. *H. pylori* are known to be able to use human lactoferrin, but not human transferrin, as its sole iron source (HUSSON et al. 1993; DHAENENS et al. 1997). A 70kDa lactoferrin binding protein (Lbp) has been recently isolated from *H. pylori* grown in iron-restricted conditions (DHAENENS et al. 1997). Human lactoferrin is found at mucosal surfaces and within human neutrophils and would thus be an accessible iron source for *H. pylori*. The genome of strain 26695, however, does not have a strong ortholog of Lbp, indicating that such a gene in *H. pylori* may have diverged from other bacterial Lbps. Interestingly, there are four FrpB orthologs (iron repressible proteins), which have weak homology with Lbps.

Siderophores. All *H. pylori* strains tested have been shown to produce extracellular siderophores (ILLINGWORTH et al. 1993). The *H. pylori* genome supports this contention, with apparently two systems: the Fec-Exb system (> 11 genes) and the Feo system (anaerobic-like ferrous iron assimilation).

Other Genes and Proteins Involved in Iron Acquisition. The genome of *H. pylori* is equipped with a clear ortholog of the ferric uptake regulator, Fur [HP1027]. In other organisms Fur usually represses transcription of genes involved in iron acquisition when iron levels are high (LITWIN and CALDERWOOD 1993). *H. pylori* also has other orthologs of periplasmic iron-binding proteins (*ceuE*; HP1561 and HP1562) which may function in iron transport into the cytoplasm. Additionally, at least two orthologs of ferritins, proteins that store iron, have been found (Pfr [HP0653] and NapA [HP0243]; FRAZIER et al. 1993; DOIG et al. 1993; EVANS et al. 1995a). NapA, however, has not been shown to contain iron (EVANS et al. 1995b), and instead may play a role in the activation of human neutrophils (see below). Given the finding that humans mount an antibody response to a 77kDa heme-containing protein from *H. pylori*, as well as several other iron-repressible outer membrane proteins, it appears that these proteins are expressed in vivo (WORST et al. 1995, 1996). The genes encoding these proteins have not yet been identified. So far, there are no reported mutants of any of the iron acquisition genes described above.

6 Vacuolating Cytotoxin and the *cag* Pathogenicity Island: Roles in Virulence

The vacuolating cytotoxin (VacA; HP0887) is a secreted and cleaved protein that is analogous (not homologous) to the secretion and cleavage of IgA1 proteases from pathogens such as *Neisseria gonorrhoeae* (SCHMITT and HAAS 1994). Culture supernatants from Tox$^+$ *H. pylori* (produce functionally active VacA) induce vacuolation in human primary gastric epithelial cells, in contrast with culture supernatants from an isogenic Tox$^-$ strain (SMOOT et al. 1996; HARRIS et al. 1996). Additionally, Tox$^+$ strains specifically inhibit epithelial cell proliferation, in contrast with Tox$^-$ strains (RICCI et al. 1996). Purified VacA or sonicates from Tox$^+$ strains, but not sonicates from isogenic Tox$^-$ strains, induce gastric epithelial cell damage in the mouse model (GHIARA et al. 1995; MARCHETTI et al. 1995). Taken together, these data indicate that VacA is an important *H. pylori* virulence factor. However, about 50% of all *H. pylori* isolates are Tox$^-$, yet still can cause gastritis (COVER 1996; LEUNK et al. 1988). Additionally, VacA activity varies by at least 30-fold across clinical isolates, perhaps due to the presence of at least five different *vacA* alleles and to the presence or absence of the *cag* pathogenicity island, as determined by epidemiological studies (COVER et al. 1997). Presence of different *vacA* alleles could potentially lead to antigenically variable forms of VacA, but most likely mark strains that have the ability to properly process and secrete an active cytotoxin. Finally, a *vacA* isogenic mutant of strain 26695 can still elicit epithelial cell vacuolation, gastritis, and can colonize the gnotobiotic piglet at levels similar to wild-type *H. pylori* (EATON et al. 1997). Thus, VacA is probably not the only cytotoxin secreted by *H. pylori*.

VacA binds to host gastric epithelial cells and is internalized within an acidic late endosomal vacuole (COVER et al. 1997; PAPINI et al. 1994). VacA, which may inhibit some intracellular vesicle trafficking (COVER et al. 1997), is then translocated to the cytosol where it probably inhibits the Na^+-K^+ ATPase of gastric epithelial cells (RICCI et al. 1993). The mechanisms behind this entire process of VacA movement are unknown.

The "cytotoxin-associated gene," *cagA*, was originally thought to be necessary for VacA vacuolating activity or expression, due to the strong correlation in clinical isolates: *cagA*$^+$ strains were Tox$^+$ (type I) and *cagA*$^-$ strains were Tox$^-$ (type II) (COVACCI et al. 1993; TUMMURU et al. 1993; XIANG 1995). However, using an isogenic *cagA* mutant, it has been shown that *cagA* is not required for expression or vacuolating activity of VacA (XIANG et al. 1995; TUMMURU et al. 1994). Both type I and type II strains contain *vacA* sequences.

Further analysis of type I versus type II strains of *H. pylori* revealed the presence of a 40kb DNA fragment in type I strains that is absent in type II strains (CENSINI et al. 1996). This fragment contains more than 25 genes and is called the *cag* pathogenicity island. 88%–100% of all isolates from patients with duodenal ulcers are *cag*$^+$, whereas only 50%–60% of isolates from patients with uncomplicated gastritis are *cag*$^+$ (COVER et al. 1990; CRABTREE et al. 1991; COVACCI et al. 1993). These findings indicate that type I (*cag*$^+$) strains are more virulent than type II (*cag*$^-$) strains, yet the presence of the *cag* pathogenicity island alone is not sufficient to confer full virulence.

The role of the *cag* pathogenicity island in *H. pylori* virulence has recently been explored (Table 1). Type I strains, but not type II strains, induce IL-8 expression and tyrosine phosphorylation of a 145-kDa protein from gastric epithelial cells (SEGAL et al. 1997; CENSINI et al. 1996). IL-8 is a well-known chemotactic factor for human neutrophils. Isogenic mutants of numerous genes within the *cag* pathogenicity island abolish IL-8 induction and tyrosine phosphorylation (*cagC*, *cagD*, *cagE* [also known as *picB*], *cagG*, *cagH*, *cagI*, *cagL*, *cagM*; TUMMURU et al. 1995; CENSINI et al. 1996; SEGAL et al. 1997). Polar effects of one mutant on adjacent genes was not ruled out in these studies. Three mutants have no effect on IL-8 induction: *cagA*, *cagF*, and *cagN* (CRABTREE et al. 1995; SHARMA et al. 1995; CENSINI et al. 1996; Table 1). Thus *cagA* per se may not be a virulence determinant, but rather a marker for the presence or absence of the *cag* pathogenicity island. Recently it has been suggested that *cagA* may be important for the expression of Lewis y-containing LPS in *H. pylori* (WIRTH et al. 1996). Finally, isogenic mutants in urease or *vacA* still retain IL-8 induction (SHARMA et al. 1995; HUANG et al. 1995). Thus, the IL-8 inducer from *H. pylori* is still unknown. However, contact of live, intact *H. pylori* with gastric epithelial cells appears to be a prerequisite for IL-8 induction (AIHARA et al. 1997; RIEDER et al. 1997).

Some of the *cag* genes are orthologous to genes that encode components of a secretion apparatus (e.g., *cagE* is orthologous to the membrane associated ATPase *virB4*, a protein involved in T-DNA transfer from *Agrobacterium tumefaciens* to plant cells). It is thus tempting to speculate that the *cag* pathogenicity island is involved in secretion of macromolecules that are encoded elsewhere in the genome and that these unknown macromolecules induce IL-8 expression. Some possible candidates are the *vacA*-related genes (HP0289, HP0610, and HP0922), discovered

Table 1. Genotypes and phenotypes of *H. pylori* strains and correlation with virulence (from Censini et al. 1996; Segal et al. 1997; Cover et al. 1997; A. Covacci, personal communication)

	Type I strains	Type II strains	*cagA*, *cagF*, or *cagN* mutant	*cagC*, -*D*, -*E*, -*G*, -*H*, -*I*, -*L*, or *cagM* mutant	Hemolysin mutant
Virulence	Duodenitis, duodenal ulcers, gastric cancer	Uncomplicated gastritis	?	?	?
Adhesion to GECs	+	+	+	+	?
IL-8 Induction in GECs	+	–	+	–	+
Tyrosine phosphorylation of GEC 145kDa	+	–	+	–	–
cag PAI present	+	–	+	+	+
Vacuolating cytotoxin activity	+	–	+	+	?
Urease activity	+	+	?	?	?

Type II strains of *H. pylori* lack the *cag* pathogenicity island. In contrast, type I strains have the *cag* pathogenicity island, which confers the ability of these strains to induce IL-8 secretion from gastric epithelial cells, contain vacuolating cytoxin activity, and to tyrosine phosphorylate host proteins. Presence of the *cag* pathogenicity island may therefore contribute to the greater virulence observed with type I strains. GECs, gastric epithelial cells; PAI, pathogenicity island.

from the complete genome sequence of *H. pylori* (Tomb et al. 1997), and hemolysins. It is clear that VacA itself is not secreted through the putative apparatus in the *cag* pathogenicity island, nor does VacA induce IL-8 expression (Huang et al. 1995; Sharma et al. 1995). Interestingly, a hemolysin mutant of *H. pylori* (specific gene not specified) cannot induce tyrosine phosphorylation of the 145kDa host protein, but still can induce IL-8 expression from a human gastric epithelial cell line, indicating that tyrosine phosphorylation and IL-8 induction are probably the result of separate signal transduction pathways (Segal et al. 1997). Part of this pathway may be activation of NK-kB, NF-B, and AP-1, which are known transcriptional activators of the IL-8 gene (Aihara et al. 1997; Sharma et al. 1998).

7 Catalase and Superoxide Dismutase: Evasion of the Human Immune Response?

H. pylori is well-known to induce an intense acute and chronic inflammatory response in the gastric mucosa. The inflammatory infiltrate is comprised largely of phagocytic cells, especially monocytes and neutrophils. Phagocytes are a nonspecific defense mechanism of the immune system. Upon phagocytosis of foreign material, an oxidative burst occurs, resulting in production of reactive oxygen metabolites, such as singlet oxygen, hydrogen peroxide (H_2O_2), superoxide anions (O_2^-), and the hydroxyl radical ($\cdot OH$). These oxygen metabolites are nonspecifically toxic to micro-organisms. However, most micro-organisms synthesize enzymes to detoxify these metabolites, namely catalase ($2\ H_2O_2 \rightarrow H_2O + O_2$) and superoxide dismutase ($O_2^- \rightarrow H_2O_2 + O_2$). These bacterial enzymes aid in intracellular survival of human pathogens within neutrophils (FRANZON et al. 1990; KANAFANI and MARTIN 1985; KHELEF et al. 1996; ZHENG et al. 1992). It has been shown that *H. pylori* contains both superoxide dismutase (SodB; HP0389) and catalase (KatA; HP0875) activities (ODENBREIT et al. 1996; PESCI and PICKETT 1994; BROIDE et al. 1996; SPIEGELHALDER et al. 1993). *katA*-deficient mutants have been reported (ODENBREIT et al. 1996; WESTBLOM et al. 1992; MARXER et al. 1995). However, a catalase-deficient mutant of *H. pylori* does not show any difference in phagocytic killing by human neutrophils, compared with the parental strain (MARXER et al. 1995). Catalase has also been shown not to play a role in the virulence of *Listeria monocytogenes* in mice (LEBLOND-FRANCILLARD et al. 1989). Finally, construction of a *sodB*-deficient mutant has not been reported. Thus, whether superoxide dismutase or catalase are *H. pylori* virulence determinants requires further study.

Reactive oxygen metabolites are also known to induce injury to the gastric mucosa, thereby potentially predisposing the tissue to ulcer formation (HAHN et al. 1997; KLINOWSKI et al. 1996; DAVIES et al. 1992). The antrum has been shown to possess more superoxide dismutase activity in *H. pylori*-infected specimens than that from uninfected biopsies (BROIDE et al. 1996) and this activity is markedly depleted at the ulcer edge (KLINOWSKI et al. 1996). However, enzyme activity derived from the host versus the bacteria in the gastric mucosa was not distinguished in these studies.

In addition to catalase and superoxide dismutase, there are several other predicted detoxification proteins in the *H. pylori* genome: catalaselike protein (HP0485); alkyl hydroperoxide reductase (HP1563), chlorohydrolase (HP0267), and thiophene and furan oxidizer GTPase (HP1452).

8 Lipopolysaccharide: Molecular Mimicry and Immune Response

The lipopolysaccharide (LPS) from *H. pylori* is known to have 1000-fold less ability to stimulate IL-8 production than LPS from *E. coli* (KIRKLAND et al. 1997). The reason for this relatively nonreactive LPS is not clear. Recently, it has been shown that the LPS of about 85% of all *H. pylori* strains is composed of Lewis x and/or Lewis y antigens (WIRTH et al. 1996; APPELMELK et al. 1996; SHERBURNE and TAYLOR 1995). These antigens are widespread on human cell surfaces and have been found on gastric mucosal epithelial cells and gastric mucin. These LPS structures stimulate a strong anti-Lewis x or anti-Lewis y response in humans (SHERBURNE and TAYLOR 1995; APPELMELK 1996). However, if patient sera are preadsorbed with *H. pylori* cells, cross-reactivity with the gastric mucosa is abolished. Thus molecular mimicry between the Lewis antigens and *H. pylori* LPS could lead to cross-reactive auto-antibodies which could contribute to gastric mucosal damage, thus implicating LPS as a potential virulence factor.

The *H. pylori* genome has numerous LPS biosynthetic genes, as expected. Perhaps the most interesting are the two orthologs of fucosyltransferases (HP0379 and HP0651), which transfer fucose residues to the growing LPS chain. This results in fucose-containing Lewis x or Lewis y LPS structures. One of these fucosyl-transferases, HP0651, was recently confirmed to be responsible for the biosynthesis of fucose-containing Lewis x LPS (GE et al. 1997; MARTIN et al. 1997). This enzyme was also shown to have a structure unique to this enzyme class (GE et al. 1997). The other putative fucosyltransferase gene, HP0379, has a polymeric cytidine within its coding region that could give rise to phase variation via DNA slipped-strand mispairing.

9 Other Potential Virulence Factors

Neutrophil activating protein (NapA) is a recently described protein from *H. pylori* that causes enhanced adhesion of *H. pylori* to human neutrophils and salivary mucin (EVANS et al. 1995b; NAMAVAR et al. 1998). The purified NapA protein was recently shown to interact with acidic glycosphingolipids and most specifically to α2,3-sialyllactosamine on human neutrophils (TENEBERG et al. 1997). However, the sequence of *napA* is most closely orthologous to bacterioferritins (EVANS et al. 1995a). Disruption of *napA* in *H. pylori* has not been reported; thus the role of *napA* in virulence remains to be determined.

A series of hemolysin genes have been cloned from *H. pylori* (DRAZEK et al. 1995). This was based on the ability of cloned genes in *E. coli* to lyse various species of red blood cells. For *H. pylori* hemolysins could theoretically lyse cytoplasmic or vacuolar membranes of phagocytic cells it encounters or damage epithelial cell membranes. There are at least two putative hemolysins in the *H. pylori* genome: HP1086 and HP1490. Whether one or both of these is identical to those described in the above report is unclear.

10 Use of the *H. pylori* Genome to Identify Novel Virulence Factors

The genome sequence availability of *H. pylori* (TOMB et al. 1997) now provides researchers a powerful tool to investigate new potential virulence factors. Indeed, some potentially interesting genes were already highlighted above. In addition, there are several interesting groups of genes and putative proteins that should probably be investigated, including (i) outer membrane proteins; (ii) virulence gene orthologs; and (iii) multidrug resistance gene orthologs. Each of these opportunities is described briefly.

Outer Membrane Proteins. The genome of *H. pylori* strain 26695 (TOMB et al. 1997) exhibits some interesting features that could represent adhesins. There are 20 predicted lipoproteins, one of which, HpaA, was described above. There is also a large family of related proteins (32 members) that are predicted to represent outer membrane proteins (OMPs). Two of these OMPs are believed to be adhesins that interact with Lewis b antigens (TOMB et al. 1997; ILVER et al. 1996). Given this large repertoire of sequence-related genes, it is conceivable that *H. pylori* can recombine different OMP genes to make new, antigenically naive chimeras, thereby avoiding the human immune response. Amazingly, nine OMPs may be phase variable through the presence of polymeric tracts (PolyCT, PolyA, or PolyT). In this scenario, having the correct multiple of repeats of a polymeric tract would place the gene in the ON position. Altering the number of repeats in these tracts is achieved by DNA slipped-strand mispairing, a mechanism known to occur for other bacterial virulence genes, such as the *opa* genes and certain lipooligosaccharide biosynthetic genes in the pathogenic *Neisseria* (BHAT et al. 1992; DANAHER et al. 1995; GOTSCHLICH 1994). Some of these OMPs have been previously characterized (HopA, HopB, HopC, HopD, and HopE) and have been shown to be porins (EXNER et al. 1995; DOIG et al. 1995). Their role as adhesins has not been addressed. Recently, two other OMPs, AlpA (omp20, HP0912) and AlpB (omp21, HP0913), have been described and appear to be proteins needed for adhesion to gastric epithelial cells (ODENBREIT et al. 1997; HAAS et al. 1997). Because there are so many potential OMPs in *H. pylori*, it may be difficult to assess the relative importance of any single OMP, as disruption of 32 related genes is probably not a feasible approach. Instead, single OMPs would have to be tested for adhesive properties in an *E. coli* (or similar) background. Another potential problem is that these OMPs are of similar molecular weights.

Virulence Gene Orthologs. The *H. pylori* genome has the following orthologs of known virulence genes from other bacteria: *virB11* (HP0525, HP1421), *virB4* (HP0017, HP0441, HP0459, HP0544), *virB10* (HP0527), *invA* (HP1228), *vapD* (HP0315 and HP0967), *vacB* (HP1248), *mviN* (HP0885). Thus, there is a good chance that one or more of these predicted proteins is involved in the pathogenesis of *H. pylori*. *invA* is a gene associated with invasion of *Bartonella bacilliformis* into human red blood cells (MITCHELL and MINNICK 1995). The InvA protein has a predicted nucleotide-binding site and may be an enzyme that cleaves nucleotides. MviN is a protein that is involved in the virulence of *Salmonella* in mice (VAN SLOOTEN et al. 1993). VacB is a protein required for virulence gene expression in *Shigella flexneri* and Enteroinvasive *E. coli* (TOBE et al. 1992). There are over 20 homologs of VacB in the public databases, and they probably encode a $3' \rightarrow 5'$ exoribonuclease II, involved in controlling mRNA turnover (ZIHAO et al. 1993). VapD has been shown to be associated with virulence in *Dichelobacter nodosus*

(KATZ et al. 1992); the *H. pylori* ortholog was recently cloned and sequenced (CAO and COVER 1997). VirB11 and VirB4 from *Bordetella pertussis* are required for pertussis toxin secretion (WEISS et al. 1993) and the homologs from *Agrobacterium* are cytoplasmic membrane ATPases required for virulence (STEPHENS et al. 1995; FULLNER et al. 1994; BERGER and CHRISTIE 1994; ZHOU and CHRISTIE 1997). Indeed, the VirB proteins are involved in transporting nucleoprotein particles to plant cells. In both examples, macromolecules are secreted via the newly described type IV secretion apparatus (CHRISTIE 1997). Interestingly, some of these *virB* orthologs are found within the *cag* pathogenicity island.

Multidrug Resistance Gene Orthologs. The genome of *H. pylori* has six genes that are predicted to be involved in resistance to multiple antimicrobial agents: HP0600 (multidrug resistance), HP0606 (*mtrC*), HP0630 (modulator of drug activity), HP1082 (multidrug resistance), HP1165 (tetracycline resistance), HP1181 (multidrug resistance efflux transporter), and HP1206 (multidrug resistance). It will be interesting to see whether any of these genes contributes to the antimicrobial resistance of *H. pylori*. Resistance to antimicrobials would contribute to the pathogenicity of bacteria, by giving the organism the opportunity to grow and spread, and by not allowing the host immune system the opportunity to kill the microbe.

11 Clinical Implications

Given the modest genome size of *H. pylori*, it is clear that the organism is highly specialized and specifically adapted to life in one niche, the human gastric mucosa. Because of this, it is important for us to understand exactly what virulence factors are expressed in this environment and play roles in colonization, avoidance of host immune response, and damage to the host. Conventional molecular biology and immunological studies previously uncovered virulence factors that are clearly critical to pathogenesis including urease (currently used as a vaccine candidate) and flagella (motility). Other factors including the vacuolating cytotoxin have been intensely investigated but may play a more subtle role in virulence. The completion of the genome sequence (TOMB et al. 1997) has now uncovered additional factors including many genes for outer membrane proteins of similar size that would have been difficult to sort out without the sequence. As well, a number of putative virulence genes including hemolysins have been found that are apparently poorly expressed in vivo and thus were difficult to characterize. In addition, the sequence has begun to give us a more clear picture of the limited metabolic pathways of the bacterium. While combinations of antimicrobial and acid suppressive therapy has provided an effective course of treatment for infected patients, the increase in antibiotic resistance among *H. pylori* strains requires that we constantly consider new targets of therapy. Our current understanding of *H. pylori* virulence factors gained at the bench in conjunction with new insights gained from the nucleotide sequence of the *H. pylori* genome now provides us with new antigens for use in vaccine development in addition to new metabolic pathways that can be targeted for inhibition. Although we still do not have a clear picture of the sequence of events in a model of pathogenesis of gastritis and peptic ulcer disease, the current body of knowledge clearly allows us to pursue effective therapies.

12 Summary

Since the discovery of *H. pylori* in 1982 (MARSHALL 1983; WARREN 1983), research on the mechanisms of virulence of *H. pylori* has advanced substantially. It is now well established that urease and flagella are virulence factors of *H. pylori*. Although known for some time to be toxic to epithelial cells in vitro, VacA has only recently been established as a virulence factor. The *cag* pathogenicity island has also emerged as another virulence contender, although the specific genes involved in virulence are still being determined. Other possible virulence factors, not yet confirmed by gene disruptions, are *hpaA*, *katA*, *sodA*, *cagA*, and iron-regulated genes. As of yet, no adhesins have been confirmed as being important for in vivo survival of *H. pylori*. With the sequence of the *H. pylori* genome in hand, it should be possible to more easily determine the role of specific genes in virulence. Genes of immediate interest are the OMPs, which may under go phase and antigenic variation and may represent adhesins. Additionally, virulence-related orthologs and *vacA*-related genes may provide some interesting findings. Once we define the genes that contribute to *H. pylori* virulence, we may be able to more easily develop novel therapeutic drugs or vaccines to treat and prevent *H. pylori* infection.

References

Aihara M, Tsuchimoto D, Takizawa H, Azuma A, Wakebe H, Ohmoto Y, Imagawa K, Kikuchi M, Mukaida N, Matsushima K (1997) Mechanisms involved in *Helicobacter pylori*-induced interleukin-8 production by a gastric cancer cell line, MKN45. Infect Immun 65:3218–3224

Altmeyer RM, McNern JK, Bossio JC, Rosenshine I, Finlay BB, Galan JE (1993) Cloning and molecular characterization of a gene involved in Salmonella adherence and invasion of cultured epithelial cells. Mol Microbiol 7:89–98

Andersen LP, Blom J, Nielsen H (1993) Survival and ultrastructural changes of *Helicobacter pylori* after phagocytosis by human polymorphonuclear leukocytes and monocytes. APMIS 101:61–72

Appelmelk BJ, Simoons-Smit I, Negrini R, Moran AP, Aspinall GO, Forte JG, deVries T, Quan H, Verboom T, Maaskant JJ, Ghiara P, Kuipers EJ, Bloemena E, Tadema TM, Townsend RR, Tyagarajan K, Crothers JM, Monteiro MA, Savio A, deGraaff J (1996) Potential role of molecular mimicry between *Helicobacter pylori* lipopolysaccharide and host Lewis blood group antigens in autoimmunity. Infect Immun 64:2031–2040

Armstrong JA, Cooper M, Goodwin CS, Robinson J, Wee SH, Burton M, Burke V (1991) Influence of soluble haemagglutinins on adherence of *Helicobacter pylori* to HEp-2 cells. J Med Microbiol 34: 181–187

Barer MR, Elliott TSJ, Berkeley D, Thomas JE, Eastham EJ (1988) Cytopathic effects of *Campylobacter pylori* urease. J Clin Pathol 41:597

Bauerfeind P, Garner R, Dunn BE, Mobley HLT (1997) Synthesis and activity of *Helicobacter pylori* urease and catalase at low pH. Gut 40:25–30

Berger BR, Christie PJ (1994) Genetic complementation analysis of the Agrobacterium tumefaciens virB operon: virB2 through virB11 are essential virulence genes. J Bacteriol 176:3646–3660

Bhat KS, Gibbs CP, Barrera O, Morrison SG, Jahnig F, Stern A, Kupschx EM, Meyer TF, Swanson J (1992) The opacity proteins of Neisseria gonorrhoeae strain MS11 are encoded by a family of 11 complete genes. Mol Microbiol 6:1073–1076

Bode G, Malfertheiner P, Ditschuneit H (1988) Pathogenic implications of ultrastructural findings in *Campylobacter pylori* related gastroduodenal disease. Scand J Gastroenterol [Suppl] 142:25–39

Borén T, Falk P, Roth KA, Larson G, Normark S (1993) Attachment of *Helicobacter pylori* to human gastric epithelium mediated by blood group antigens. Science 262:1892–1895

Broide E, Klinowski E, Varsano R, Eschar J, Herbert M, Scapa E (1996) Superoxide dismutase activity in *Helicobacter pylori*-positive antral gastritis in children. J Ped Gastroenterol Nutr 23:609–613

Cao P, Cover TL (1997) High-level genetic diversity in the vapD chromosomal region of *Helicobacter pylori*. J Bacteriol 179:2852–2856

Censini S, Lange C, Xiang Z, Crabtree JE, Ghiara P, Borodovsky M, Rappuoli R, Covacci A (1996) Cag, a pathogenicity island of *Helicobacter pylori*, encodes type-I-specific and disease-associated virulence factors. Proc Natl Acad Sci USA 93:14648–14653

Chmiela M, Lelwala-Guruge J, Wadström T (1994) Interaction of cells of *Helicobacter pylori* with human polymorphonuclear leucocytes: possible role of haemagglutinins. FEMS Immunol Med Microbiol 9:41–48

Chmiela M, Paziak-Domanska B, Rudnicka W, Wadström T (1995a) The role of heparan sulphate-binding activity of *Helicobacter pylori* bacteria in their adhesion to murine macrophages. APMIS 103:469–474

Chmiela M, Paziak-Domanska B, Wadström T (1995b) Attachment, ingestion and intracellular killing of *Helicobacter pylori* by human peripheral blood mononuclear leucocytes and mouse peritoneal inflammatory macrophages. FEMS Immunol Med Microbiol 10:307–316

Christie PJ (1997) The Agrobacterium tumefaciens T-complex transport apparatus: a paradigm for a new family of multifunctional transporters in eubacteria. J Bacteriol 179:3085–3094

Clayton CL, Pallen MJ, Kleanthous H, Wren BW, Tabaqchali S (1990) Nucleotide sequence of two genes from *Helicobacter pylori* encoding for urease subunits. Nucleic Acids Res 18:362

Clyne M, Drumm B (1993) Adherence of *Helicobacter pylori* to primary human gastrointestinal cells. Infect Immun 61:4051–4057

Cornelissen CN, Sparling PF (1994) Iron piracy: acquisition of transferrin-bound iron by bacterial pathogens. Mol Microbiol 14:843–850

Covacci A, Censini S, Bugnoli M, Petracca R, Burroni D, Macchia G, Massone A, Papini E, Xiang Z, Figura N et al. (1993) Molecular characterization of the 128-kDa immunodominant antigen of *Helicobacter pylori* associated with cytotoxicity and duodenal ulcer. Proc Natl Acad Sci USA 90:5791–5795

Cover TL, Dooley CP, Blaser MJ (1990) Characterization of and human serologic response to proteins in *Helicobacter pylori* broth culture supernatants with vacuolizing cytotoxin activity. Infect Immun 58:603–610

Cover TL (1996) The vacuolating cytotoxin of *Helicobacter pylori*. Mol Microbiol 20:241–246

Cover TL, Berg DE, Blaser MJ (1997) VacA and the cag Pathogenicity Island of H pylori. In: Ernst PB, Michetti P, Smith PD (eds) The immunobiology of *Helicobacter pylori*: from pathogenesis to prevention. Lippincott-Raven, Philadelphia, pp 75–90

Crabtree JE, Farmery SM, Lindley IJD, Figura N, Peichl P, Tompkins DS (1994) CagA/cytotoxic strains of *Helicobacter pylori* and interleukin-8 in gastric epithelial cell lines. J Clin Pathol 47:945–950

Crabtree JE, Taylor JD, Wyatt JI, Heatley RV, Shallcross TM, Tompkins DS, Rathbone BJ (1991) Mucosal IgA recognition of *Helicobacter pylori* 120 kDa protein, peptic ulceration, and gastric pathology. Lancet 338:332–335

Crabtree JE, Xiang Z, Lindley IJ, Tompkins DS, Rappuoli R (1995) Induction of interleukin-8 secretion from gastric epithelial cells by a cagA isogenic mutant of *Helicobacter pylori*. J Clin Pathol 48:967–969

Craig PM, Territo MC, Karnes WE, Walsh JH (1992) *Helicobacter pylori* secretes a chemotactic factor for monocytes and neutrophils. Gut 33:1020–1023

Danaher RJ, Levin JC, Arking D, Burch CL, Sandlin R, Stein DC (1995) Genetic basis of Neisseria gonorrhoeae lipooligosaccharide antigenic variation. J Bacteriol 177:7275–7279

Davies GR, Simmonds NJ, Stevens TR, Grandison A, Blake DR, Rampton DS (1992) Mucosal reactive oxygen metabolite production in duodenal ulcer disease. Gut 33:1467–1472

Dhaenens L, Szczebara F, Husson MO (1997) Identification, characterization, and immunogenicity of the lactoferrin-binding protein from *Helicobacter pylori*. Infect Immun 65:514–518

Dick JD (1990) Helicobacter (Campylobacter) pylori: a new twist to an old disease. Annu Rev Microbiol 44:249–269

Doig P, Austin JW, Trust TJ (1993) The *Helicobacter pylori* 19.6-kilodalton protein is an iron-containing protein resembling ferritin. J Bacteriol 175:557–560

Doig P, Austin JW, Kostrzynska M, Trust TJ (1992) Production of a conserved adhesin by the gastro-duodenal pathogen *Helicobacter pylori*. J Bacteriol 174:2539–2547

Doig P, Exner MM, Hancock RE, Trust TJ (1995) Isolation and characterization of a conserved porin protein from *Helicobacter pylori*. J Bacteriol 177:5447–5452

Drazek ES, Dubois A, Holmes RK, Kersulyte D, Akopyants NS, Berg DE, Warren RL (1995) Cloning and characterization of hemolytic genes from *Helicobacter pylori*. Infect Immun 63:4345–4349

Dunn BE, Campbell GP, Perez-Perez GI, Blaser MJ (1990) Purification and characterization of urease from *Helicobacter pylori*. J Biol Chem 265:9464–9469

Dunn BE, Vakil NB, Schneider BG, Miller MM, Zitzer JB, Peutz T, Phadnis SH (1997) Localization of *Helicobacter pylori* urease and heat shock protein in human gastric biopsies. Infect Immun 65: 1181–1188

Dwarakanath AD, Tsai HH, Sunderland D, Hart CA, Figura N, Crabtree JE, Rhodes JM (1995) The production of neuraminidase and fucosidase by *Helicobacter pylori*: their possible relationship to pathogenicity. FEMS Immunol Med Microbiol 12:213–216

Eaton KA, Brooks CL, Morgan DR, Krakowka S (1991) Essential role of urease in pathogenesis of gastritis induced by *Helicobacter pylori* in gnotobiotic piglets. Infect Immun 59:2470–2475

Eaton KA, Cover TL, Tummuru MKR, Blaser MJ, Krakowka S (1997) Role of vacuolating cytotoxin in gastritis due to *Helicobacter pylori* in gnotobiotic piglets. Infect Immun 65:3462–3464

Eaton KA, Krakowka S (1994) Effect of gastric pH on urease-dependent colonization of gnotobiotic piglets by *Helicobacter pylori*. Infect Immun 62:3604–3607

Eaton KA, Morgan DR, Krakowka S (1989) Campylobacter virulence factors in gnotobiotic piglets. Infect Immun 57:1119–1125

Eaton KA, Morgan DR, Krakowka S (1992) Motility as a factor in the colonisation of gnotobiotic piglets by *Helicobacter pylori*. J Med Microbiol 37:123–127

Eaton KA, Suerbaum S, Josenhans C, Krakowka S (1996) Colonization of gnotobiotic piglets by *Helicobacter pylori* deficient in two flagellin genes. Infect Immun 64:2445–2448

Emödy L, Carlsson Å, Ljungh Å, Wadström T (1988) Mannose-resistant haemagglutinin by *Campylobacter pylori*. Scand J Infect Dis 20:353–354

Evans DG, Evans DJ, Mould JJ, Graham DY (1988) N-acetylneuraminyllactose-binding fibrillar hem-agglutinin of *Campylobacter pylori*: a putative colonization factor antigen. Infect Immun 56: 2896–2906

Evans DG, Karjalainen TK, Evans DJ, Graham DY, Lee C-H (1993) Cloning, nucleotide sequence, and expression of a gene encoding an adhesin subunit protein of *Helicobacter pylori*. J Bacteriol 175: 674–683

Evans DJ, Evans DG, Kirkpatrick SS, Graham DY (1991) Characterization of the *Helicobacter pylori* urease and purification of its subunits. Microb Pathog 10:15–26

Evans DJ, Evans DG, Lampert HC, Nakano H (1995a) Identification of four new prokaryotic bacte-rioferritins, from *Helicobacter pylori*, Anabaena variabilis, Bacillus subtilis and Treponema pallidum. Gene 153:123–127

Evans DJ, Evans DG, Takemura T, Nakano H, Lampert HC, Graham DY, Granger DN, Kvietys PR (1995b) Characterization of a *Helicobacter pylori* neutrophil-activating protein. Infect Immun 63:2213–2220

Exner MM, Doig P, Trust TJ, Hancock RE (1995) Isolation and characterization of a family of porin proteins from *Helicobacter pylori*. Infect Immun 63:1567–1572

Falk P, Roth KA, Borén T, Ulf Westblom T, Gordon JI, Normark S (1993) An in vitro adherence assay reveals that *Helicobacter pylori* exhibits cell lineage-specific tropism in the human gastric epithelium. Proc Acad Natl Sci USA 90:2035–2039

Falk PG, Bry L, Holgersson J, Gordon JI (1995) Expression of a human alpha-1,3/4-fucosyltransferase in the pit cell lineage of FVB/N mouse stomach results in production of Leb-containing glycoconjugates: a potential transgenic mouse model for studying *Helicobacter pylori* infection. Proc Natl Acad Sci USA 92:1515–1519

Falkow S (1988) Molecular Koch's postulates applied to microbial pathogenicity. Rev Infect Dis 10 [Suppl 2]:S274–S276

Falkow S (1991) Bacterial entry into eukaryotic cells. Cell 65:1099–1102

Falkow S (1997) What is a pathogen? ASM News 63:359–365

Fox JG, Batchelder M, Marini R, Yan L, Handt L, Li X, Shames B, Hayward A, Campbell J, Murphy JC (1995) Helicobacter pylori-induced gastritis in the domestic cat. Infect Immun 63:2674–2681

Franzon VL, Arondel J, Sansonetti PJ (1990) Contribution of superoxide dismutase and catalase activities to Shigella flexneri pathogenesis. Infect Immun 58:529–535

Frazier BA, Pfeifer JD, Russell DG, Falk P, Olsen AN, Hammar M, Westblom TU, Normark SJ (1993) Paracrystalline inclusions of a novel ferritin containing nonheme iron, produced by the human gastric pathogen Helicobacter pylori: evidence for a third class of ferritins. J Bacteriol 175:966–972

Fullner KJ, Stephens KM, Nester EW (1994) An essential virulence protein of Agrobacterium tumefaciens, VirB4, requires an intact mononucleotide binding domain to function in transfer of T-DNA. Mol Gen Genet 245:704–715

Garner RM, Fulkerson JF, Mobley HLT (1998) Helicobacter pylori glutamine synthetase lacks features associated with transcriptional and posttranslational regulation. Infect Immun 66:1839–1847

Ge Z, Chan NW, Palcic MM, Taylor DE (1997) Cloning and heterologous expression of an alpha 1,3-fucosyltransferase gene from the gastric pathogen Helicobacter pylori. J Biol Chem 272:21357–21363

Geis G, Leying H, Suerbaum S, Mai U, Opferkuch W (1989) Ultrastructure and chemical analysis of Campylobacter pylori flagella. J Clin Microbiol 27:436–441

Geis G, Suerbaum S, Forsthoff B, Leying H, Opferkuch W (1993) Ultrastructure and biochemical studies of the flagellar sheath of Helicobacter pylori. J Med Microbiol 38:371–377

Ghiara P, Marchetti M, Blaser MJ, Tummuru MKR, Cover TL, Segal ED, Tompkins LS, Rappuoli R (1995) Role of the Helicobacter pylori virulence factors vacuolating cytotoxin, cagA, and urease in a mouse model of disease. Infect Immun 63:4154–4160

Goodwin CS, Armstrong JA, Marshall BJ (1986) Campylobacter pyloridis, gastritis, and peptic ulceration. J Clin Pathol 39:353–365

Gotschlich EC (1994) Genetic locus for the biosynthesis of the variable portion of Neisseria gonorrhoeae lipooligosaccharide. J Exp Med 180:2181–2190

Haas R, Odenbreit S, Till M, Hofreuter D (1997) Genetic and functional characterisation of the alpAB gene locus essential for adhesion of Helicobacter pylori to gastric epithelial cells. Accession no Z82988 (unpublished observation)

Hahn KB, Park IS, Kim YS, Cho SW, Lee SI, Youn JK (1997) Role of rebamipide on induction of heat-shock proteins and protection against reactive oxygen metabolite-mediated cell damage in culture gastric mucosa cells. Free Radic Biol Med 22:711–716

Harris PR, Cover TL, Crowe DR, Orenstein JM, Graham MF, Blaser MJ, Smith PD (1996) Helicobacter pylori cytotoxin induces vacuolation of primary human mucosal epithelial cells. Infect Immun 64:4867–4871

Hazell SL, Lee A (1986) Campylobacter pyloridis, urease, hydrogen ion back diffusion, and gastric ulcers. Lancet 2:15–17

Hazell SL, Mendz GL (1993) The metabolism and enzymes of Helicobacter pylori: function and potential virulence effects. In: Goodwin CS, Worsley BW (eds) Helicobacter pylori: biology and clinical practice. CRC Press, London, pp 115–142

Hirno S, Utt M, Ringnér M, Wadström T (1995) Inhibition of heparan sulphate and other glycosaminoglycans binding to Helicobacter pylori by various polysulphated carbohydrates. FEMS Immunol Med Microbiol 10:301–306

Hu L-T, Mobley HLT (1990) Purification and N-terminal analysis of urease from Helicobacter pylori. Infect Immun 58:992–998

Huang J, O'Toole PW, Doig P, Trust TJ (1995) Stimulation of interleukin-8 production in epithelial cell lines by Helicobacter pylori. Infect Immun 63:1732–1738

Huang J, Smyth CJ, Kennedy NP, Arbuthnott JP, Keeling PWN (1988) Haemagglutinating activity of Campylobacter pylori. FEMS Microbiol Let 56:109–112

Husson MO, Legrand D, Spik G, Leclerc H (1993) Iron acquisition by Helicobacter pylori: importance of human lactoferrin. Infect Immun 61:2694–2697

Illingworth DS, Walter KS, Griffiths PL, Barclay R (1993) Siderophore production and iron-regulated envelope proteins of Helicobacter pylori. Zentralbl Bakteriol 280:113–119

Ilver D, Arnquist A, Frick I-M et al. (1996) The Helicobacter pylori blood group antigen binding adhesin. Gut 39:A55

Jackson CJ, Kelly DJ, Clayton CL (1995) The cloning and characterisation of chemotaxis genes in *Helicobacter pylori*. Gut 37 [Suppl 1]:A18

Jones AC, Logan RPH, Foynes S, Cockayne A, Wren BW, Penn CW (1997) A flagellar sheath protein of *Helicobacter pylori* is identical to HpaA, a putative N-acetylneuraminyllactose-binding hemagglutinin, but is not an adhesin for AGS cells. J Bacteriol 179:5643–5647

Josenhans C, Labigne A, Suerbaum S (1995a) Comparative ultrastructural and functional studies of *Helicobacter pylori* and Helicobacter mustelae flagellin mutants: both flagellin subunits, FlaA and FlaB, are necessary for full motility in Helicobacter species. J Bacteriol 177:3010–3020

Josenhans C, Labigne A, Suerbaum S (1995b) Reporter gene analyses show that expression of both *H. pylori* flagellins is dependent on growth phase. Gut 37 [Suppl 1]:A62

Kanafani H, Martin SE (1985) Catalase and superoxide dismutase activities in virulent and nonvirulent Staphylococcus aureus isolates. J Clin Microbiol 21:607–610

Karita M, Kouchiyama T, Okita K, Nakazawa T (1991) New small animal model for human gastric *Helicobacter pylori* infection: success in both nude and euthymic mice. Am J Gastroenterol 86: 1596–1603

Katz ME, Strugnell RA, Rood JI (1992) Molecular characterization of a genomic region associated with virulence in Dichelobacter nodosus. Infect Immun 60:4586

Khelef N, DeShazer D, Friedman RL, Guiso N (1996) In vivo and in vitro analysis of Bordetella pertussis catalase and Fe-superoxide dismutase mutants. FEMS Microbiol Lett 142:231–235

Kirkland T, Viriyakosol S, Perez-Perez GI, Blaser MJ (1997) *Helicobacter pylori* lipopolysaccharide can activate 70Z/3 cells via CD14. Infect Immun 655:604–608

Klinowski E, Broide E, Varsano R, Eschar J, Scapa E (1996) Superoxide dismutase activity in duodenal ulcer patients. Eur. J Gastroenterol Hepatol 8:1151–1155

Kostrzynska M, Betts JD, Austin JW, Trust TJ (1991) Identification, characterization, and spatial localization of two flagellin species in *Helicobacter pylori* flagella. J Bacteriol 173:937–946

Krakowka S, Eaton KA, Rings DM (1995) Occurrence of gastric ulcers in gnotobiotic piglets colonized by *Helicobacter pylori*. Infect Immun 63:2352–2355

Krakowka S, Morgan DR, Kraft WG, Leunk RD (1987) Establishment of gastric *Campylobacter pylori* infection in the neonatal gnotobiotic piglet. Infect Immun 55:2789–2796

Labigne A, Cussac V, Courcoux P (1991) Shuttle cloning and nucleotide sequences of *Helicobacter pylori* genes responsible for urease activity. J Bacteriol 173:1920–1931

Leblond-Francillard M, Gaillard JL, Berche P (1989) Loss of catalase activity in Tn1545-induced mutants does not reduce growth of Listeria monocytogenes in vivo. Infect Immun 57:2569–2573

Lee WK, An YS, Kim KH, Kim SH, Song JY, Ryn BD, Choi YJ, Yoon YH, Baik SC, Rhee KH, Cho MJ (1997) Construction of a *Helicobacter pylori–Escherichia coli* shuttle vector for gene transfer in *Helicobacter pylori*. Appl Environ Microbiol 63:4866–71

Lelwala-Guruge J, Ljungh Å, Wadström T (1992) Haemagglutination patterns of *Helicobacter pylori*. APMIS 100:908–913

Leninger E, Roberts M, Kenimer JG, Charles IG, Fairweather N, Novotny P, Brennan MJ (1991) Pertactin, an Arg-Gly-Asp containing Bordetella pertussis surface protein that promotes adherence to mammalian cells. Proc Natl Acad Sci USA 88:345–349

Leunk RD, Johnson PT, David BC, Kraft WG, Morgan DR (1988) Cytotoxic activity in broth-culture filtrates of *Campylobacter pylori*. J Med Microbiol 26:93–99

Leying H, Suerbaum S, Geis G, Haas R (1992) Cloning and genetic characterization of a *Helicobacter pylori* flagellin gene. Mol Microbiol 6:2863–2874

Lingwood CA, Huesca M, Kuksis A (1992) The glycerolipid receptor for *Helicobacter pylori* (and Exoenzyme S) is phosphatidylethanolamine. Infect Immun 60:2470–2474

Lingwood CA, Wasfy G, Han H, Huesca M (1993) Receptor affinity purification of a lipid-binding adhesin from *Helicobacter pylori*. Infect Immun 61:2474–2478

Litwin CM, Calderwood SB (1993) Role of iron in regulation of virulence genes. Clin Microbiol Rev 6:137–149

Luke CJ, Penn CW (1995) Identification of a 29kDa flagellar sheath protein in *Helicobacter pylori* using a murine monoclonal antibody. Microbiology 141:597–604

Mai UEH, Perez-Perez GI, Allen JB, Wahl SM, Blaser MJ, Smith PD (1992) Surface proteins from *Helicobacter pylori* exhibit chemotactic activity for human leukocytes and are present in gastric mucosa. J Exp Med 175:517–525

Mai UEH, Perez-Perez GI, Wahl LM, Wahl SM, Blaser MJ, Smith PD (1991) Soluble surface proteins from *Helicobacter pylori* activate monocytes/macrophages by lipopolysaccharide-independent mechanism. J Clin Invest 87:894–900

Marchetti M, Arico B, Burroni D, Figura N, Rappuoli R, Ghiara P (1995) Development of a mouse model of *Helicobacter pylori* infection that mimics human disease. Science 267:1655–1658

Marshall B (1983) Unidentified curved bacilli on gastric epithelium in active chronic gastritis. Lancet i:1273–1275

Marshall BJ, Barrett LJ, Prakesh C, McCallum RW, Guerrant RL (1988) Protection of *Campylobacter pylori*dis but not Campylobacter jejuni against acid susceptibility by urea. In: Kaijser B, Falsen E (eds) Capylobacter IV. University of Goteborg, Goteborg, pp 402–403

Martin SL, Edbrooke MR, Hodgman TC, van den Eijnden DH, Bird MI (1997) Lewis X biosynthesis in *Helicobacter pylori*. Molecular cloning of an alpha (1,3)-fucosyltransferase gene. J Biol Chem 272:21349–21356

Marxer M, Farzam F, Spiegelhalder C et al. (1995) Interaction of a katalase- and a urease-negative mutant of *Helicobacter pylori* with polymorphonuclear granulocytes. Gut 37 [Suppl 1]:A21

McColm AA, Bagshaw JA, O'Malley CF (1993) Development of a ^{14}C-urea breath test in ferrets colonized with Helicobacter mustelae: effect of treatment with bismuth, antibiotics, and urease inhibitors. Gut 34:181–186

Mendz GL, Hazell SL (1996) The urea cycle of *Helicobacter pylori*. Microbiology 142:2959–2967

Mitchell SJ, Minnick MF (1995) Characterization of a two-gene locus from Bartonella bacilliformis associated with the ability to invade human erythrocytes. Infect Immun 63:1552

Mobley HLT, Island MD, Hausinger RP (1995) Molecular biology of ureases. Microbiol Rev 59:451–480

Moran AP, Valkonen K, Wadström T (1995) Identification of the lectin-like laminin-binding protein of *Helicobacter pylori*. Gut 37 [Suppl 1]:A1

Nakazawa T, Ishibashi M, Konishi H, Takemoto T, Shigeeda M, Kochiyama T (1989) Hemagglutinating activity of *Campylobacter pylori*. Infect Immun 57:989–991

Namavar F, Sparrius M, Veerman EC, Appelmelk BJ, Vandenbroucke-Grauls CM (1998) Neutrophil-activating protein mediates adhesion of *Helicobacter pylori* to sulfated carbohydrates on high-moleular-weight salivary mucin. Infect Immun 66:444

Neilands JB (1995) Siderophores: structure and function of microbial iron transport compounds. J Biol Chem 270:26723–26726

Nielsen P, Anderson LP (1992) Activation of human phagocytic oxidative metabolism by *Helicobacter pylori*. Gastroenterology 103:1747–1753

Noach LA, Rolf TM, Tytgat GNJ (1994) Electron microscopic study of association between *Helicobacter pylori* and gastric and duodenal mucosa. J Clin Pathol 47:699–704

Odenbreit S, Till M, Hofreuter D, Haas R (1997) Outer membrane proteins AlpA and AlpB are involved in *Helicobacter pylori* binding to gastric epithelial cells. Gut 41 [Suppl 1]:10/391

Odenbreit S, Wieland B, Haas R (1996) Cloning and genetic characterization of *Helicobacter pylori* catalase and construction of a catalase-deficient mutant strain. J Bacteriol 178:6960–6967

O'Toole PW, Janzon L, Doig P, Huang J, Kostrzynska M, Trust TJ (1995) The putative neuraminyl-lactose-binding hemagglutinin HpaA of *Helicobacter pylori* CCUG 17874 is a lipoprotein. J Bacteriol 177:6049–6057

O'Toole PW, Kostrzynska, Trust TJ (1994) Non-motile mutants of *Helicobacter pylori* and Helicobacter mustelae defective in flagellar hook production. Mol Microbiol 14:691–703

Owen RJ, Martin SR, Borman P (1985) Rapid urea hydrolysis by gastric Campylobacters. Lancet i:111

Papini E, de Bernard M, Milia E, Bugnoli M, Zerial M, Rappuoli R, Montecucco C (1994) Cellular vacuoles induced by *Helicobacter pylori* originate from late endosomal compartments. Proc Acad Natl Sci USA 91:9720–9724

Pepe JC, Miller VL (1993) Yersinia enterocolitica invasin: a primary role in the initiation of infection. Proc Natl Acad Sci USA 90:6473–6477

Pesci EC, Pickett CL (1994) Genetic organization and enzymatic activity of a superoxide dismutase from the microaerophilic human pathogen, *Helicobacter pylori*. Gene 143:111–116

Phadnis SH, Parlow MH, Levy M, Ilver D, Caulkins CM, Connors JB, Dunn BE (1996) Surface localization of *Helicobacter pylori* urease and heat shock protein homolog requires bacterial autolysis. Infect Immun 64:905–912

Piotrowski J, Slomiany A, Murty VLN, Fekete Z, Slomiany BL (1991) Inhibition of *Helicobacter pylori* colonization by sulfated gastric mucins. Biochem Int 24:749–756

Ricci V, Sommi P, Cova E, Fiocca R, Romano M, Ivey KJ, Solcia E, Ventura U (1993) Na+,K(+)-ATPase of gastric cells. A target of *Helicobacter pylori* cytotoxic activity. FEBS Lett 334:158–160

Ricci V, Ciacci C, Zarrilli R, Sommi P, Tummuru MK, Del Vecchio, Blanco C, Bruni CB, Cover TL, Blaser MJ, Romano M (1996) Effect of *Helicobacter pylori* on gastric epithelial cell migration and proliferation in vitro: role of VacA and CagA. Infect Immun 64:2829–2833

Rieder G, Hatz RA, Moran AP, Walz A, Stolte M, Enders G (1997) Role of adherence in interleukin-8 induction in *Helicobacter pylori*-associated gastritis. Infect Immun 65:3622–3630

Ringnér M, Valkonen KH, Wadström T (1994) Binding of vitronectin and plasminogen to Helicobacter pylor. FEMS Immunol Med Microbiol 9:29–34

Robinson J, Goodwin CS, Cooper M, Burke V, Mee BJ (1990) Soluble and cell-associated haemagglutinins of Helicobacter (Campylobacter) pylori. J Med Microbiol 33:277–284

Schmitt W, Haas R (1994) Genetic analysis of the *Helicobacter pylori* vacuolating cytotoxin: structural similarities with the IgA protease type of exported protein. Mol Microbiol 12:307–319

Schmitz A, Josenhans C, Suerbaum S (1997) Cloning and characterization of the *Helicobacter pylori* flbA gene, which encodes for a membrane protein involved in coordinated expression of flagellar genes. J Bacteriol 179:987–997

Segal ED, Falkow S, Tompkins LS (1996) *Helicobacter pylori* attachment to gastric cells induces cytoskeletal rearrangements and tyrosine phosphorylation of host cell proteins. Proc Natl Acad Sci USA 93:1259–1264

Segal ED, Lange C, Covacci A, Tompkins LS, Falkow S (1997) Induction of host signal transduction pathways by *Helicobacter pylori*. Proc Natl Acad Sci USA 94:7595–7599

Sharma SA, Tummuru MKR, Blaser MJ, Kerr LD (1998) Activation of IL-8 gene expression by *Helicobacter pylori* is regulated by transcription factor nuclear factor-B in gastric epithelial cells. J Immunol 160:2401–2407

Sharma SA, Tummuru MK, Miller GG, Blaser MJ (1995) Interleukin-response of gastric epithelial cell lines to *Helicobacter pylori* stimulation in vitro. Infect Immun 63:1681–1687

Sherburne R, Taylor DE (1995) *Helicobacter pylori* expresses a complex surface carbohydrate, Lewis X. Infect Immun 63:4564–4568

van Slooten JC, Okada T, Kutsukake K, Pechere JC, Harayama S (1993) Two close but independently transcribed genes at 23 min on the chromosome of S. typhimurium are involved in the mouse virulence (unpublished observation); accession no Z26133

Smoot DT, Mobley HLT, Chippendale GR, Lewison JF, Resau JH (1990) *Helicobacter pylori* urease activity is toxic to human gastric epithelial cells. Infect Immun 58:1992–1994

Smoot DT, Resau JH, Naab T, Desborges BC, Gilliam T, Henry KB, Curry SB, Nidiry J, Sewchand J, Mills-Robertson K, Frontin K, Abebe E, Dillon M, Chippendale GR, Phelps PC, Scott VF, Mobley HLT (1993) Adherence of *Helicobacter pylori* to cultured human gastric epithelial cells. Infect Immun 61:350–355

Smoot DT, Resau JH, Earlington MH, Simpson M, Cover TL (1996) Effects of *Helicobacter pylori* vacuolating cytotoxin on primary cultures of human gastric epithelial cells. Gut 39:795–799

Spielgelhalder C, Gerstenecker B, Kersten A, Schiltz E, Kist M (1993) Purification of *Helicobacter pylori* superoxide dismutase and cloning and sequencing of the gene. Infect Immun 61:5315–5325

Stephens KM, Roush C, Nester E (1995) Agrobacterium tumefaciens VirB11 protein requires a consensus nucleotide-binding site for function in virulence. J Bacteriol 177:27

Suerbaum S (1995) The complex flagella of gastric Helicobacter species. Trends Microbiol 3:168–170

Suerbaum S, Josenhans C, Labigne A (1993) Cloning and genetic characterization of the *Helicobacter pylori* and Helicobacter mustelae flaB flagellin genes and construction of H pylori flaA- and flaB-negative mutants by electroporation-mediated allelic exchange. J Bacteriol 175:3278–3288

Takahashi S, Igarashi H, Nakamura K, Masubuchi N, Saito S, Aoyagi T, Itoh T, Hirata I (1993) *Helicobacter pylori* urease activity-comparative study between urease positive and urease negative strain. Jpn J Clin Med 51:3149–3153

Tarkkanen J, Kosunen TU, Saksela E (1993) Contact of lymphocytes with *Helicobacter pylori* augments natural killer cell activity and induces production of gamma interferon. Infect Immun 61:3012–3016

Teneberg S, Miller-Podraza H, Lampert HC, Evans DJ, Evans DG, Danielsson D, Karlsson KA (1997) Carbohydrate binding specificity of the neutrophil-activating protein of *Helicobacter pylori*. J Biol Chem 272:19067–19071

Tobe T, Sasakawa C, Okada N, Honma Y, Yoshikawa M (1992) vacB, a novel chromosomal gene required for expression of virulence genes on the large plasmid of Shigella flexneri. J Bacteriol 174:6359–6367

Tomb J-F, White O, Kerlavage AR, Clayton RA, Sutton GG, Fleischmann RD, Ketchum KA, Klenk HP, Gill S, Dougherty BA, Nelson K, Quackenbush J, Zhou L, Kirkness EF, Peterson S, Loftus B, Richardson D, Dodson R, Khalak HG, Glodek A, McKenney K, Fitzgerald LM, Lee N, Adams MD, Hickey EK, Berg DE, Gocayne JD, Utterback TR, Peterson JD, Kelley JM, Cotton MD, Weidman JM, Fujii C, Bowman C, Watthey L, Wallin E, Hayes WS, Borodovsky M, Karp PD, Smith

HO, Fraser CM, Venter JC (1997) The complete genome sequence of the gastric pathogen *Helicobacter pylori*. Nature 388:539–547

Trust TJ, Doig P, Emödy L, Kienle Z, Wadström T, O'Toole P (1991) High-affinity binding of the basement membrane proteins collagen Type IV and laminin to the gastric pathogen *Helicobacter pylori*. Infect Immun 59:4398–4404

Tsuda M, Karita M, Morshed MG, Okita K, Nakazawa T (1994) A urease-negative mutant of *Helicobacter pylori* constructed by allelic exchange mutagenesis lacks the ability to colonize the nude mouse stomach. Infect Immun 62:3586–3589

Tummuru MK, Cover TL, Blaser MJ (1993) Cloning and expression of a high-molecular-mass antigen of *Helicobacter pylori*: evidence of linkage to cytotoxin production. Infect Immun 61:1799–1809

Tummuru MK, Cover TL, Blaser MJ (1994) Mutation of the cytotoxin-associated cagA gene does not affect vacuolating cytotoxin activity of *Helicobacter pylori*. Infect Immun 62:2609–2613

Tummuru MK, Sharma SA, Blaser MJ (1995) *Helicobacter pylori* picB, a homologue of the Bordetella pertussis toxin secreted protein, is required for induction of IL-8 in gastric epithelial cells. Mol Microbiol 18:867–876

Tzouvelekis L, Mentis AF, Makris AM, Spiliadis C, Blackwell C, Weir DM (1991) In vitro binding of *Helicobacter pylori* to human gastric mucin. Infect Immun 59:4252–4254

Valkonen KH, Wadström T, Moran AP (1994) Interaction of lipopolysaccharides of *Helicobacter pylori* with basement membrane protein laminin. Infect Immun 62:3640–3648

Valkonen KH, Wadström T, Moran AP (1997) Identification of the N-acetylneuraminyllactose-specific laminin-binding protein of *Helicobacter pylori*. Infect Immun 65:916–923

Vanet A, Labigne A (1998) Evidence for specific secretion rather than autolysis in the release of some *Helicobacter pylori* proteins. Infect Immun 66:1023–1027

Warren JR (1983) Unidentified curved bacilli on gastric epithelium in active chronic gastritis. Lancet i:1273–1275

Weiss AA, Johnson FD, Burns DL (1993) Molecular characterization of an operon required for pertussis toxin secretion. Proc Natl Acad Sci USA 90:2970–2974

Westblom TU, Phadnis S, Langenberg W, Yoneda K, Madan E, Midkiff BR (1992) Catalase negative mutants of *Helicobacter pylori*. Eur J Clin Microbiol Infect Dis 11:522–526

Wirth HP, Yang M, Karita M, Blaser MJ (1996) Expression of the human cell surface glycoconjugates Lewis x and Lewis y by *Helicobacter pylori* isolates is related to cagA status. Infect Immun 64:4598–4605

Worst DJ, Otto BR, de Graaff J (1995) Iron-repressible outer membrane proteins of *Helicobacter pylori* involved in heme uptake. Infect Immun 63:4161–4165

Worst DJ, Sparrius M, Kuipers EJ, Kusters JG, de Graaff J (1996) Human serum antibody response against iron-repressible outer membrane proteins of *Helicobacter pylori*. FEMS Microbiol Let 144:29–32

Wu CW, Chung WW, Chi CW, Kao HL, Lui WY, P'eng FK, Wang SR (1996) Immunohistochemical study of arginase in cancer of the stomach. Virchows Arch 428:325–331

Xiang Z, Censini S, Bayeli PF, Telford JL, Figura N, Rappuoli R, Covacci A (1995) Analysis of expression of CagA and VacA virulence factors in 43 strains of *Helicobacter pylori* reveals that clinical isolates can be divided into two major types and that cagA is not necessary for expression of the vacuolating cytotoxin. Infect Immun 63:94–98

Xu J-K, Goodwin CS, Cooper M, Robinson J (1990) Intracellular vacuolization caused by the urease of *Helicobacter pylori* J Infect Dis 161:1302–1304

Zheng H, Hasset DJ, Bean K, Cohen MS (1992) Regulation of catalase in Neisseria gonorrhoeae. Effects of oxidant stress and exposure to human neutrophils. J Clin Invest 90:1000–1006

Zihao R, Camelo L, Arraiano CM (1993) DNA sequencing and expression of the gene rnb encoding Escherichia coli ribonuclease II. Mol Microbiol 8:43–51

Zhou X-R, Christie PJ (1997) Suppression of mutant phenotypes of Agrobacterium tumefaciens VirB11 ATPase by overproduction of VirB proteins. J Bacteriol 179:5835–5842

Host Response and Vaccine Development to *Helicobacter pylori* Infection

T.G. BLANCHARD, S.J. CZINN, and J.G. NEDRUD

1 Introduction/Background

Infection of humans by *Helicobacter pylori* can have various outcomes (Fig. 1). In virtually all cases a state of chronic/active gastritis results from an infection by *H. pylori*, but whether this gastritis progresses to more severe disease states such as duodenal or gastric ulcers or serves as a precursor to gastric cancer appears to be influenced by both the host response and bacterial virulence determinants. Bacterial virulence factors have been reviewed elsewhere in this volume ("Mechanisms of

Departments of Pathology and Pediatrics, 10900 Euclid Avenue, Case Western Reserve University, Cleveland, OH 44106, USA

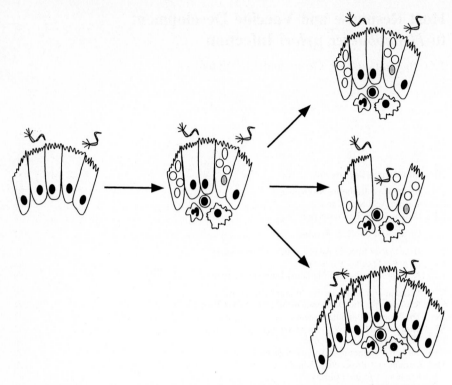

Fig. 1. Clinical outcomes associated with chronic *H. pylori* infection. The environmental niche of *H. pylori* is in the mucus coat overlying the gastric epithelium. The interaction of *H. pylori* with the gastric epithelium (*left*) results in proinflammatory events attracting neutrophils and monocytes (*center*). Ultimately, chronic infection can result in one of three different clinical manifestations. Over time the interaction between the bacterial virulence factors and the host response can result in either chronic gastritis (*top right*), peptic ulcer disease (*middle right*) or the development of gastric adenocarcinoma (*bottom right*)

Helicobacter pylori Infection: Bacterial Factors"); this chapter focuses on the host response to *Helicobacter* infections in the context of these virulence factors.

In order to evaluate host responses to an infectious pathogen there are several approaches which can be taken. The first approach is to simply obtain tissue biopsies from infected and uninfected individuals and to analyze them histologically. In addition, various in vitro tests either with or without stimulation by live or killed/fractionated *Helicobacter* organisms might also be performed on these biopsies. This approach has been utilized extensively to investigate *Helicobacter* infections and the salient findings are summarized here. The second approach is to do challenge studies in humans or to identify naturally occurring acute infections and to monitor host responses over time as in the first approach. There are ethical issues which make challenge studies in humans difficult to perform and therefore information is limited. Furthermore, since acute natural *Helicobacter* infections may not display any overt symptoms, it is difficult to identify acutely infected individuals. The final approach is to use animal models for *Helicobacter* infections to evaluate the host response. The advantage of animal models is that the challenge organism and onset of infection are fixed by the investigator so that a defined infection can be followed over time. In addition, infected animals can be manipulated in various ways to discern the effects of various host factors on the infection. A disadvantage of animal models is the fact that they are models and may not accurately predict the human host response to infection by a similar or even identical organism. The reader is referred to "Animal Models of *Helicobacter* Gastritis" (this volume) for an extensive discussion of *Helicobacter* animal models; selected animal host responses to *Helicobacter* infections are briefly summarized here.

The human response to chronic *H. pylori* infection appears to be an antral-predominant gastritis composed of both neutrophils and mononuclear cells. By itself this gastritis cannot explain either the development of duodenal or gastric ulcers or a predisposition towards gastric cancer. Since historical data predating the discovery of *H. pylori* as well as more contemporary data suggests that duodenal ulcers seem to "protect" against gastric cancer, it also seems paradoxical that *H. pylori* infection is a confirmed risk factor for both entities. As summarized in "Mechanisms of *Helicobacter pylori* Infection: Bacterial Factors" (this volume), it is unlikely that differing bacterial factors can explain this paradox as CagA$^+$, VacA$^+$, so-called "type I" strains of *H. pylori* are associated with both peptic ulcer disease and gastric cancer. In addition, CagA , VacA , type II strains have been isolated from ulcer patients. Variation in the host response to infection, perhaps due to genetic and/or environmental factors, therefore appears to be critical in determining the outcome of a *Helicobacter* infection.

2 Innate Host Response Mechanisms

2.1 Gastric Acid Secretion

One host factor which may in part be genetically determined and which appears to be important in determining disease outcome is acid secretion. In general, patients with duodenal ulcers tend to hyper secrete gastric acid. Gastric acid secretion is controlled by factors including parietal cell numbers and differences in the sensitivity of parietal cells to hormonal stimulation by gastrin. It has also been suggested that *H. pylori* infection may affect the secretion of gastric acid. Studies performed in healthy subjects with and without *H. pylori* infection have shown a significant increase in gastrin levels, a powerful stimulant for gastric acid secretion, in healthy, asymptomatic subjects infected with *H. pylori* (PETERSON et al. 1993). However, it has been difficult to confirm that the enhanced gastrin levels result in an increase in gastric acid secretion in the population of asymptomatic patients infected with *H. pylori*. In contrast, enhanced gastrin levels are associated with elevated levels of gastric acid in the population of *H. pylori* infected individuals with duodenal ulcers (PETERSON et al. 1993). Interestingly, once *H. pylori* has been eradicated from these subjects, serum gastrin and gastric acid abnormalities are no longer present (Moss and CALAM 1993). This suggests that the elevated serum gastrin levels associated with duodenal ulcers may be a primary result of the associated *H. pylori* infection and promotes the development of duodenal ulcers.

Although *H. pylori* urease can buffer gastric acidity, *H. pylori* is still somewhat acid sensitive and tends to localize in areas of the stomach with low acid secretion. In individuals with "normal" levels of stomach acid, *H. pylori* is found predominantly in the antrum which does not contain acid secreting parietal cells. It has also been suggested that the level of acid secretion may ultimately determine which part of the stomach is predominantly inflamed in *H. pylori* infected individuals. Several studies have shown that acid suppressive therapy with proton pump inhibitors increases the degree of corpus gastritis associated with *H. pylori* infection (KUIPERS et al. 1996). Thus, the relationship between acid secretion and chronic *H. pylori* infection may play a critical role in determining the clinical course of chronic *H. pylori* infection.

ADRIAN LEE and coworkers (1995) have proposed a hypothesis that goes one step further, suggesting that the level of gastric acid secretion at the time of initial *H. pylori* infection can predict the ultimate clinical course and outcome. Under conditions of low acid secretion *H. pylori* infection is localized to the gastric corpus. With long-term acid suppression, the number of organisms found in the antrum decreases whereas the number of *H. pylori* organisms in the corpus increases resulting in worsening corpus gastritis. This then evolves to gastric atrophy promoting the development of gastric cancer. This theory suggests that *H. pylori* associated gastritis is primarily found in the gastric antrum only in individuals with normal or increased acid secretion. This category of patient would then be at increased risk for the development of gastric metaplasia within the duodenum which in turn promotes the migration of *H. pylori* into the duodenum favoring the development of peptic ulcer disease. Although generally useful, this hypothesis cannot account for the development of duodenal ulcers in the face of normal or low gastric acid secretion, nor can it explain the development of gastric adenocarcinoma in patients with acid hyper secretion.

DAVID GRAHAM and colleagues have recently updated the Lee hypothesis in an attempt to account for these situations (GRAHAM 1997). GRAHAM and others suggest that in addition to acid secretion, bacterial virulence factors may determine disease outcome. In an individual infected with nonvirulent, *cagA-*, *H. pylori* the inflammatory response results in an antral predominant gastritis. Such a scenario promotes the development of a duodenal ulcer only if the patient hyper secretes acid. Whereas patients infected with *cagA*$^+$ (virulent) strains of *H. pylori* are at risk for the development of a duodenal ulcer in the presence of "normal" or high acid secretion. Based on this hypothesis, the development of gastric cancer requires infection with a virulent strain of *H. pylori* in the presence of hyposecretion or active suppression of acid. In this case the inflammatory response is concentrated in the body of the stomach which over time can result in the development of atrophic gastritis. As a result of this atrophy, parietal cells are depleted and replaced with mucous gland metaplasia further limiting the acid secreting capacity of the stomach. Ultimately, the presence of atrophic gastritis promotes the replacement of normal gastric mucosa with intestinal type mucosa. The development of intestinal metaplasia is a precursor lesion associated with the development of gastric cancer. This scenario based on host acid secretion and bacterial virulence factors is one possible approach to explain disease outcome as a result of chronic *H. pylori* infection.

In summary there is some evidence to suggest that *H. pylori* infection results in elevations of serum and fasting gastrin levels when patients are infected with *H. pylori* infection. However, it is unclear whether this results in enhanced gastric acid secretion. The increased basal gastric acid output noted in patients with duodenal ulcer disease also appears to be related to *H. pylori* infection since eradication of the infection normalizes the basal acid output. It is unclear why *H. pylori* infection is associated with elevated basal acid outputs in duodenal ulcer patients but not in healthy subjects infected with *H. pylori*. Infection with a virulent strain of *H. pylori* in combination with acid hypersecretion tends to result in antral gastritis and the development of peptic ulcer disease. *H. pylori* infection in the presence of acid suppression tends to result in inflammation of the corpus, gastric atrophy and the development of gastric adenocarcinoma. The interaction between bacterial virulence factors and the host gastric acid response appear to more fully predict the clinical outcomes associated with chronic *H. pylori* infection.

2.2 Gastric Cytokine Production

Irrespective of the possible role of gastric acid as a component of the host response to *H. pylori* infection, one prominent feature of the host response which has been observed by many investigators is the enhanced presence of the neutrophil-activating chemokine interleukin (IL) 8 in the gastric mucosa of infected individuals (BODGER and CRABTREE 1998; CRABTREE et al. 1994; MOSS et al. 1994; YAMAOKA et al. 1995). IL-8 production by *H. pylori* infected gastric epithelium has been extensively studied both in vivo and in vitro. In vivo, the magnitude of the IL-8 response has been correlated with the severity of the gastritis (CRABTREE 1996). In vitro experiments indicate that *H. pylori* adherence to gastric epithelial cells appears to be required for induction of IL-8 since bacteria separated from epithelial cells by a permeable membrane filter fail to induce IL-8 production (RIEDER et al. 1997). Many putative *H. pylori* adhesins have been described; for details on the nature of these adhesins the reader is referred to "Mechanisms of *Helicobacter pylori* Infection: Bacterial Factors" (this volume). Adherence of live or sodium azide treated *H. pylori* induce Il-8 secretion. Alternatively, heat killed *H. pylori*, *H. pylori* extracts, isolated proteins, and membrane fractions could not induce IL-8 secretion (RIEDER et al. 1997; SHARMA et al. 1995). Additional in vitro studies indicated that adherence of *H. pylori* to gastric epithelial cells resulted in reorganization of host cytoskeletal proteins and tyrosine phosphorlyation of a 145kDa host cell protein (SEGAL et al. 1996). Another laboratory has shown *H. pylori* induction of IL-8 expression in endothelial cells which also appears to be tyrosine kinase dependent

(DING et al. 1997). Although tyrosine phosphorylation is often associated with signal transduction, subsequent studies with various kinase inhibitors showed a partial dissociation between host protein phosphorlylation and IL-8 production, suggesting multiple pathways for IL-8 induction (SEGAL et al. 1997).

Bacterial virulence factors are also important in regulating the magnitude of the IL-8 response. Analysis of human gastric biopsies has shown that *cagA* positive strains of *H. pylori* are associated with increased levels of IL-8 mRNA and protein expression as well as heightened inflammatory responses and peptic ulceration (PEEK et al. 1995; YAMAOKA et al. 1996, 1997). In vitro studies by many investigators have confirmed the correlation between CagA$^+$, VacA$^+$ type I *H. pylori* strains and stimulation of enhanced IL-8 secretion using cultured gastric epithelial cells. Studies using isogenic *H. pylori* mutants have shown, however, that neither the *cagA* or *vacA* genes are directly involved in regulating IL-8 induction (CRABTREE et al. 1995; SHARMA et al. 1995). Rather, it appears that other genes within the cagA pathogenicity island are responsible (SEGAL et al. 1997; TUMMURU et al. 1995). While the pathways are still being defined, activation of the transcription factor NF-κB is an important intermediate mediator of IL-8 induction by these bacterial gene products (KEATES et al. 1997; MUNZENMAIER et al. 1997; SHARMA et al. 1998).

In addition to IL-8, efforts are underway to identify the dominant inflammatory cytokines produced by gastric lymphocytes from patients suffering from histological gastritis. Independent of *H. pylori* status, IFN-γ (a proinflammatory TH1 cytokine) and tumor-necrosis factor (TNF) have been the primary cytokines that appear to be upregulated when gastritis is present (D'ELIOS et al. 1997; FAN et al. 1993, 1994; KARTTUNEN et al. 1990, 1995, 1997). A recent report by BODGER et al. (1997) confirms the finding that in *H. pylori* positive patients gastric TNF levels are closely correlated with the degree of gastric inflammation. Equally interesting is that these investigators also found elevated levels of IL-10, a cytokine thought to be involved in protection from *H. pylori* infection.

Alternatively, both TH1 and TH2 cytokines may be involved in the pathogenesis of this chronic infection. In support of a role for TH1 cytokines in the pathogenesis of *H. pylori*-associated gastritis, a recent study demonstrated that mRNA for the TH1 inducing cytokine IL-12 was observed at a higher frequency and concentration in gastric tissues from *H. pylori* positive versus *H. pylori* negative patients (KARTTUNEN et al. 1997). In addition to inflammatory TH1 cytokines, one group has reported the presence of T cell clones from infected patients with mild disease with a TH0 cytokine profile (producing IFN-γ in addition to IL-4 and/or IL-5; D'ELIOS et al. 1997). In addition to those cytokines mentioned above, adherence of *H. pylori* to epithelial cells has also been demonstrated to directly induce the production of a number of proinflammatory cytokines such as granulocyte-macrophage colony-stimulating factor (GM-CSF), monocyte chemoattractant protein-1 (MCP-1), TNF, and NF-κ B (BEALES and CALAM 1997; JUNG et al. 1997). BEALES and CALAM (1997) hypothesize that GM-CSF may initiate as well as promote the development of *H. pylori* associated gastritis. Finally, a recent pediatric study has also confirmed the presence of elevated levels of TNF and IL-6 in children with *H. pylori* associated gastric inflammation (KUTUKCULER et al. 1997). Thus, in total *H. pylori* contact with epithelial cells activates a number of "innate" pro-inflammatory pathways.

3 Genetics of the Host Response

Information on the influence of genetic factors upon the host response to *H. pylori* infections in humans comes from epidemiological studies. One widely quoted study of Swedish monozygotic versus dizygotic twins reared together or apart showed that the presence or absence of *H. pylori* infection was more concordant in monozygotic twins, suggesting an influence of genetics upon susceptibility to *H. pylori* infection (MALATY et al. 1994). A series of other studies have examined the frequency of some class II major histocompatability genes in patients with *H. pylori* associated diseases such as duodenal ulcer and gastric adenocarcinoma. While some DQA_1 alleles appeared to be associated with resistance or susceptibility to these diseases (AZUMA et al. 1995, 1998), other investigators have suggested that although susceptibility to gastric cancer may be related to HLA DQ alleles, this HLA association may not be related to *H. pylori* infection status (LEE et al. 1996).

Although data are sparse for humans, in murine animal models utilizing both *H. pylori* and *H. felis* the magnitude and character of *Helicobacter*-associated gastric inflammation is regulated by host genetics (LEE et al. 1997; MOHAMMADI et al. 1996; SAKAGAMI et al. 1996, 1997). For instance, when infected with *H. felis*, BALB/c and CBA mice exhibited only mild inflammation. C57BL/6 mice, in contrast, developed more severe inflammation and marked thickening of the gastric mucosa accompanied by replacement of parietal cells with mucus secreting cells (MOHAMMADI et al. 1996; SAKAGAMI et al. 1996). *H. felis* infected C3H/He mice also developed a more severe form of gastritis which appeared to depend, at least in part, upon host responses to bacterial LPS (SAKAGAMI et al. 1997). It has also been suggested that the differences observed in *H. felis*-associated inflammation of these strains of mice may be related to their phospholipase A_2 genotypes and apoptosis of gastric epithelial cells after infection (WANG et al. 1998).

These genetic studies have been accomplished in mice which have several advantages as animal models. First the availability of inbred strains of mice and rats allows free exchange of cells and tissues between individual animals. Second, there is a wealth of reagents available for rodents. Finally, there are large numbers of transgenic and gene targeted ("knock out") mice available that can be used to study the contribution of various host factors to the overall host-pathogen relationship. In spite of these powerful tools, it has been difficult to translate rodent genetic studies directly to humans for several reasons. First, the nature of the gastritis observed in animals often has a different character than that observed in humans with variable degrees of neutrophil involvement (for details, the reader is referred to "Animal Models of *Helicobacter* Gastritis," this volume). Second, in the case of *Helicobacter* induction of IL-8 discussed above, there is no direct homologue of the neutrophil chemokine IL-8 in rodents. Thus mouse and rat studies on this important mediator of human *Helicobacter*-associated gastritis cannot be carried out. Third, most of the *H. pylori* rodent models which have been described exhibit only low to moderate levels of gastritis and atrophy. *H. felis*, which has been extensively used as an alternate model does induce high levels of gastritis in some strains of mice (MOHAMMADI et al. 1996; SAKAGAMI et al. 1996). However, the absence of the pathogenicity island and VacA from *H. felis* precludes its use for studying the interaction of these bacterial factors with the host responses. Thus while a genetic component to the human host response is probably important in *H. pylori* infections, deficiencies in existing animal models have hampered progress in this area. For the moment we are left with descriptive and/or in vitro studies of *H. pylori* interaction with human tissues and imperfect animal models.

4 *Helicobacter*-Specific Adaptive Immune Response

In addition to the role that gastric acid and epithelial or monocyte derived cytokines may play in determining the location, character, and severity of gastritis in *H. pylori* infected individuals, an additional host factor which appears to play a role in the severity of *Helicobacter* disease and which may also offer hope for controlling the disease (see "Vaccines," below) is the adaptive immune response.

4.1 *H. pylori*-Specific Antibodies

Within one to two years after the isolation and discovery of *H. pylori*, reports on specific antibody responses began to appear (JONES et al. 1986; MARSHALL et al. 1984). The presence of both systemic and local antibody responses in infected individuals was reported (CRABTREE et al. 1991; KIST 1991; RATHBONE et al. 1986). When analyzed by western blot, these antibodies bound a large number of bacterial antigens including many putative virulence factors such as urease, VacA, and CagA (CRABTREE et al. 1991; CZINN et al. 1989; KIST 1991). However, since it is thought that infected individuals rarely clear an infection on their own, these antibody responses appeared to play little or no role in controlling the infection. Although antigen-antibody immune complexes within the gastric mucosa could conceivably be immunopathological, most of the gastric antibodies seem to be of the IgA isotype which do not fix complement well. Nevertheless, one recent study has demonstrated the presence of both C3b and elements of the complement membrane attack complex in gastric biopsies of *H. pylori* infected individuals (BERSTAD et al. 1997) leading to the possibility, at least, of immune complex disease in infected individuals.

Another possible role for antibodies in *Helicobacter* associated disease was suggested by the discovery in 1991 that serum from infected individuals or immunized mice and some *H. pylori* specific monoclonal antibodies could bind to normal mouse or human gastric tissue (NEGRINI et al. 1991). Thus was born the "molecular mimicry" theory of *H. pylori* gastritis which suggested that shared antigens between gastric tissue and *H. pylori* might provoke an autoimmune reaction. This theory has been bolstered by more recent evidence showing that *H. pylori* LPS shares epitope(s) with the human blood group Lewis x or Lewis y glycoantigens which may also be present on the beta chain of the gastric parietal cell proton pump, H/K-ATPase (APPELMELK et al. 1996; ASPINALL et al. 1996; SIMOONS SMIT et al. 1996; WIRTH et al. 1996). Further suggestions of autoimmunity have come from a recent animal model where mice made transgenic for another Lewis blood group antigen were found to develop antiparietal cell antibodies after infection with *H. pylori* (GURUGE et al. 1998). Description of autoimmune gastritis in humans featuring antiparietal cell antibodies predates the discovery of *H. pylori*. However, while *H. pylori* infection is quite common, human autoimmune gastritis is relatively rare. Furthermore, the putative role of *H. pylori* LPS in autoimmune gastritis stands in marked contrast to the low biological activity of *H. pylori* LPS reported by others (KIRKLAND et al. 1997; MUOTIALA et al. 1992; PEREZ-PEREZ et al. 1995) Thus, the significance of shared epitopes between gastric tissue and *H. pylori* requires further investigation before concluding that *H. pylori* can provoke a functional autoimmune reaction.

4.2 *H. pylori*-Specific Cell-Mediated Immune Response

Cell-mediated immune responses in *H. pylori* infected individuals have been a controversial topic. Some investigators have detected *Helicobacter*-specific proliferative response by peripheral blood lymphocytes (PBLs) from infected patients (KLUGE et al. 1993; TOSI et al. 1992). Other investigators have shown, however, that PBLs from *H. pylori* sero-negative individuals (presumably uninfected but perhaps previously exposed?) proliferated at an equal or greater magnitude than did PBLs from seropositive patients in response to *H. pylori* antigens (BIRKHOLZ et al. 1993; DI TOMMASO et al. 1995; FAN et al. 1994; KARTTUNEN et al. 1990; SHARMA et al. 1994). This result has led to the suggestion that either the host or *H. pylori* itself may be down-regulating cell-mediated immune responses in order to limit inflammatory damage to the host, or to help *H. pylori* evade bacterial clearance mechanisms.

Another way to monitor cell-mediated immune responses is to measure "spontaneous" or antigen induced T cell cytokines in PBLs or gastric biopsies from uninfected or *H. pylori* infected individuals. IFN-γ, an inflammatory Th1 cytokine has been a predominant cytokine and the Th2 cytokines IL-4 and IL-5 have been virtually absent when gastric lymphocytes from *H. pylori* infected patients were evaluated (D'ELIOS et al. 1997; FAN et al. 1993, 1994; KARTTUNEN et al. 1990, 1995, 1997; BAMFORD et al. 1998; HAEBERLE et al. 1997; BAMFORD 1998). In some cases, either IFN-γ or its mRNA have also been detected in inflamed gastric mucosa from persons without *H. pylori*, perhaps suggesting a common pathway to gastric inflammation as a result of either *H. pylori* infection or other causes (FAN et al. 1993; HAEBERLE et al. 1997; KARTTUNEN et al. 1997). As mentioned above, TH0 cells have been cloned from infected patients with mild disease (D'ELIOS et al. 1997).

A non-T cell cytokine produced by macrophages and other cells but which can positively regulate the generation of Th1 cellular immune responses is IL-12. This cytokine or its mRNA has been detected in gastric biopsies from *H. pylori* infected patients and its synthesis by PBL cultures has been shown to be selectively induced by live *H. pylori* (HAEBERLE et al. 1997; KARTTUNEN et al. 1997). Collectively these results suggest that *H. pylori* infection induces Th1 cellular immune responses which can contribute to the gastric inflammation in infected individuals.

This conclusion is also supported by research in the mouse model. *H. felis* infected C57BL/6 mice develop severe gastric inflammation and both spleen cells and gastric lymphocytes from these mice produce IFN-γ but no IL-4 or IL-5 (MOHAMMADI et al. 1996a,b). Furthermore when infected mice are treated with neutralizing anti-IFN-γ antibodies gastric inflammation is significantly reduced (MOHAMMADI et al. 1996). In a related study, when *H. felis*-specific TH1 cell lines were adoptively transferred into recipient mice which were then infected with *H. felis*, the recipient animals demonstrated enhanced gastric inflammation (MOHAMMADI et al. 1997). A transferred TH2 cell line also exacerbated inflammation but to a lesser degree. Finally, when BALB/c mice are infected with *H. felis*, they develop much milder gastritis which is significantly increased when infected mice are treated with IL-12 (MOHAMMADI et al. 1996). Thus both human data and research in animal models supports the hypothesis that a Th1 cellular immune response may contribute to *Helicobacter*, associated disease. While the antigens which these T cells recognize have not been completely defined, research in both mice, (MOHAMMADI, CZINN, and NEDRUD, unpublished) and humans (D'ELIOS et al. 1997) indicate that a spectrum of *Helicobacter* antigens including urease, CagA, VacA, and *Helicobacter* heat shock proteins are recognized.

5 Vaccination and Protective Immunity to *H. pylori*

In addition to the contribution of the host immune response towards *Helicobacter*-associated inflammation, several animal model studies have demonstrated that protective immunity can be achieved by proper stimulation of the adaptive immune response. As described in detail below, there is now much data to support the development of a vaccine for the cure or prevention of *H. pylori* in humans. Significant advances have been made in the selection of protective antigens, experimental adjuvants and delivery vehicles, and optimal route of administration. The animal studies that have made these advances possible have also begun to shed some light on the mechanisms of immunity that are playing the most important roles in providing protection. Most data indicate that just as the cell-mediated immune response may play a significant role in the disease progression by influencing the inflammatory response, the cell-mediated immune response is also responsible for protective immunity.

5.1 Rationale for the Development of an *H. pylori* Vaccine

Since an effective "triple antimicrobial therapy" has been developed for the treatment of *H. pylori*, one might justifiably challenge the need to spend a great amount of time, effort and capital on vaccine development. However, close examination of the consequences of triple therapy on both the individual and global level provide the rationale for such an endeavor. Current antimicrobial therapies are complicated and demanding on the patient, requiring the ingestion of multiple agents several times a day for up to 3 weeks (SOLL 1996). Although the success of this therapy can be as high as 90%, ultimately the lack of patient compliance reduces its efficacy. Additionally, treatment can be accompanied by such adverse effects as nausea, diarrhea, abdominal pain, and pseudomembranous colitis (BELL et al. 1992; RAUWS 1993) resulting in loss of appeal for continued ingestion of the pharmaceuticals and a consequent failure to eradicate the *H. pylori* infection. The high cost of antimicrobial therapy is also prohibitive in many developing nations where *H. pylori* infection is endemic with rates of infection as high as 80%–90%. However, even if an inexpensive antimicrobial therapy were available, widespread treatment of *H. pylori* could result in the development of antibiotic resistant strains. Antibiotic resistance in *H. pylori* has already been observed in patients treated with triple therapy who failed to cure infection (JORGENSEN et al. 1996; MEGRAUD 1997). It also bears considering that such widespread use of these antimicrobials to treat *H. pylori* could result in the selection of other antibiotic resistant pathogens.

There are at least two other major considerations to be made regarding the effectiveness of antimicrobial therapy in controlling *H. pylori* infection and disease. First, there is no evidence to date to suggest that antibiotic cure results in protective resistance to subsequent reinfection with *H. pylori*. Although several studies have demonstrated that successful eradication of *H. pylori* with triple therapy results in extremely low rates of reinfection (WALSH and PETERSON 1995), this observation may be attributed to a lack of subsequent exposure to *H. pylori*. In fact, several long-term studies performed in developing nations where the incidence of infection is much higher indicate infection rates of 10%–13% following eradication of *H. pylori* with antimicrobial therapy. Whether these statistics represent true reinfection or recrudescence remains a topic of debate (VAN DER ENDE et al. 1997). However, it has been reported that successfully treated patients can become reinfected by accidental endoscopic transmission (LANGENBERG et al. 1990). Lack of resistance to subsequent challenge following successful antimicrobial therapy has been demonstrated in several animal models. Following eradication of gastric *Helicobacter* infection by antimicrobial therapy, both ferrets and mice could be readily reinfected by their respective *Helicobacter* species (CHEN et al. 1993; CZINN et al. 1996; Fox et al. 1994).

Second, pharmaceutical cure of *H. pylori* infection does not address the particular need of those nonsymptomatic individuals who might go on to develop gastric adenocarcinoma. If *H. pylori* plays a role in gastric carcinogenesis, patients need to be identified and cured prior to the initiation of events that may take decades to manifest themselves as gastric adenocarcinoma. As mentioned above, most patients remain asymptomatic despite the presence of histologic gastritis. This chronic inflammation is considered to be a risk factor for the development of gastric cancer (CORREA 1992).

Immune-based therapies would provide an inexpensive and convenient solution to widespread *H. pylori* infection with the added benefit of providing long lived protective immunity from future exposure to the pathogen. Childhood vaccination could, in theory, not only prevent adult gastritis and peptic ulcer disease but also reduce the incidence of gastric cancer later in life. Although the complications associated with antibiotic therapy mentioned above could be avoided by immune therapy, as discussed below, perhaps the most compelling reason to pursue an *H. pylori* vaccine is that it seems so very possible.

Approximately 10 years passed between the initial description by WARREN and MARSHALL (1983) of the culturing of *H. pylori* from patient biopsies and the first report by CZINN and NEDRUD (CZINN et al. 1993) of successful vaccination of mice against *H. felis* by oral immunization. In the years since, vaccine research has advanced at a rapid rate and clinical trials have already begun (Table 1). Although 10 years may seem a disproportionate length of time for the development of a prototype vaccine to be developed in animals, several significant obstacles had to be overcome before these initial experiments could be performed. The nature of gastrointestinal immunity, the development of suitable animal models, and the selection of a candidate antigen (s) were and continue to be the main challenges towards vaccine development.

5.2 The Mucosal Immune System

Although *H. pylori* permanently colonizes the gastric mucosa, strictly speaking it is a noninvasive bacterium. As such it is never exposed to the immune effector mechanisms which typically eradicate infectious diseases from the host tissue. It is generally held that resistance to micro-organisms which invade at the mucosa is optimally provided by the mucosal immune system. To adequately understand the progress and future challenges for *H. pylori* vaccine development, a cursory understanding of the common mucosal immune system as it relates to the gastrointestinal tract is necessary.

In recent years it has become increasingly evident that both the components and the mechanisms employed to induce and effect an adaptive immune response at mucosal tissues are phenotypically and functionally distinct from those classically described for systemic immunity (reviewed in KRAEHENBUHL and NEUTRA 1992;

Table 1. Significant events in the advancement of *H. pylori* vaccine research

Year	Event	References
1988–1990	Description of *H. mustelae*/ferret model	(Fox et al. 1988, 1990)
1990	Description of *H. felis*/mouse model	(Lee et al. 1990)
1991	Development of oral immunization protocol using *Helicobacter* lysate and CT	(Czinn and Nedrud 1991)
1993	Protective immunity against *H. felis* by prophylactic immunization using *H. felis* lysate and CT	(Chen et al. 1993; Czinn et al. 1993)
1994	Protective prophylactic immunization against *H. felis* using urease and CT	(Ferrero 1994; Michetti et al. 1994)
1994–1995	Description of *H. pylori*/mouse model	(Karita et al. 1994; Marchetti et al. 1995; McColm et al. 1995)
1995	Protective prophylactic immunization against *H. felis* using groES and CT, multisubunit vaccine gives complete protection	(Ferrero et al. 1995)
1995	Protective prophylactic immunization against *H. pylori* using VacA and LT	(Marchetti et al. 1995)
1995	Therapeutic immunization against *H. felis* with urease B and CT	(Corthesy-Theulaz et al. 1995)
1996	Long-term immunity in *H. felis*/mouse model	(Radcliff et al. 1996)
1996	Therapeutic immunization of ferrets against *H. mustelae*	(Cuenca et al. 1996)
1997	Phase II clinical trials of therapeutic immunization in humans using urease and LT	(Michetti et al. 1997)
1997	Therapeutic immunity to *H. pylori* in the mouse by oral immunization with VacA or CagA with a nontoxic derivative of LT	(Ghiara et al. 1997)
1997–1998	Prophylactic immunity to *H. felis* infection by intranasal immunization	(Corthesy-Theulaz et al. 1998; Kleanthous et al. 1998; Weltzin et al. 1997)
1998	Prophylactic immunity to *H. pylori* in the mouse using VacA or CagA with a nontoxic mutant of LT	(Marchetti et al. 1998)
1998	Prophylactic immunity to *H. pylori* in the mouse by intranasal immunization using recombinant *S. typhimurium*	(Corthesy-Theulaz et al. 1998)
1998	Prophylactic immunity to *H. pylori* in the mouse by oral immunization with a single dose of recombinant *S. typhimurium*	(Gomez-Duarte et al. 1998)
1998	Prophylactic immunity to *H. pylori* in the mouse by systemic immunization	(Guy et al. 1998)

Mestecky and McGhee 1987). The gastrointestinal tract represents an enormous surface area ($400m^2$) in continual contact with dietary elements, normal and pathogenic bacterial flora, and allergins. A single layer of columnar epithelium is all that separates the body from potential harm while providing an appropriate surface for the absorption of nutrients and water. Although many innate immune mechanisms are present at the intestinal mucosa, frequent exposure to opportunistic pathogens and the ease with which the integrity of the mucosa can be compromised make it essential that adaptive immunity be able to service this tissue.

The lymphatic tissue of the intestine consists of both organized mucosa-associated lymphoid tissue (O-MALT) and diffuse mucosa-associated lymphoid tissue

(D-MALT; KRAEHENBUHL and NEUTRA 1992). In general it is believed that O-MALT represent the sites of antigen sampling and lymphocyte activation. This is accomplished via the PEYER'S patches which are dispersed throughout the lumenal surface. Specialized epithelial cells called M cells (microfold cells) on the surface of the PEYER'S patches serve as professional antigen samplers by endocytosing antigens and microbes from the lumen and shuttling them across the cell. When the antigens are released from the basolateral membrane, they have been transported across the epithelium and deposited within highly organized lymph tissue containing professional antigen presenting cells and lymphocytes. The relevant T and B lymphocytes (precommitted to a secretory IgA response) are activated, and circulate throughout the body as they differentiate. Eventually the cells "home" back to the original tissue but also disseminate to other exocrine tissues by interaction of specific homing receptors and addressins present on the lymphocytes and endothelium that distinguish the tissue as mucosal. Thus, acquired immunity can be disseminated amongst many mucosal tissues although stimulated locally. This "seeding" of the lamina propria is optimally accomplished through the activation of mucosal lymphocytes and not very efficiently by systemic immunization.

The effector mechanisms of an adaptive mucosal immune response are performed throughout the length of the mucosa by the D-MALT, populations of cells within the mucosal epithelium and lamina propria. Greater than 60% of the lamina propria lymphocytes are T cells with $CD4^+$ cells outnumbering $CD8^+$ cells by a factor of 2:1. The T cells play pivotal roles in immune regulation of B cells and other T cells via cytokine production and eliminating viral infections by cytotoxicity. An additional T cell component of the D-MALT include intraepithelial lymphocytes (IEL). The IELs are predominantly $CD8^+$ and have cytotoxic activity. They consist of an unusually high proportion of $\gamma\delta$ T cells whose stimulation and activation requirements are distinct from $\alpha\beta$ T cells but less well understood. Although the detailed relationship between the IELs, enterocytes, and lamina propria lymphocytes (LPLs) has not been delineated, it is clear these cell types all play crucial roles in either actively down-regulating or amplifying antigen specific immunity.

Although the role of the T cells is undoubtedly of paramount importance in a mucosal immune response the best described and well-known effector mechanism of mucosal immunity is the active secretion of antigen-specific IgA and IgM into the lumen (MAZANEC et al. 1993). Plasma cells that populate the lamina propria actively secrete polymeric IgA (pIgA) and IgM which bind to the polymeric immunoglobulin receptor (pIgR) on the basolateral membrane of the enterocytes. Antibodies which bind the pIgR are endocytosed and transported to the apical surface where the extracellular domain of the pIgR is cleaved, releasing the IgA. Thus an antigen specific antibody response can be mounted at the lumen without compromising the integrity of the epithelial cell barrier or resulting in a loss of plasma cells. However, because the IgA secreted into the lumen becomes lost due to enzymes and peristalsis it is necessary for the body to continually produce large amounts of IgA. In fact, more IgA is produced daily than all other isotypes combined (MESTECKY and MCGHEE 1987). Successful local stimulation of the mucosal immune system can dictate the specificity of these antibodies thus allowing a barrier of immune exclusion against specific pathogens.

As mentioned above, activation of specific lymphocytes at one region of the intestine can lead to an immune response at distal locations. Immunologists have taken advantage of this mechanism for the testing of many oral vaccines for the induction of immunity against oral, respiratory, genital, and ocular pathogens (LIANG et al. 1989; MICHALEK et al. 1976; MONTGOMERY et al. 1983; NEDRUD et al. 1987; NICHOLS et al. 1978). However, most protein antigens are not very immunogenic by the oral route. Complications include stomach acid, poor delivery to the M cells and/or limited uptake by M cells, and the need for large amounts of antigen. Therefore, several mechanisms have been developed to optimize the immunogenicity of antigens delivered by the oral route. As discussed below, several of these mechanisms were employed to test the potential role of oral immunization for the induction of protective immunity in the stomach against *Helicobacter*.

Examination of the healthy stomach reveals no O-MALT in the gastric mucosa and only limited numbers of LPLs and IELs. Additionally, pIgR expression is low with correspondingly low levels of pIgA secretion (ISAACSON 1982; VALNES et al. 1984, 1990). Given the lack of organized lymph tissue and low levels of IgA found at its surface one might wonder whether the common mucosal immune system can be taken advantage of for vaccination against *H. pylori*. Although infection of the gastric mucosa with *H. pylori* is accompanied by the recruitment of antigen specific effector lymphocytes and the production of significant levels of secreted *H. pylori*-specific IgA, the degree to which this response is induced and mediated by mucosal mechanisms remains unclear. In fact the immune response to infection by *H. pylori* may strictly be the result of a local inflammatory response to persistent infection acting independently of our understanding of mucosal immunity. Thus the problems of antigenic delivery to the mucosal immune system, and inducing an adaptive immune response at a mucosa lacking important effector cells had to be overcome for the development of a vaccine.

5.3 Early Prophylactic Vaccine Studies

Prior to the description of a small laboratory animal model for *Helicobacter* infection, our laboratory began investigating the potential role of mucosal immunity for vaccination of *H. pylori* by developing a protocol which would favor the production of *Helicobacter*-specific IgA by the gut mucosa. By employing an oral immunization regime similar to that previously described for use against Sendai virus infection in mice (NEDRUD et al. 1987), CZINN and NEDRUD (1991) were able to use *H. pylori* lysates in combination with the mucosal adjuvant CT to successfully generate *H. pylori*-specific serum IgG and IgA and intestinal IgA antibodies in both mice and ferrets. These antibodies were observed in the gastric washes as well, although the source of these antibodies (gastric and/or salivary) was not determined.

As the immunization protocol described above was being developed by CZINN and NEDRUD (CZINN et al. 1992, 1993), several small animal models of *Helicobacter* infection were described which now allowed for the safety and protective efficacy of vaccination against *Helicobacter* to be determined, most notably the *H. felis*/mouse (LEE et al. 1990), and *H. mustelae*/ferret (Fox et al. 1991) models. CZINN and NEDRUD applied their oral immunization protocol and were able to provide protective immunity against challenge with live *H. felis* in 80% of experimental animals by using *H. felis* whole cell sonicate and cholera toxin (CT) (CZINN et al. 1992, 1993). Thus, it was demonstrated that the stomach could benefit from the common mucosal immune system as an effector site. CHEN et al. almost simultaneously made similar observations using an oral immunization protocol based upon that described above (CHEN et al. 1992, 1993).

Within several years many major contributions were made towards vaccine development using the mouse model of *H. felis* infection (Table 1). Without exception all of these studies employed the use of oral immunization and the mucosal adjuvant CT. CHEN et al. demonstrated that while immunization-induced immunity was protective, mice which had previously been infected with *H. felis* and subsequently cured by antimicrobial therapy were not resistant to reinfection, thus demonstrating a distinction between the immune response generated by infection and immunization (CHEN et al. 1993; CZINN et al. 1996; Fox et al. 1994). Two independent groups employed the first subunit vaccines consisting of recombinant *H. pylori* urease B subunit and achieved protection ranging from 25%–80% against challenge with *H. felis* (FERRERO 1994; MICHETTI et al. 1994). SELLMAN et al. (1995) described the induction of a *Helicobacter*-specific IgA response at the gastric mucosa following challenge of immunized mice and several groups reported that mice protected from challenge generated a gastric inflammatory response despite the absence of detectable organisms. It was also determined that by using a combination of purified *H. pylori* antigens, 100% protection could be achieved against challenge with *H. felis* (FERRERO et al. 1995). When recombinant heat shock protein A and urease B subunit were given in combination with CT, complete protection was achieved, whereas immunization with either protein individually generated protection in approximately 80% of the mice. Thus a subunit vaccine was developed with an efficacy equal to that of the whole cell sonicate employed by other groups. Finally, prophylactic immunity was shown to be long-lived in mice which had been immunized 15\months prior to challenge (RADCLIFF et al. 1996). When immunized with whole cell lysate and CT 100% immunity was achieved.

5.4 Therapeutic Vaccine Studies

The advance towards human clinical *H. pylori* vaccine trials was greatly facilitated by the prophylactic immunization studies described above. However, the success of prophylactic immunization suggested that such a vaccine might be administered therapeutically as well. During natural infection *H. pylori* is able to persist in the face of a vigorous immune response, yet immunization could successfully prevent chronic infection of the gastric mucosa. This was of interest because the induced immune response was no higher than that of infected animals (BLANCHARD et al.

1996; SELLMAN et al. 1995). One possible explanation for the success of vaccination was that the chronology of the immune response in relation to infection might be responsible for protection. However, as mentioned above, mice and ferrets previously cured of an infection by antimicrobial therapy can be readily reinfected despite the presence of the immune response generated to the initial infection. Thus, another plausible explanation was that oral immunization somehow presented the relevant antigen to the host in such a way as to induce a qualitatively different, and therefore protective, immune response. Based on such an assumption, several groups administered the vaccine to infected animals as a therapeutic vaccine.

The *H. felis*/mouse model was initially employed by two different groups. Experimentally infected mice were immunized with either whole cell sonicate (DOIDGE et al. 1994) or purified recombinant *H. pylori* urease B subunit (CORTHESY-THEULAZ et al. 1995) plus CT. Approximately 50% of the mice could effectively resolve their *H. felis* infections following immunization. A third group of investigators tested a similar immunization in the *H. mustelae*/ferret model. The ferret model possesses several advantages over the murine models in that it represents a natural host-pathogen relationship with disease progression similar to *H. pylori* infection of humans (Fox 1988; Fox et al. 1988, 1990, 1991). Additionally, the size of the animal allows for periodic endoscopy and gastric biopsy collection for continued monitoring of the same animals without sacrifice. CUENCA et al. achieved eradication of *H. mustelae* in approximately one third of the ferrets receiving therapeutic immunization consisting of five doses of 0.1–10mg purified *H. pylori* urease holoenzyme plus 60µg CT. All mock immunized ferrets remained infected. Since the homology between *H. mustelae* and *H. pylori* urease is not as extensive as between *H. felis* and *H. pylori* urease, these results were particularly encouraging. However, in contrast to prophylactic immunization of mice which develop postimmunization gastritis following challenge, eradication was accompanied by a significant reduction in the degree of gastritis.

Several groups have now developed murine models of *H. pylori* infection (KLEANTHOUS et al. 1998; MARCHETTI et al. 1995; McCOLM et al. 1995; RADCLIFF et al. 1997). Although the degree and character of inflammation in these models is often less than satisfactory, such models are invaluable for testing the efficacy of prototype *H. pylori* vaccine candidates. GHIARA et al. (1997) have used a mouse adapted *H. pylori* isolate to test the effects of therapeutic vaccination against *H. pylori* in mice. When recombinant *H. pylori* VacA or CagA were administered orally with a mucosal adjuvant, 92% and 70% eradication was achieved respectively. Furthermore, clearance of *H. pylori* with VacA immunization resulted in protection against subsequent challenge in 70% of the mice.

Successful eradication of chronic *Helicobacter* infections in these three animal models is encouraging since greater than half of the world's population is chronically infected with *H. pylori*. Considering the cost and potential complications of administering antimicrobial therapies to these populations, therapeutic vaccination seems a most desirable alternative. The most advanced clinical trial performed to date was an oral therapeutic vaccine consisting of recombinant *H. pylori* urease apoenzyme in combination with LT. Although complete eradication of the bacteria was not observed in any patients, reductions in the bacterial load were observed in the majority of the subjects (Michetti et al. 1997).

5.5 Subunit Vaccines and Antigen Selection

Most early vaccination experiments were performed in mice and pigs and employed either whole cell sonicates of *H. felis* (Chen et al. 1992, 1993; Czinn et al. 1992, 1993) or whole killed *H. pylori* (Eaton and Krakowka 1992). Several groups have continued to use whole cell sonicates of *H. felis* to optimize vaccination strategies, investigate immune mechanisms, and further characterize pathogenesis (Blanchard et al. 1998; Doidge et al. 1994; Lee and Chen 1994; Mohammadi et al. 1996a,b, 1997). However, a similar immunization strategy would be improbable in humans for several reasons. First, it would be extremely impractical to produce the amount of *H. pylori* lysate needed to serve the human population in need. Second, the use of uncharacterized lysates opens the possibility for the inclusion of potentially pathogenic antigens to be present within the preparation. Third, it is likely that some if not many of these uncharacterized antigens would induce an immune response that cross-reacts with other potentially helpful intestinal flora. To circumvent these potential problems several laboratories have made concerted efforts towards the development of subunit vaccines.

A subunit vaccine consisting of the urease enzyme was the most logical place to begin. It is surface exposed, represents up to 6% of the total cell mass (Hu and Mobley 1990), and is highly conserved among gastric *Helicobacter* species. Additionally, studies using the pig model of *H. pylori* infection have demonstrated that urease is an essential colonization factor (Eaton et al. 1991). Michetti et al. (1994) made the first demonstration that purified *H. pylori* urease could be used to provide prophylactic immunity to *H. felis* infection in mice. Several other groups have subsequently employed this model as either a biochemically purified product of *H. pylori* or as a purified recombinant subunit. Lee et al. (1995) have performed a series of immunizations in which it was demonstrated that as little as 5µg doses of recombinant *H. pylori* urease can be used to induce protective immunity. Consistent with these findings, Blanchard et al. (1995) have demonstrated that preincubation of *H. felis* with monoclonal antibodies specific for the B subunit of urease prevents the bacteria from infecting the gastric mucosa of mice.

The successful use of the urease apoenzyme in animals has advanced to its use in human clinical trials (Michetti et al. 1997). Early trials with urease in humans have shown it to be safe (Kreiss et al. 1996). However, its effectiveness in animal models is typically about 80%. Ferrero et al. addressed this problem by performing oral immunizations with a combination of recombinant *H. pylori* heat shock protein A and urease in mice. By combining the two antigens, 100% protection from challenge with *H. felis* could be achieved where as either component individually induced only 80% protection (Ferrero et al. 1995). As mentioned above, an initial phase II clinical trial in humans using recombinant urease and LT for therapeutic immunization reduced the bacterial load but did not completely eradicate the *H. pylori* (MICHETTI et al. 1997). It may be that in addition to urease a second or third component will have to be added to achieve acceptable efficacy.

In addition to the urease enzyme and heat shock protein A described above several groups have begun to characterize other *H. pylori* antigens for use as subunit vaccines. In the first description of chronic *H. pylori* infection in the mouse, MARCHETTI et al. (1995) employed the vacuolating cytotoxin (VacA) protein to achieve protective efficacy equivalent to that of urease. Although the two molecules were not tested in the same preparation, consistent with earlier observations employing subunit vaccines, neither one individually protected 100% of challenged mice. This group has continued to employ VacA as an antigen in mouse studies designed for the development of an improved mucosal adjuvant for human use. However, they have also utilized recombinant CagA in both prophylactic and therapeutic immunizations with success in both reports (GHIARA et al. 1997; MARCHETTI et al. 1998). LEE et al. have demonstrated that purified *H. pylori* catalase is an efficient vaccine in mice against challenge with either *H. felis* or *H. pylori* (RADCLIFF et al. 1997) and our lab is currently investigating the efficacy of a novel low molecular weight nickel binding protein. Given the recent results of clinical therapeutic vaccination trials and the many animal model studies employing subunit vaccines, it is likely that a subunit vaccine for use in humans will require several different antigens.

5.6 Current and Prospective Adjuvants

The difficulty of stimulating a mucosal immune response has been appreciated since early studies describing the common mucosal immune system. In general, to induce an immune response the antigen had to be administered orally in large doses. Alternatively, if the antigen had specificity for the intestinal mucosa (streptococcal M protein, reovirus, lectins) small doses could achieve the same result. Since most protein antigens, including *Helicobacter* proteins, are poor immunogens when given by the oral route, the search for a "mucosal adjuvant" has been one of the most intensely researched areas of mucosal immunity. When used in low doses, CT is the most effective mucosal adjuvant described to date, and at least for laboratory animal studies, has greatly facilitated our understanding of mucosal immunology.

The widespread use in animal models of the oral immunization protocol developed by CZINN and NEDRUD which employed CT as a mucosal adjuvant has been described above (CZINN and NEDRUD 1991). It has also been demonstrated that in the absence of CT, oral *Helicobacter* vaccination is unsuccessful (EATON and KRAKOWKA 1992; LEE and CHEN 1994). Oral or intranasal vaccination studies in mice and pigs in the absence of an adjuvant or in ferrets using muramyl dipeptide as an adjuvant did not protect from *Helicobacter* infection (CHEN et al. 1993; EATON and KRAKOWKA 1992; LEE et al. 1995; PALLEY et al. 1993; WELTZIN et al. 1997). And a human phase I clinical trial employing *H. pylori* infected patients, has demonstrated that oral administration of recombinant *H. pylori* urease without an adjuvant is well tolerated but does not reduce the incidence of *H. pylori* infection (KREISS et al. 1996).

These studies clearly establish the need for a mucosal adjuvant in a *Helicobacter* vaccine when administered by the oral or nasal route but the toxicity of CT and *E. coli* heat-labile toxin (LT) molecules preclude their use in humans. In fact, during a recent phase II clinical study where recombinant urease was given to subjects in combination with LT 66% of the subjects experienced significant diarrhea, although a modest decline in bacterial infection was noted in those volunteers who received the vaccine (MICHETTI et al. 1997). Several approaches are now being developed to make bacterial endotoxins suitable for human use or to find viable alternatives.

To appreciate the challenge involved in generating a nontoxic CT adjuvant an understanding of the structure and biology of CT/LT is important (reviewed in SPANGLER 1992). These toxins are composed of two protein subunits. The pentameric B subunit (ca. 12kDa) forms a donut-like structure that binds to GM_1 ganglioside present on epithelial cells. The single A subunit (ca 28kDa) projects through the B subunit pentamer. When the B subunit binds to target cells, entry of the A subunit into the cell's cytoplasm is facilitated. Inside the cell, the A subunit separates into a the A_1 peptide which possesses enzymatic activity, and the A_2 peptide, which forms the tail-like anchor to the B subunits. Transfer of ADP-ribose from NAD to a G protein which is part of the adenyl cyclase complex is catalyzed by the A_1 peptide. The result is an irreversible activation of adenyl cyclase which leads to an intracellular accumulation of cAMP. The accumulation of cAMP promotes the efflux of water and electrolytes from the cell. The mechanisms by which these toxins achieve mucosal adjuvanticity are poorly understood but no doubt multifactorial (reviewed in HOLMGREN et al. 1993). However, several strategies have been deduced by which these molecules might be used safely in humans.

One plausible mechanism might be to take advantage of the carrier potential of the B subunit (CTB) to deliver antigens to the gut epithelium. This concept was suggested by one of the earliest CT adjuvant studies in which horse radish peroxidase was covalently coupled to CTB and found to induce enhanced mucosal IgA responses after oral immunization (MCKENZIE and HALSEY 1984). Numerous investigators have attempted to use CTB or LTB as a mucosal carrier in other systems (reviewed in ELSON and DERTZBAUGH 1994; HOLMGREN et al. 1993). This theme has recently been taken one step further by genetically replacing the toxic A_1 domain of the A subunit with foreign antigen which is then linked to the B pentamer by the A_2 tail (HAJISHENGALLIS et al. 1995).

Many studies have also been performed in which biochemically purified CTB has been used as an adjuvant in place of CT holotoxin. Interpretations of these studies are complicated by the fact that commercially purified CTB is typically contaminated with small amounts of holotoxin which may synergize with CTB (HASHIGUCCI et al. 1996; TAMURA et al. 1994; WILSON et al. 1990). Two studies using the *H. felis* rodent model have indicated that whereas commercially prepared CTB could enhance protection versus *Helicobacter* infection, holotoxin free recombinant CTB does not possess adjuvant activity (BLANCHARD et al. 1997; LEE and CHEN 1994). Thus, one possibility may be to covalently or genetically couple a *Helicobacter* antigen to recombinant CTB or LTB to take advantage of its carrier function and administer the conjugate with a low, nontoxic but synergistic dose of holotoxin.

Another approach is to reduce or eliminate the toxicity of the A subunit genetically by introducing mutations into the CT or LT molecules that would preserve adjuvant activity. To date over two dozen such mutant CT and LT molecules have been described by a number of laboratories around the world (BURNETTE et al. 1991; CIEPLAK et al. 1995; DICKINSON and CLEMENTS 1995; DOUCE et al. 1995; YAMAMOTO et al. 1997). Testing for the adjuvanticity of all these mutant molecules has not been completed and most often the test antigens are model proteins with no infectious challenge model. Although the oral adjuvanticity is reduced or lost in some of these mutants, some mutants are active intranasally. Such adjuvants may hold significant promise since intranasal immunization has been employed successfully as an effective means of *Helicobacter* immunization in mice (WELTZIN et al. 1997; KLEANTHOUS 1997; CORTHESY-THEULAZ 1998). Recently, a mutant LT molecule has been developed which has been found to be effective in immunizing against *H. pylori* in the mouse models both prophylactively and therapeutically (GHIARA et al. 1997; MARCHETTI et al. 1998). This molecule is deficient in cleavage of the A_1 and A_2 peptides of the A subunit of LT.

Thus, although toxicity of CT and LT are significant problems to be overcome in the quest for an effective but safe adjuvant for an *H. pylori* vaccine, a number of ongoing experimental approaches are addressing this issue. The probability that one or more of these approaches will be successful is high, but will require definitive testing in clinical trials in humans. Several other alternatives to bacterial endotoxins are being explored for use as mucosal adjuvants. Several groups have explored the use of oral muramyl dipeptide which has significant adjuvant properties for systemic immunizations. When used in ferrets no protection was achieved (WHARY et al. 1997) and ferrets actually suffered from increased pathological gastritis upon challenge. It is important to remember that adjuvants which fail to elicit mucosal immunity by oral immunization could possibly be successful when administered by alternative routes (see below).

Until recently one potential solution for a *Helicobacter* vaccine which has been relatively ignored is the use of attenuated recombinant bacterial strains to deliver *Helicobacter* antigens to the gut mucosa. Enteric pathogens such as *Salmonella typhimurium* and *Shigella flexneri* have been exploited in vaccine research against other pathogens by cloning the genes for foreign proteins into attenuated strains which can cause a limited infection in the host. Thus, these bacteria serve as carriers to deliver the proteins of interest directly to the mucosal immune system. As immunity is developed to these strains, immunity is concurrently developed against the recombinant protein. GOMEZ-DUARTE et al. have used an attenuated strain of *S. typhimurium* expressing *H. pylori* urease A and B subunits to achieve protective immunity against challenge with *H. pylori* in mice as determined by urease activity of gastric biopsies (GOMEZ-DUARTE et al. 1998). Of extreme interest was the ability to achieve protection with only one dose of bacteria. If such an observation were consistently obtained, the problem of host immunity to the delivery vehicle which might proclude subsequent use for booster immunizations could be avoided. COTHESY-THEULAZ et al. have also employed an attenuated *S. typhimurium* recombinant vaccine expressing *H. pylori* urease A and B subunits (CORTHESY-THEULAZ et al. 1998). After two intranasal doses of bacteria, greater than 50% of mice were protected from challenge with *H. pylori* as indicated by both urease activity of gastric biopsies and direct visualization of bacteria in histological sections. It is likely that as yet unreported experiments are currently being conducted to explore the utility of other bacterial carrier systems, novel biochemical adjuvants, and mucosal lectins for eventual use with *Helicobacter* antigens.

5.7 Route of Vaccine Delivery

Most childhood vaccines are administered intramuscularly. The ensuing adaptive immune response is suitable to provide memory throughout the entire body. As discussed above, the bodies mucosal tissues are poorly protected by this type of immunization but can be immunized locally. Several early studies demonstrated that a systemic immunization might be inadequate to provide protective immunity against *Helicobacter* infections in animal models while oral and intragastric immunizations, when given with a suitable mucosal adjuvant provide protective immunity. Despite the seeming success by the oral route, recent findings suggest that it may be worth reexamining other routes of immunization. For several reasons, it may be better to immunize via alternative mucosal routes or even systemically.

First, recent evidence suggests that protective immunity against *H. felis* in the mouse model might be incomplete. Although *H. felis* cannot be detected several weeks following challenge, the postimmunization gastritis that accompanies the challenge is frequently of higher magnitude than natural infection and persists for months. We and others have observed a significant decrease in this postimmunization gastritis following antimicrobial therapy, indicating that inflammation in "protected" mice is driven by levels of bacteria below our level of detection (ERMAK et al. 1997). We have also observed this postimmunization gastritis using the *H. pylori* mouse model (unpublished observations).

Second, the phase II clinical trial discussed above, in which *H. pylori* positive subjects were treated with an oral therapeutic vaccine consisting of *H. pylori* urease apoenzyme and *E. coli* LT did not eradicate the bacteria in any of the test subjects despite a reduction in bacterial load (MICHETTI et al. 1997). Additionally, the toxic effects of the LT were manifest in 66% of the patients, an effect which may not be of concern when administered by other routes. Third, protective prophylactic immunization against *Helicobacter* has not been accomplished in any animal model other than the mouse by this route. These models include *H. mustelae*/ferret, *H. pylori*/cat, *H. pylori*/nonhuman primates, and *H. pylori*/pigs. Thus the success observed in the mouse model might be attributed to the size of the animal, trophism of the bacteria for the tissue, or some other unknown factor. Fourth, many novel nontoxic bacterial endotoxin adjuvants retain adjuvanticity by other routes but not necessarily the stomach. Finally, it is possible that much smaller doses of both antigen and adjuvant could be administered by alternative routes.

Recently, a comprehensive study was performed comparing the immunogenicity of CT when administered by the oral, gastric, rectal, and vaginal routes (HANEBERG et al. 1994). Each delivery route stimulated an optimal response in defined mucosal tissues. Surprisingly, the best gastrointestinal response was stimulated by immunization via the rectum. In another study designed to determine the optimal route of delivery for a *Helicobacter* urease vaccine with LT, similar routes were examined (KLEANTHOUS et al. 1998). Again, rectal and intranasal delivery of the vaccine generated a better immune response and protection against challenge with *H. felis*.

The study of *Helicobacter* immunity has challenged our understanding of mucosal immunity. As discussed below, protective immunity can be achieved not only in the absence of secretory IgA, but in the absence of any immunoglobulin at all (NEDRUD et al. 1998). Such an observation forces us to consider novel effector mechanism of mucosal immunity. In their initial description of oral immunization against *H. felis* in the mouse model, CHEN et al. (1993) compared the efficacy of parenteral immunization with oral immunization. They demonstrated that despite the induction of systemic antibody by intravenous immunization, no protection was achieved. However, intraperitoneal immunization resulted in protection of 55% of the challenged mice. The success of their oral immunization, published simultaneously with a similar report by CZINN et al. (1993) and the earlier observation that systemic immunization was nonprotective in the *H. pylori*/pig model (EATON and KRAKOWKA 1992) have caused most laboratories to focus almost exclusively on oral immunization.

Recent reports however, are demonstrating that protective efficacy can be achieved by several other routes. At least three separate laboratories have successfully employed intranasal immunization to protect and/or cure mice from *H. pylori* infection. Ghiaria used their nontoxic derivative of LT, previously shown to be an effective oral adjuvant, to protect and cure mice from *H. pylori* using CagA and VacA (MARCHETTI et al. 1998). WELTZIN et al. (1997) have also demonstrated protective efficacy against challenge with *H. pylori* but were able to accomplish this using wild-type LT. In another report demonstrating an advance not only in route of administration but in delivery vehicles, CORTHESY-THEULAZ et al. (1998) gave two doses of *S. typhimurium* expressing Urease subunits A and B and achieved protection from challenge with *H. pylori*. These uniform results are encouraging and suggest a means of vaccinating humans against *H. pylori* without the problems of traversing the harsh gastric environment or inducing diarrhea. However, the extent of the protection has not been definitively determined. Although some studies have demonstrated a lack of bacteria and therefore theoretically complete protection, histology in which postchallenge inflammation is recorded has not been published.

In one of the most surprising reports a separate group was able to achieve significant reductions in bacterial load in mice challenged with *H. pylori* by systemic immunization (GUY et al. 1998). Although such results are contrary to our notion of mucosal immunity, they may indicate that our knowledge of *H. pylori* pathology needs to be reexamined. Although novel adjuvants were employed in that study our own experiments have indicated that intraperitoneal or subcutaneous injection of antigen with alum, complete Freund's adjuvant, and incomplete Freund's adjuvant are capable of inducing protective immunity against *H. felis* infection of the mouse (unpublished observations).

6 Mechanisms of Protective Immunity

6.1 Protective Immunity and the Humoral Immune Response

Although several groups are actively immunizing animals against *Helicobacter* infections, the mechanism by which protective immunity to *Helicobacter* infections is established remain largely unknown. As described above, there are many mechanisms which can contribute to adaptive immunity at the mucosal tissues. It is generally believed that antigen-specific IgA forms a protective barrier which prohibits the binding of pathogens to the mucosa. Several groups have directly addressed the role of antibodies in the protective immune response against *Helicobacter* species in animals, but preexisting *Helicobacter*-specific mucosal IgA antibodies have not been reproducibly correlated with protection from infection. To date no immunological markers which can reliably predict whether the host will be protected against challenge have been described (MICHETTI et al. 1994).

Our own studies using the *H. felis*/mouse model have indicated a potential role for antibodies in protective immunity. When IgA or IgG anti-urease monoclonal antibodies were incubated with *H. felis* prior to inoculation of mice by gastric intubation, infection was prevented (BLANCHARD et al. 1995; CZINN et al. 1993). Interestingly, IgG was as effective as IgA in preventing infection. Further evidence comes from ELISA data demonstrating that although challenge of immunized mice does not result in quantitatively higher levels of *Helicobacter*-specific antibodies in the gastric mucosa (BLANCHARD et al. 1998; SELLMAN et al. 1995) immunization prior to challenge does induce a qualitative difference in antigenic specificity. Immunoblotting analysis with samples from infected or immunized/protected mice have revealed potentially significant qualitative differences between the two groups (BLANCHARD et al. 1996).

However, our studies in gene targeted "knock out" mice indicate that cell-mediated immunity may be more important than antibodies. IgA deficient knockout mice immunized with bacterial sonicate and CT as described above can be protectively immunized using the *H. felis*/mouse model (NEDRUD et al. 1996). The oral vaccine was equally effective in the IgA knock out animals and the immunocompetent control mice. Examination of *Helicobacter*-specific antibodies in mucosal secretions revealed that immunized IgA deficient mice had high levels of *H. felis*-specific IgM in mucosal secretions. Since both IgA and IgM are polymeric immunoglobulins which can be transported into mucosal secretions by the polymeric immunoglobulin receptor, it is possible that IgM could be mediating a protective function versus *Helicobacter* infection in these mice. Our subsequent experiments in μMT antibody deficient mice have revealed that protective immunity can be achieved in the absence of any antibody (NEDRUD et al. 1998). In fact, as in our IgA knockout mice, the efficacy of vaccination was equivalent to wild-type immunocompetent control mice. Thus, while antibodies may be playing a role in protection, they are not necessary to achieve protection.

6.2 Protective Immunity and Cell-Mediated Immune Responses

Recent evidence suggests that TH2 cell-mediated immune responses may play a role in protection from infection. All of this data has been generated from immunization studies using CT or LT as a mucosal adjuvant for oral immunization. Observations supporting a role for TH2 based immunity are consistent with the known activities of mucosal adjuvants such as CT or LT of *E. coli* (HÖRNQVIST and LYCKE 1993; TAKAHASHI et al. 1996; XU-AMANO et al. 1993).

Observations in our laboratory demonstrate that in infected C57BL/6 mice (predisposed to an IFN-γ mediated immune responses) a predominantly TH1 response developed. IFN-γ levels correlated with the level of inflammation in individual mice. Additionally, the magnitude of the inflammation was reduced if mice were treated with anti-IFN-γ antibodies (MOHAMMADI et al. 1996). Of more interest was the observation that, in immunized/challenged mice, anti-IFN-γ treatment revealed the production of IL-4 by lymphocytes from immunized mice, however, indicating that immunization did induce a TH2 response (MOHAMMADI et al. 1996). Furthermore, when spleen cells from immunized/protected mice (containing IL-4 producing lymphocytes) or a *Helicobacter*-specific TH2 cell line were adoptively transferred into naive C57BL/6 recipients, there was a striking drop in bacterial load subsequent to challenge with live *H. felis* (MOHAMMADI et al. 1996). No such reduction in bacterial load was observed in mice which received cells from infected but nonimmunized animals or a TH1 cell line. The hypothesis that TH2 cells are important in bacterial clearance or protection from infection is also supported by recent experiments in gene targeted IL-4 knock out mice. *H. felis* infected IL-4 knock out mice exhibited a higher bacterial load than wild-type infected mice (MOHAMMADI et al. 1996) whereas orally immunized IL-4 deficient mice were not well protected from *H. felis* infection (RADCLIFF et al. 1996). Collectively these data point to a critical role for TH2 cells in mediating the protective effects of oral immunization versus *Helicobacter* organisms.

7 Summary

Studies in both humans and animals demonstrate that *H. pylori* is capable of illiciting an innate response that in part is regulated by the genetic makeup of the host. These innate responses includes stimulating immune effector mechanisms at the cellular and biochemical level resulting in the influx of neutrophils into the lamina propria and have even been shown to modify gastric acid secretion.

The availability of good animal models of chronic *Helicobacter* infection has also allowed investigators to begin to examine how the adaptive host immune response prevents and/or exacerbates *Helicobacter*-induced gastroduodenal disease. The experimental *H. felis*/mouse model has been utilized by a number of laboratories to investigate mechanisms of host defense against chronic *Helicobacter* infection. This model and the more recently developed *H. pylori* rodent model has not only allowed investigators to confirm the feasibility of immunotherapy to prevent and/or cure *Helicobacter* infection but also to begin to examine how the host immune response prevents and/or exacerbates *Helicobacter*-induced gastroduodenal disease.

Based on these studies a hypothesis is emerging that suggests that protection and/or cure from *Helicobacter* infection is mediated primarily by an upregulated cellular immune response which may act via an antibody independent mechanism. Paradoxically, following natural infection with *H. pylori*, a component of the cellular immune response also promotes chronic gastric inflammation without clearance of the organism. The recent development of reliable and reproducible *H. pylori*/rodent models of disease and the availability of numerous inbred strains, transgenic and knockout animals, will allow investigators to continue to explore the role the host cellullar and humoral immune response plays in promoting or preventing this infection.

References

Appelmelk BJ, Simoons-Smit I, Negrini R, Moran AP, Aspinall GO, Forete JG, De Vries T, Quan H, Verboom T, Maaskant JJ, Ghiara P, Kuipers EJ, Bloemena E, Tadema TM, Townsend RR, Tyagarajan K, Crothers JMJ, Monteiro MA, Savio A, De Graaff J (1996) Potential role of molecular mimicry between *Helicobacter pylori* lipopolysaccharide and host Lewis blood group antigens in autoimmunity. Infect Immun 64:2031
Aspinall GO, Monteiro MA, Pang H, Walsh EJ, Moran AP (1996) Lipopolysaccharide of the *Helicobacter pylori* type strain NCTC 11637 (ATCC 43504): structure of the O antigen and core oligosaccharide regions. Biochemistry 35:2489
Azuma T, Ito S, Sato F, Yamazaki Y, Miyaji H, Ito Y, Suto H, Kuriyama M, Kato T, Kohli Y (1998) The role of the HLA-DQA1 gene in resistance to atrophic gastritis and gastric adenocarcinoma induced by *Helicobacter pylori* infection. Cancer 82:1013
Azuma T, Ito Y, Miyaji H, Dojyo M, Tanaka Y, Hirai M, Ito S, Kato T, Kohli Y (1995) Immunogenetic analysis of the human leukocyte antigen DQA1 locus in patients with duodenal ulcer or chronic atrophic gastritis harbouring *Helicobacter pylori*. Eur J Gastroenterol Hepatol 7[Suppl 1]:S71
Beales IL, Calam J (1997) *Helicobacter pylori* stimulates granulocyte-macrophage colony-stimulating factor (GM-CSF) production from cultured antral biopsies and a human gastric epithelial cell line. Eur J Gastroenterol Hepatol 9:451
Bell GD, Powell K, Burridge SM, Pallecaros A, Jones PH, Gant PW, Harrison G, Trowell JE (1992) Experience with 'triple' anti-*Helicobacter* eradication therapy: side effects and the importance of testing the pre-treatment bacterial isolate for metronidazole resistance. Aliment Pharmacol Ther 6:427

Berstad AE, Brandtzaeg P, Stave R, Halstensen TS (1997) Epithelium related deposition of activated complement in *Helicobacter pylori* associated gastritis. Gut 40:196

Birkholz S, Knipp U, Opferkuch W (1993) Stimulatory effects of *Helicobacter pylori* on human peripheral blood mononuclear cells of *H. pylori* infected patients and healthy blood donors. Zentralbl Bakteriol 280:166

Blanchard TG, Czinn SJ, Maurer R, Thomas WD, Soman G, Nedrud JG (1995) Urease-specific monoclonal antibodies prevent *Helicobacter felis* infection in mice. Infect Immun 63:1394

Blanchard TG, Lycke N, Czinn SJ, Nedrud JG (1998) Recombinant cholera toxin B subunit is not an effective mucosal adjuvant for oral immunization of mice against *H. felis*. Immunology 94:22

Blanchard TG, Nedrud JG, Czinn SJ (1996) Qualitative and quantitative differences in the local immune response to *Helicobacter* in mice and humans following immunization or infection. Gastroenterology 110:A867

Blanchard TG, Nedrud JG, Reardon E, Czinn SJ (1998) Qualitative and quantitative analysis of the local and systemic antibody responses in mice and humans with *Helicobacter* immunity and infection (submitted for publication)

Bodger K, Crabtree JE (1998) *Helicobacter pylori* and gastric inflammation. Br Med Bull 54:139

Bodger K, Wyatt JI, Heatley RV (1997) Gastric mucosal secretion of interleukin-10: relations to histopathology, *Helicobacter pylori* status, and tumour necrosis factor-alpha secretion. Gut 40:739

Burnette WN, Mar VL, Platler BW, Schlotterbeck JD, McGinley MD, Stoney KS, Rohde MF, Kaslow HR (1991) Site-specific mutagenesis of the catalytic subunit of cholera toxin: substituting lysine for arginine 7 causes loss of activity. Infect Immun 59:4266

Chen M, Lee A, Hazell S (1992) Immunisation against gastric helicobacter infection in a mouse/*Helicobacter felis* model. Lancet 339:1120

Chen M, Lee A, Hazell S, Hu P, Li Y (1993) Immunisation against gastric infection with *Helicobacter* species: first step in the prophylaxis of gastric cancer? Zentralbl Bakteriol 280:155

Cieplak WJ, Mead DJ, Messer RJ, Grant CCR (1995) Site-directed mutagenic alteration of potential active-site residues of the A subunit of *Escherichia coli* Heat-labile enterotoxin. J Biol Chem 270:30545

Correa P (1992) Human gastric carcinogenesis: a multistep and multifactorial process-first American Cancer Society award lecture on cancer epidemiology and prevention. Cancer Res 52:6735

Corthesy-Theulaz I, Porta N, Glauser M, Saraga E, Vaney A-C, Haas R, Kraehenbuhl JP, Blum AL, Michetti P (1995) Oral immunization with *Helicobacter pylori* urease B subunit as a treatment against *Helicobacter* infection in mice. Gastroenterology 109:115

Corthesy-Theulaz IE, Hopkins S, Bachmann D, Saldinger PF, Porta N, Haas R, Zheng-Xin Y, Meyer T, Bouzourene H, Blum AL, Kraehenbuhl JP (1998) Mice are protected from *Helicobacter pylori* infection by nasal immunization with attenuated Salmonella typhimurium phoPc expressing urease A and B subunits. Infect Immun 66:581

Crabtree JE (1996) Gastric mucosal inflammatory responses to *Helicobacter pylori*. Aliment Pharmacol Ther 10[Suppl 1]:29

Crabtree JE, Taylor JD, Wyatt JI, Heatley RV, Shallcross TM, Tompkins DS, Rathbone BJ (1991) Mucosal IgA recognition of *Helicobacter pylori* 120 kDa protein, peptic ulceration, and gastric pathology. Lancet 338:332

Crabtree JE, Wyatt JI, Trejdosiewicz LK, Peichl P, Nichols PH, Ramsay N, Primrose JN, Lindley IJD (1994) Interleukin-8 expression in *Helicobacter pylori* infected, normal, and neoplastic gastroduodenal mucosa. J Clin Pathol 47:61

Crabtree JE, Xiang Z, Lindley IJD, Tompkins DS, Rappuoli R, Covacci A (1995) Induction of interleukin-8 secretion from gastric epithelial cells by a cagA negative isogenic mutant of *Helicobacter pylori*. J Clin Pathol 48:967

Cuenca R, Blanchard TG, Czinn SJ, Nedrud JG, Monath TP, Lee CK, Redline RW (1996) Therapeutic immunization against *Helicobacter mustelae* infection in naturally infected ferrets. Gastroenterology 110:1770

Czinn S, Cai A, Nedrud J (1992) Oral immunization protects germ-free mice against infection from *Helicobacter felis*. Gastroenterology 102:A611

Czinn SJ, Bierman JC, Diters RW, Blanchard TJ, Leunk RD (1996) Characterization and therapy for experimental infection by *Helicobacter mustelae* in ferrets. Helicobacter 1:43

Czinn SJ, Cai A, Nedrud JG (1993) Protection of germ-free mice from infection by *Helicobacter felis* after active oral or passive IgA immunization. Vaccine 11:637

Czinn SJ, Carr H (1987) Rapid diagnosis of *Campylobacter pyloridis*-associated gastritis. J Pediatr 110:569

Czinn SJ, Carr H, Sheffler L, Aronoff S (1989) Serum IgG antibody to the outer membrane proteins of *Campylobacter pylori* in children with gastroduodenal disease. J Infect Dis 159:586

Czinn SJ, Nedrud JG (1991) Oral immunization against *Helicobacter pylori*. Infect Immun 59:2359

D'Elios MM, Manghetti M, Almerigogna F, Amedei A, Costa F, Burroni D, Baldari CT, Romagnani S, Telford JL, Del Prete G (1997) Different cytokine profile and antigen-specificity repertoire in *Helicobacter pylori*-specific T cell clones from the antrum of chronic gastritis patients with or without peptic ulcer. Eur J Immunol 27:1751

D'Elios MM, Manghetti M, De Carli M, Costa F, Baldari CT, Burroni D, Telford JL, Romagnani S, Del Prete G (1997) T helper 1 effector cells specific for *Helicobacter pylori* in the gastric antrum of patients with peptic ulcer disease. J Immunol 158:962

Di Tommaso A, Xiang Z, Bugnoli M, Pileri P, Figura N, Bayeli PF, Rappuoli R, Abrignani S, De Magistris MT (1995) *Helicobacter pylori*-specific CD4[1] T-cell clones from peripheral blood and gastric biopsies. Infect Immun 63:1102

Dickinson BL, Clements JD (1995) Dissociation of Escherichia coli heat-labile enterotoxin adjuvanticity from ADP-ribosyltransferase activity. Infect Immun 63:1617

Ding SZ, Cho CH, Lam SK (1997) *Helicobacter pylori* induces interleukin-8 expression in endothelial cells and the signal pathway is protein tyrosine kinase dependent. Biochem Biophys Res Commun 240:561

Doidge C, Gust I, Lee A, Buck F, Hazell S, Manne U (1994) Therapeutic immunization against *Helicobacter* infection (letter). Lancet 343:913

Douce G, Trucotte C, Cropley I, Roberts M, Pizza M, Domenighini M, Rappuoli R, Dougan G (1995) Mutants of *Escherichia coli* heat labile toxin lacking ADP-ribosyltransferase activity act as nontoxic, mucosal adjuvants. Proc Natl Acad Sci USA 92:1644

Eaton KA, Brooks CL, Morgan DR, Krakowka S (1991) Essential role of urease in pathogenesis of gastritis induced by *Helicobacter pylori* in gnotobiotic piglets. Infect Immun 59:2470

Eaton KA, Krakowka S (1992) Chronic active gastritis due to *Helicobacter pylori* in immunized Gnotobiotic piglets. Gastroenterology 103:1580

Elson CO, Dertzbaugh MT (1994) Mucosal adjuvants. In: Ogra PL, Mestecky J, E LM, Strober W, McGhee JR, Bienenstock J (eds) Handbook of mucosal immunology, San Diego

Ermak TH, Ding R, Ekstein B, Hill J, Myers GA, Lee CK, Pappo J, Kleanthous HK, Monath TP (1997) Gastritis in urease-immunized mice after *Helicobacter felis* challenge may be due to residual bacteria. Gastroenterology 113:1118

Fan XJ, Chua A, O'Connell MA, Kelleher D, Keeling PWN (1993) Interferon-gamma and tumour necrosis factor production in patients with *Helicobacter pylori* infection. Ir J Med Sci 162:408

Fan XJ, Chua A, Shahi CN, McDevitt J, Keeling PWN, Kelleher D (1994) Gastric T lymphocyte responses to *Helicobacter pylori* colonisation. Gut 35:1379

Ferrero RL, Thiberge J-M, Huerre M, Labigne A (1994) Recombinant antigens prepared from the urease subunits of *Helicobacter* spp: evidence of protection in a mouse model of gastric infection. Infect Immun 62:4981

Ferrero RL, Thiberge J-M, Kansau I, Wuscher N, Huerre M, Labigne A (1995) The groES homolog of *Helicobacter pylori* confers protective immunity against mucosal infection in mice. Proc Natl Acad Sci USA 92:6499

Fox JG (1988) Systemic diseases. In: Fox JG (ed) Biology and diseases of the ferret, Philadelphia

Fox JG, Batchelder M, Hayward A, Yan L, Palley L, Murphy JC, Shames B (1994) Prior *Helicobacter mustelae* infection does not confer protective immunity against experimental reinfection in ferrets. Am J Gastroenterol 89:1318

Fox JG, Cabot EB, Taylor NS, Laraway R (1988) Gastric colonization by *Campylobacter pylori* subsp *mustelae* in ferrets. Infect Immun 56:2994

Fox JG, Correa P, Taylor NS, Lee A, Otto G, Murphy JC, Rose R (1990) *Helicobacter mustelae*-associated gastritis in ferrets: an animal model of *Helicobacter pylori* gastritis in humans. Gastroenterology 99:352

Fox JG, Otto G, Taylor NS, Rosenblad W, Murphy JC (1991) *Helicobacter mustelae*-induced gastritis and elevated gastric pH in the ferret (Mustela putorius furo). Infect Immun 59:1875

Ghiara P, Rossi M, Marchetti M, Di Tommaso A, Vindigni C, Ciampolini F, Covacci A, Telford JL, De Magistris MT, Pizza M, Rappuoli R, Del Giudice G (1997) Therapeutic intragastric vaccination against *Helicobacter pylori* in mice eradicates an otherwise chronic infection and confers protection against reinfection. Infect Immun 65:4996

Gomez-Duarte OG, Lucas B, Yan ZX, Panthel K, Haas R, Meyer TF (1998) Protection of mice against gastric colonization by *Helicobacter pylori* by single oral dose immunization with attenuated Salmonella typhimurium producing urease subunits A and B. Vaccine 16:460

Graham DY (1997) *Helicobacter pylori* infection in the pathogenesis of duodenal ulcer and gastric cancer: a model. Gastroenterology 113:1983

Guruge JL, Falk PG, Lorenz RG, Dans M, Wirth HP, Blaser MJ, Berg DE, Gordon JI (1998) Epithelial attachment alters the outcome of *Helicobacter pylori* infection. Proc Natl Acad Sci USA 95:3925

Guy B, Hessler C, Fourage S, Haensler J, Vialon-Lafay E, Rokbi B, Millet M-JQ (1998) Systemic immunizatin with urease protects mice against *Heliocbacter pylori* infection. Vaccine 16:850

Haeberle HA, Kubin M, Bamford KB, Garofalo R, Graham DY, El-Zaatari F, Karttunen R, Crowe SE, Reyes VE, Ernst PB (1997) Differential Stimulation of Interleukin-12 and IL-10 by live and killed *Helicobacter pylori* in vitro and association of IL-12 production with gamma interferon-producing T cells in the human gastric mucosa. Infect Immun 65:4229

Hajishengallis G, Hollingshead SK, Koga T, Russell MW (1995) Mucosal immunization with a bacterial protein antigen genetically coupled to cholera toxin A2/B subunits. J Immunol 154:4322

Haneberg B, Kendall D, Amerongen HM, Apter FM, Kraehenbuhl J-P, Neutra MR (1994) Induction of specific immunoglobulin A in the small intestine, colon-rectum, and vagina measured by a new method for collection of secretions from mucosal surfaces. Infect Immun 62:15

Hashigucci K, Ogawa H, Ishidate T, Yamashita R, Kamiya H, Watanabe K, Hattori N, Sato T, Suzuki Y, Nagamine T, Aizawa C, Tamura S, Kurata T, Oya A (1996) Antibody responses in volunteers induced by nasal influenza vaccine combined with *Escherichia coli* heat-labile enterotoxin B subunit containing a trace amount of the holotoxin. Vaccine 14:113

Holmgren J, Lycke N, Czerkinsky C (1993) Cholera toxin and cholera B subunit as oral-mucosal adjuvant and antigen vector systems. Vaccine 11:1179

Hörnqvist E, Lycke N (1993) Cholera toxin adjuvant greatly promotes antigen priming of T cells. Eur J Immunol 23:2136

Hu L-T, Mobley LT (1990) Purification and N-terminal analysis of urease from *Helicobacter pylori*. Infect Immun 58:992

Isaacson P (1982) Immunoperoxidase study of the secretory Immoglobulin system and lysozyme in normal and diseased gastric mucosa. Gut 23:578

Jones DM, Eldridge J, Fox AJ, Sethi P, Whorwell PJ (1986) Antibody to the gastric campylobacter-like organism (*"Campylobacter pyloridis"*) – clinical correlations and distribution in the normal population. J Med Microbiol 22:57

Jorgensen M, Daskalopoulos G, Warburton V, Mitchell HM, Hazell SL (1996) Multiple strain colonization and metronidazole resistance in *Helicobacter pylori*-infected patients: identification from sequential and multiple biopsy specimens. J Infect Dis 174:631

Jung HC, Kim JM, Song IS, Kim CY (1997) *Helicobacter pylori* induces an array of pro-inflammatory cytokines in human gastric epithelial cells: quantification of mRNA for interleukin-8, -1 alpha/beta, granulocyte-macrophage colony-stimulating factor, monocyte chemoattractant protein-1 and tumour necrosis factor-alpha. J Gastroenterol Hepatol 12:473

Karita M, Li Q, Cantero D, Okita K (1994) Establishment of a small animal model for human *Helicobacter pylori* infection using germ-free mouse. Am J Gastroenterol 89:208

Karttunen R, Andersson G, Poiikonen K, Kosunen TU, Karttunen T, Juutinen K, Niemela S (1990) *Helicobacter pylori* induces lymphocyte activation in peripheral blood cultures. Clin Exp Immunol 82:485

Karttunen R, Karttunen T, Ekre H-PT, MacDonald TT (1995) Interferon gamma and interleukin 4 secreting cells in the gastric antrum in *Helicobacter pylori* positive and negative gastritis. Gut 36:341

Karttunen RA, Karttunen TJ, Yousfi MM, El-Zimaity H, Graham DY, El-Zaatari F (1997) Expression of mRNA for interferon-gamma, interleukin-10, and interleukin-12 (p40) in normal gastric mucosa and in mucosa infected with *Helicobacter pylori*. Scand J Gastroenterol 32:22

Keates S, Hitti YS, Upton M, Kelly CP (1997) *Helicobacter pylori* infection activates NF-kappa B in gastric epithelial cells. Gastroenterology 113:1099

Kirkland T, Viriyakosol S, Perez-Perez GI, Blaser MJ (1997) *Helicobacter pylori* lipolysaccharide can activate 70Z/3 cells via CD14. Infect Immun 65:604

Kist M (1991) Immunology of *Helicobacter pylori*. In: Marshall BJ, McCallum RW, Guerrant RL (eds) *Helicobacter pylori* in peptic ulceration and gastritis, Boston

Kleanthous H, Myers GA, Georgakopoulos KM, Tibbitts TJ, Ingrassia JW, Gray HL, Ding R, Zhang ZZ, Lei W, Nichols R, Lee CK, Ermak TH, Monath TP (1998) Rectal and intranasal immunizations with recombinant urease induce distinct local and serum immune responses in mice and protect against *Helicobacter pylori* infection. Infect Immun 66:2879

Kluge A, Mielke M, Volkheimer G, Niedobitek F, Hahn H (1993) Role of the systemic cellular immune response in the pathogenesis of *Helicobacter pylori*-associated duodenal ulcer. Zentralbl Bakteriol 280:177

Kraehenbuhl JP, Neutra M (1992) Molecular and cellular basis of immune protection of mucosal surfaces. Physiol Rev 72:853

Kreiss C, Buclin T, Cosma M, Corthesy-Theulaz I, Michetti P (1996) Safety of oral immunisation with recombinant urease in patients with *Helicobacter pylori* infection (letter). Lancet 347:1630

Kuipers EJ, Lundell L, Klinkenberg-Knol EC, Havu N, Festen HP, Liedman B, Lamers CB, Jansen JB, Dalenback J, Snel P, Nelis GF, Meuwissen SG (1996) Atrophic gastritis and *Helicobacter pylori* infection in patients with reflux esophagitis treated with omeprazole or fundoplication. N Engl J Med 334:1018

Kutukculer N, Aydogdu S, Goksen D, Caglayan S, Yagcyi RV (1997) Increased mucosal inflammatory cytokines in children with *Helicobacter pylori*-associated gastritis. Acta Paediatr 86:928

Langenberg W, Rauws EAJ, Oudbier JH (1990) Patient-to-patient transmission of *Campylobacter pylori* infection by fiberoptic gastroduodenoscopy and biopsy. J Infect Dis 161:507

Lee A, Chen M (1994) Successful immunization against gastric infection with *Helicobacter* species: use of a cholera toxin B-subunit-whole-cell vaccine. Infect Immun 62:3594

Lee A, Dixon MF, Danon SJ, Kuipers E, Megraud F, Larsson H, Mellgard B (1995) Local acid production and *Helicobacter pylori*: a unifying hypothesis of gastroduodenal disease. Eur J Gastroenterol Hepatol 7:461

Lee A, Fox JG, Otto G, Murphy J (1990) A small animal model of human *Helicobacter pylori* active chronic gastritis. Gastroenterology 99:1315

Lee A, O'Rourke J, De Ungria MC, Robertson B, Daskalopoulos G, Dixon MF (1997) A standardised mouse model of *Helicobacter pylori* infection. Introducing the Sydney strain. Gastroenterology 112:1386

Lee CK, Weltzin R, Thomas WDJ, Kleanthous H, Ermak TH, Soman G, Hill JE, Ackerman SK, Monath TP (1995) Oral Immunization with recombinant *Helicobacter pylori* urease induces secretory IgA antibodies and protects mice from challenge with *Helicobacter felis*. J Infect Dis 172:161

Lee JE, Lowy AM, Thompson WA, Lu M, Loflin PT, Skibber JM, Evans DB, Curley SA, Mansfield PF, Reveille JD (1996) Association of gastric adenocarcinoma with the HLA class II gene DQB1 * 0301. Gastroenterology 111:426

Liang X, Lamm ME, Nedrud JG (1989) Cholera toxin as a mucosal adjuvant for respiratory antibody responses in mice. Reg Immunol 2:244

Malaty HM, Engstrand L, Pedersen NL, Graham DY (1994) *Helicobacter pylori* infection: genetic and environmental influences. A study of twins. Ann Intern Med 120:982

Marchetti M, Arico B, Burroni D, Figura N, Rappuoli R, Ghiara P (1995) Development of a mouse model of *Helicobacter pylori* infection that mimics human disease. Science 267:1655

Marchetti M, Rossi M, Giannelli V, Giuliani MM, Pizza M, Censini S, Covacci A, Massari P, Pagliaccia C, Manetti R, Telford JL, Douce G, Dougan G, Rappuoli R, Ghiara P (1998) Protection against *Helicobacter pylori* infection in mice by intragastric vaccination with *H. pylori* antigens is achieved using a non-toxic mutant of *E. coli* heat-labile enterotoxin (LT) as adjuvant. Vaccine 16:33

Marshall BJ, McGechie DB, Francis GJ, Utley PJ (1984) Pyloric campylobacter serology. Lancet ii:281

Mazanec MB, Nedrud JG, Kaetzel CS, Lamm ME (1993) A three-tiered view of IgA's role in mucosal defense. Immunol Today 14:430

McColm AA, Bagshaw J, Wallis J, McLaren A (1995) Screening of anti-*Helicobacter* therapies in mice colonized with H. *pylori*. Gut 37:A92

McKenzie SJ, Halsey JF (1984) Cholera toxin B subunit as a carrier protein to stimulate a mucosal immune response. J Immunol 133:1818

Megraud F (1997) Resistance of *Helicobacter pylori* to antibiotics. Aliment Pharmacol Ther 11 [Suppl1]: 43

Mestecky J, McGhee JR (1987) Immunoglobulin A (IgA): molecular and cellular interactions involved in IgA biosynthesis and immune response. Adv Immunol 40:153

Michalek SM, McGhee JR, Mestecky J, Arnold RR, Bozzo L (1976) Ingestion of Streptococcus mutants induces secretory immunoglobulin A and carries immunity. Science 192:1238

Michetti P, Corthesy-Thelaz I, Davin C, Haas R, Vaney A-C, Heitz M, Bille J, Kraehenbuhl JP, Saraga E, Blum AL (1994) Immunization of Balb/c mice against *Helicobacter felis* infection with *Helicobacter pylori* urease. Gastroenterology 107:1002

Michetti P, Kreiss C, Kotloff K, Porta N, Blanco JL, Bachman D, Sadlinger PF, Corthesy-Theulaz I, Losonsky G, Nichols R, Stolte M, Monath T, Ackerman S, Blum A (1997) Oral immunization of *H. pylori* infected adults with recombinant urease and LT adjuvant (abstract). Gastroenterology 112:A1042

Mohammadi M, Czinn S, Redline R, Nedrud J (1996a) *Helicobacter*-specific cell-mediated immune responses display a predominant TH1 phenotype and promote a DTH response in the stomachs of mice. J Immunol 156:4729

Mohammadi M, Nedrud J, Czinn S (1996b) IL-12 treatment induces susceptibility to *Helicobacter*-associated gastritis in the resistant BALB/c mouse strain (abstract). Gut 39[Suppl 2]:A59

Mohammadi M, Nedrud J, Redline R, Lycke N, Czinn S (1997) Murine CD4 T cell responses to *Helicobacter* infection: TH1 cells enhance gastritis and TH2 cells reduce bacterial load. Gastroenterology 113:1848

Mohammadi M, Redline R, Nedrud J, Czinn S (1996) Role of the host in pathogenesis of *Helicobacter*-associated gastritis: *H. felis* infection of inbred and congenic mouse strains. Infect Immun 64:238

Montgomery PC, Ayyildiz A, Lemaitre-Coelho IM, Vaerman J-P, Rockey JH (1983) Induction and expression of antibodies in secretions: the ocular immune system. Ann NY Acad Sci 409:428

Moss SF, Calam J (1993) Acid secretion and sensitivity to gastrin in patients with duodenal ulcer: effect of eradication of *Helicobacter pylori*. Gut 34:888

Moss SF, Legon S, Davies J, Calam J (1994) Cytokine gene expression in *Helicobacter pylori* associated antral gastritis. Gut 35:1567

Munzenmaier A, Lange C, Glocker E, Covacci A, Moran A, Bereswill S, Baeuerle PA, Kist M, Pahl HL (1997) A secreted/shed product of *Helicobacter pylori* activates transcription factor nuclear factor-kappa B. J Immunol 159:6140

Muotiala A, Helander IM, Pyhälä L, Kosunen TU, Moran AP (1992) Low biological activity of *Helicobacter pylori* lipopolysaccharide. Infect Immun 60:1714

Nedrud J, Blanchard T, Czinn S, Harriman G (1996) Orally-immunized IgA deficient mice are protected against *H. felis* infection (abstract). Gut 39[Suppl 2]:A45

Nedrud JG, Blanchard TG, Redline R, Sigmund N, Czinn SJ (1998) Orally immunized μMT antibody-deficient mice are protected against *H. felis* infection (abstract). Gastroenterology 114:A1049

Nedrud JG, Liang X, Hague N, Lamm ME (1987) Combined oral/nasal immunization protects mice from Sendai virus infection. J Immunol 139:3484

Negrini R, Lisato L, Zanella I, Cavazzini L, Gullini S, Villanacci V, Poiesi C, Albertini A, Ghielmi S (1991) *Helicobacter pylori* infection induces antibodies cross-reacting with human gastric mucosa. Gastroenterology 101:437

Nichols RL, Murray ES, Nisson PE (1978) Use of enteric vaccines in protection against chlamydial infections of the genital tract and the eye of guinea pigs. J Infect Dis 138:742

Palley LS, Murphy J, Yan Y, Taylor N, Polidoro D, Fox J (1993) The effects of an oral immunization scheme using muramyl dipeptide as an adjuvant to prevent gastric *Helicobacter mustelae* infection of ferrets. Acta Gastroenterol Belg 56[Suppl]:54

Peek RM, Miller GG, Tham KT, Perez-Perez GI, Zhao X, Atherton JC, Blaser MJ (1995) Heightened inflammatory response and cytokine expression in vivo to cagA+ *Helicobacter pylori* strains. Lab Invest 73:760

Perez-Perez GI, Shepherd VL, Morrow JD, Blaser MJ (1995) Activation of human THP-1 cells and rat bone marrow-derived macrophages by *Helicobacter pylori* lipopolysaccharide. Infect Immun 63:1183

Peterson WL, Barnett CC, Evans DJ Jr, Feldman M, Carmody T, Richardson C, Walsh J, Graham DY (1993) Acid secretion and serum gastrin in normal subjects and patients with duodenal ulcer: the role of *Helicobacter pylori*. Am J Gastroenterol 88:2038

Radcliff FJ, Chen M, Lee A (1996) Protective immunization against *Helicobacter* stimulates long-term immunity. Vaccine 14:780

Radcliff FJ, Hazell SL, Kolesnikow T, Doidge C, Lee A (1997) Catalase, a novel antigen for *Helicobacter pylori* vaccination. Infect Immun 65:4668

Radcliff FJ, Ramsay AJ, Lee A (1996) Failure of immunisation against *Helicobacter* infection in IL-4 deficient mice: evidence for a TH2 immune response as the basis for protective immunity. Gastroenterology 110:A997

Rathbone BJ, Wyatt JI, Worsley BW, Shires SE, Trejdosiewicz LK, Heatley RV, Losowsky MS (1986) Systematic and local antibody responses to gastric *Campylobacter pyloridis* in non-ulcer dyspepsia. Gut 27:642

Rauws EAJ (1993) Reasons for failure of *Helicobacter pylori* treatment. Eur J Gastroenterol Hepatol 5[Suppl 2]:S92

Rieder G, Hatz RA, Moran AP, Walz A, Stolte M, Enders G (1997) Role of adherence in interleukin-8 induction in *Helicobacter pylori*-associated gastritis. Infect Immun 65:3622

Sakagami T, Dixon M, O'Rourke J, Howlett R, Alderuccio F, Vella J, Shimoyama T, Lee A (1996) Atrophic gastric changes in both H. *felis* and H. *pylori* infected mice are host dependent and seperate from antral gastritis. Gut 39:639

Sakagami T, Vella J, Dixon MF, O'Rourke J, Radcliff F, Sutton P, Shimoyama T, Beagley K, Lee A (1997) The endotoxin of *Helicobacter pylori* is a modulator of host-dependent gastritis. Infect Immun 65:3310

Segal ED, Falkow S, Tompkins LS (1996) *Helicobacter pylori* attachment to gastric cells induces cytoskeltal rearrangements and tyrosine phosphorylation of host cell proteins. Proc Natl Acad Sci USA 93:1259

Segal ED, Lange C, Covacci A, Tompkins LS, Falkow S (1997) Induction of host signal transduction pathways by *Helicobacter pylori*. Proc Natl Acad Sci USA 94:7595

Sellman S, Blanchard TG, Nedrud JG, Czinn SJ (1995) Vaccine Strategies for prevention of *Helicobacter pylori* infections. Eur J Gastroenterol Hepatol 7[Suppl 1]:S1

Sharma SA, Miller GG, Perez-Perez GI, Gupta RS, Blaser MJ (1994) Humoral and cellular immune recognition of *Helicobacter pylori* proteins are not concordant. Clin Exp Immunol 97:126

Sharma SA, Tummuru MKR, Blaser MJ, Kerr LD (1998) Activation of IL-8 gene expression by *Helicobacter pylori* is regulated by transcription factor nuclear factor-B in gastric epithelial cells. J Immunol 160:2401

Sharma SA, Tummuru MR, Miller GG, Blaser MJ (1995) Interleukin-8 response of gastric epithelial cell lines to *Helicobacter pylori* stimulation in vitro. Infect Immun 63:1681

Simoons Smit IM, Appelmelk BJ, Verboom T, Negrini R, Penner J, Aspinall G, Moran A, Fei S, Shi B, Rudnica W, Savio A, de Graaff J (1996) Typing of *Helicobacter pylori* with monoclonal antibodies against Lewis antigens in lipopolysaccharide. J Clin Microbiol 34:2196

Soll AH (1996) Medical treatment of peptic ulcers disease: practice guidelines. J Am Med Assoc 275:622

Spangler BD (1992) Structure and function of cholera toxin and the related *Escherichia coli* heat-labile enterotoxin. Microbiol Rev 56:622

Takahashi I, Marinaro M, Kiyono H, Jackson RJ, Nakagawa I, Fujihashi K, Hamada S, Clements JD, Bost KL, McGhee JR (1996) Mechanisms for mucosal immunogenicity and adjuvancy of *Escherichia coli* labile enterotoxin. J Infect Dis 173:627

Tamura S-i, Yamanaka A, Shimohara M, Tomita T, Komase K, Tsuda Y, Suzuki Y, Nagamine T, Kawahara K, Danbara H, Aizawa C, Oya A, Kurata T (1994) Synergistic action of cholera toxin B subunit (and *Escherichia coli* heat-labile toxin B subunit) and a trace amount of cholera whole toxin as an adjuvant for nasal influenza vaccine. Vaccine 12:419

Tosi MF, Sorensen RU, Czinn SJ (1992) Cell-mediated immune responsiveness to *Helicobacter pylori* in healthy seropositive and seronegative adults. Immunol Infect Dis 2:133

Tummuru MK, Sharma SA, Blaser MJ (1995) *Helicobacter pylori* picB, a homolog of the *Bordetella pertussis* toxin secretion protein, is required for induction of IL-8 in gastric epithelial cells. Mol Microbiol 18:867

Valnes K, Brandtzaeg P, Elgjo K, Stave R (1984) Specific and nonspecific humoral defense factors in the epithelium of normal and inflamed gastric mucosa. Gastroenterology 86:402

Valnes K, Huitfeldt HS, Brandtzaeg P (1990) Relation between T cell number and epithelial HLA class II expression quantified by image analysis in normal and inflamed human gastric mucosa. Gut 31:647

Van der Ende A, Van der Hulst RWM, Dankert J, Tytgat GNJ (1997) Reinfection versus recrudescence in *Helicobacter pylori* infection. Aliment Pharmacol Ther 11:55

Walsh JH, Peterson WL (1995) The treatment of *Helicobacter pylori* infection in the management of peptic ulcer disease. N Engl J Med 333:984

Wang TC, Goldenring JR, Dangler C, Ito S, Mueller A, Jeon WK, Koh TJ, Fox JG (1998) Mice lacking secretory phospholipase A2 show altered apoptosis and differentiation with *Helicobacter felis* infection. Gastroenterology 114:675

Warren JR, Marshall BJ (1983) Unidentified curved bacilli on gastric epithelium in active chronic gastritis. Lancet i:1273

Weltzin R, Kleanthous H, Guirdkhoo F, Monath TP, Lee CK (1997) Novel intranasal immunization techniques for antibody induction and protection of mice against gastric *Helicobacter felis* infection. Vaccine 15:370

Whary MT, Palley LS, Batchelder M, Murphy JC, Yan L, Taylor NS, Fox JG (1997) Promotion of ulcerative duodenitis in young ferrets by oral immunization with *Helicobacter mustelae* and muramyl dipeptide. *Helicobacter* 2:65

Wilson AD, Clarke CJ, Stokes CR (1990) Whole cholera toxin and B subunit act synergistically as an adjuvant for the mucosal immune response of mice to keyhole limpet haemocyanin. Scand J Immunol 31:443

Wirth H-P, Yang M, Karita M, Blaser MJ (1996) Expression of the human cell surface glycoconjugates Lewis X and Lewis Y by *Helicobacter pylori* isolates is related to cagA status. Infect Immun 64:4598

Xu-Amano J, Kiyono H, Jackson R, Staats HF, Fujihashi K, Burrows PD, Elson CO, Pillai S, McGhee JR (1993) Helper T cell subsets for Immunoglobulin A responses: oral immunization with tetanus toxoid and cholera toxin as adjuvant selectively induces Th2 cells in mucosa associated tissues. J Exp Med 178:1309

Yamamoto S, Takeda Y, Yamamoto M, Kurazono H, Imaoka K, Yamamoto M, Fujihashi K, Noda M, Kiyono H, McGhee JR (1997) Mutants in the ADP-ribosyltransferase cleft of cholera toxin lack diarrheagenicity but retain adjuvanticity. J Exp Med 185:1203

Yamaoka Y, Kita M, Kodama T, Sawai N, Imanishi J (1996) *Helicobacter pylori* cagA gene and expression of cytokine messenger RNA in gastric mucosa. Gastroenterology 110:1744

Yamaoka Y, Kita M, Kodama T, Sawai N, Kashima K, Imanishi J (1995) Expression of cytokine mRNA in gastric mucosa with *Helicobacter pylori* infection. Scand J Gastroenterol 30:1153

Yamaoka Y, Kita M, Kodama T, Sawai N, Kashima K, Imanishi J (1997) Induction of various cytokines and development of severe mucosal inflammation by cagA gene positive *Helicobacter pylori* strains. Gut 41:442

Diagnosis of *Helicobacter pylori* Infection

T.U. Westblom and B.D. Bhatt

1 Introduction

Success in diagnosing a disease depends to a large extent upon the choice of diagnostic techniques. Nowhere is this more obvious than in the case of gastroduodenal infection with *Helicobacter pylori*. *H. pylori* had been observed in the gastric mucosa by several independent investigators since the beginning of the twentieth century (Krienitz 1906; Luger and Neuberger 1921; Doenges 1939; Freedberg and Barron 1940), yet its existance was often doubted by the experts of the time. In 1954 Palmer reported a large study of more than 1000 patients undergoing suction biopsies of their stomachs. Palmer had specifically looked for the "spirochetes" observed by others, but found none and concluded that these organisms were just "simple contamination of the mucosal surface by swallowed spirochetes." Palmer missed the opportunity to discover *H. pylori* by using an inappropriate diagnostic test. He stained his biopsies with the commonly used H&E stain. This

Department of Internal Medicine, College of Medicine, Texas A&M University, Central Texas Veterans Health Care System, Temple, Texas, USA stain is excellent for displaying tissue morphology but can be a relatively poor stain for visualizing *H. pylori*. Twenty-five years later WARREN in Australia was studying gastric mucosa using a Warthin-Starry silver stain (MARSHALL 1989). This stain shows the bacteria very well, and soon he and MARSHALL surprised the scientific community by reporting the presence of "unidentified curved bacilli on gastric epithelium in active chronic gastritis" (WARREN and MARSHALL 1983).

Since the first successful isolation of *H. pylori* (MARSHALL et al. 1984) multiple tests have become available to determine whether a patient is infected with the organism. Initially they all required invasive procedures such as endoscopy and mucosal biopsy. Although combinations of histology, culture, and/or rapid urease tests still may be considered the gold standard, they suffer from being labor intensive and expensive. Depending on the clinical situation they may also be unnecessarily invasive, particularly for patients who have become asymptomatic following antibiotic treatment. Noninvasive tests offer convenience and lower costs but have the drawback of being only indirect measures of the presence of *H. pylori*. There may also be limitations to their usefulness, such as in the case of serology, which loses its specificity in the period following antibiotic treatment. Many questions still remain regarding the most cost-efficient work-up for the patient with dyspeptic symptoms or peptic ulcer disease. To a large extent the choice of diagnostic tests still depends on the decision whether to use endoscopy. If endoscopy is performed, histology, culture, and a rapid urease test should be carried out.

2 Histological Methods

Histological staining of gastric biopsies is still considered one of the gold standards for diagnosing *H. pylori* infection. In addition to visualizing the organism, histology can also give important information about the surrounding tissues and degree of inflammation. Many suitable histological stains are available, and the choice of one is often influenced by local expertise. Warthin-Starry stain was originally recommended by WARREN and MARSHALL 1983). It is excellent at visualizing *H. pylori* but is time consuming and expensive. Other silver stains, such as Steiner and HpSS, have also been used with very high sensitivity (DOGLIONI et al. 1997; FALLONE et al. 1995). The most commonly used nonsilver stains are Giemsa and hemotoxylin and eosin. The Giemsa stain was first described for *H. pylori* diagnosis by GRAY et al. (1986) and has traditionally been recommended for routine use because of its simplicity and low cost (MADAN et al. 1988). H&E does not stain the organism as distinctly as silver stains and Giemsa, and historically it performed poorly in the early studies, and the organisms were frequently missed. As experience with *H. pylori* has increased most pathologist today have no trouble identifying *H. pylori* in an H&E stain. It now has a sensitivity that is comparable to other stains but a slightly lower specificity (LAINE et al. 1997; FALLONE et al. 1997). The Genta stain represents a hybrid between silver and traditional stains. It combines Alcian blue, Steiner, and H&E into one stain that can both visualize *H. pylori* and give histopathological information about the gastric mucosa (GENTA et al. 1994).

Other stains that have been reported to perform well but are currently not in wide use include Cohen's combination of PAS, Feulgen, Mayer's hematoxylin, and methylene blue (COHEN et al. 1997), Gimenez stain (MCMULLEN et al. 1987), carbol fuchsin (ROCHA et al. 1989), acridine orange (WALTERS et al. 1986), modified Wright stain (BUTLER 1994), toluidine O (SLATER 1990), Wayson (ANDREICA et al. 1990), Löffler methylene blue (GROULS 1988), Cresyl fast violet (BURNETT et al. 1987), and Brown-Hopps (WESTBLOM et al. 1988b; ROBEY-CAFFERTY et al. 1989). Although many different stains have been tried over the years, the Giemsa stain still remains the stain of choice for routine diagnosis due to its simplicity and low cost (GRAY et al. 1986; MADAN et al. 1988; AYMARD et al. 1988; LAINE et al. 1997). However, as with most histological stains, it requires the traditional preparation of blocks and sectioning. If rapid presumptive diagnosis is important direct microscopy can be an alternative.

Direct microscopy with modified gram staining is a simple and rapid diagnostic test for fresh biopsy specimens. In the hands of an experienced technician this stain can be a highly accurate diagnostic test (MONTGOMERY et al. 1988; VAN HORN and DWORKIN 1990). Touch or brush cytology can also give rapid microscopic diagnosis (TREVISANI et al. 1997; NARVAEZ RODRIGUEZ et al. 1995; CARMONA et al. 1995; PINTO et al. 1991; SCHNADIG et al. 1990; MENDOZA et al. 1993). Another old diagnostic technique that has found a new use in *H. pylori* diagnosis is the use of frozen sections. In a recent study from Finland toluidine blue staining of frozen biopsy sections gave the diagnosis in 20min, with a sensitivity and specificity of 98% (SALMENKYLA et al. 1997).

Histological examination has the drawback of requiring costly invasive tests such as endoscopy. However, it has the advantage of simultaneous assessment of severity of the gastritis and the presence of intestinal metaplasia and atrophy. It is important to remember that histological examination is highly dependent on the experience and accuracy of the examining pathologist (KOLTS et al. 1993). There can be high interobserver variation between pathologists (PEURA 1995). *H. pylori* is widely distributed throughout the gastric mucosa, although its presence can be patchy (HAZELL et al. 1987b; MORRIS et al. 1989). Other things that may influence the accuracy of the histological diagnosis are recent treatments with antimicrobials or proton-pump inhibitors. They may lower the number of bacteria and improve the histological appearance without neccessarily curing the infection.

3 Culture Diagnosis

Even though culture is not the most sensitive way of diagnosing *H. pylori* infection, it is highly specific, and it is essential for selecting therapy based on antimicrobial susceptibilities. The appropriate techniques for culturing *H. pylori* from endoscopic biopsies of the stomach and duodenum have been extensively reviewed elsewhere (WESTBLOM 1991; HOLTON 1997; SANG et al. 1991; TEE et al. 1991; VEENENDAAL et al. 1993; XIA et al. 1993; KEHLER et al. 1994; VAN DER HULST et al. 1996; WESTBLOM et al. 1991a,b; ANSORG et al. 1991; AXON et al. 1997). There are many different culture media in use. Most of these are equivalent in terms of performance, provided they are sufficiently fresh (no older than 2 weeks), and the choice therefore depends more on the experience and preferences of the local laboratory. Regardless of the basic composition of the media it is recommended that both a selective and nonselective medium be used (AXON et al. 1997). Selective media contain antibiotics such as vancomycin, nalidixic acid, cefsulodin, and amphotericin B to prevent overgrowth of other micro-organisms.

H. pylori is a slow growing organism on all media and cultures take 2–5 days to become positive. Identification is made by typical morphology on Gram stain as well as positive reactions for urease, catalase, and oxidase. H. pylori is often difficult to grow in culture because of its fastidious nature, and recovery rates are reduced after prior treatment with antibiotics or proton-pump inhibitors (SJÖSTROM et al. 1997; DAW et al. 1991). If the biopsy has not been handled properly during transportation to the laboratory, culture yield can decline (AXON et al. 1997). A negative culture therefore does not rule out H. pylori infection. However, an experienced laboratory can achieve sensitivities as high as 90% or above (NICHOLS et al. 1991; DELTENRE et al. 1989). The major advantage of using culture as a diagnostic tool is that isolation of the organism can assist in the choice of antibiotic treatment. The major drawback is that it requires endoscopy, but if the patient is already having an invasive procedure as part of his evaluation, culture should always be performed.

4 Rapid Urease Tests

In 1985 OWEN et al. (1985) reported that H. pylori exhibited a rapid urease hydrolysis that could distinguish it from other bacteria. Within a few months a rapid diagnostic test based on this phenomenon was reported by McNULTY and WISE (1985). Rapid urease tests detect the production of ammonia by the urease enzyme in H. pylori. Increased levels of ammonia elevate the pH, which can be detected by an indicator such as phenol red (MARSHALL et al. 1987).

Several kits are now commercially available. They require a gastric mucosal biopsy to be added to a urea substrate and a pH sensitive marker. The test is then observed for a change in color indicating the presence of H. pylori. The first commercial urease test was the CLO test, named after H. pylori's common name at the time (Campylobacter-like organism) (MARSHALL et al. 1987). Many variations on the basic formula has been reported over the years, often utilizing in-house modifications of the basic media (WESTBLOM et al. 1988a; HAZELL et al. 1987a; DAS et al. 1987; CZINN and CARR 1987; RIARD et al. 1989; KHANNA et al. 1990), urea concentrations (VAIRA et al. 1988; YEUNG et al. 1990; THILLAINAYAGAM et al. 1991; BOYANOVA et al. 1996) or incubation temperatures (LAINE et al. 1996a; WESTBLOM et al. 1988a; VAIRA et al. 1988; CZINN and CARR 1987; RIARD et al. 1989).

Recently two new commercial tests have come onto the market, PyloriTek (YOUSFI et al. 1996, 1997; PUETZ et al. 1997; ELITSUR et al. 1998; LAINE et al. 1996b; YOUSFI et al. 1996) and Hpfast (LAINE et al. 1996b; WOO et al. 1996). PyloriTek is a rapid reagent strip with sensitivity and specificity similar to those of the CLO test (PUETZ et al. 1997; ELITSUR et al. 1998; LAINE et al. 1996b; YOUSFI et al. 1996), provided the test is read at 1 h. When read after more than 1h many false-positive results are seen and specificity falls to 68% (YOUSFI et al. 1997). However, the required short reading time is a distinct advantage over the other tests. When CLO test, PyloriTek, and Hpfast were compared in a single group of patients, they had very similar sensitivity (88%–92%) and specificity (99%–100%), but the mean time to a positive test for PyloriTek was 0.5h, compared to 2.0h for CLO test and 2.2h for Hpfast (LAINE et al. 1996b). Another new rapid urease test, HUT test, has been evaluated in two German studies (MALFERTHEINER et al. 1996; LABENZ et al. 1996) and found to be comparable to CLO test but with a shorter mean time to a positive reading of 104 min (MALFERTHEINER et al. 1996).

All rapid urease tests are accurate and easy to perform but have the drawback of requiring endoscopy. It is important to keep in mind that test sensitivity can be affected by recent use of antibacterials, proton-pump inhibitors, and bismuth-containing compounds. Still, the rapid urease tests remain important diagnostic tools that often can identify *H. pylori* infection before the patient has left the endoscopy suite.

5 Serological Tests

Infection with *H. pylori* results in production of both local and systemic antibodies. The first diagnostic antibody test used complement fixation and showed a strong correlation between antibodies and infection with *H. pylori* (JONES et al. 1984). Since then many other antibody tests have been developed, most notably enzyme-linked immunosorbent assays (ELISAs). Although their choice of antigens may vary, most ELISAs have good sensitivity (in the 90%–100% range) but their specificity is often lower (VAN DE WOUW et al. 1996; WILCOX et al. 1996; FELDMAN et al. 1995). It has been shown that antibody response differs in various populations. Titers are usually lower in children and in adult patients of northern European origin (WESTBLOM et al. 1992, 1993b; GOOSSENS et al. 1992). It is therefore important that these tests be validated locally in the population to be tested.

Several rapid antibody tests have been developed for use in an office setting. These tests can have results within 5–10min but give only a qualitative answer. Their sensitivity and specificity typically are lower than those of regular ELISAs (WESTBLOM et al. 1992, 1993a; STONE et al. 1997; JONES et al. 1997; CHEN et al.

1997; HUELIN et al. 1996; CHEY et al. 1998), and some of them are unsuitable for pediatric patients due to the lower antibody response in children (WESTBLOM et al. 1992; ELITSUR et al. 1997). A new rapid test, FlexSure HP, using a solid-phase immunochromatographic technique has recently been introduced (SCHRIER et al. 1998). This test requires only 4 min of incubation before it is read. Several investigators have found FlexSure HP to perform equally well as regular ELISA (SHARMA et al. 1997; ANDERSON et al. 1997; KROSER et al. 1998; GRAHAM et al. 1996), but in asymptomatic children the specificity is too low for use in routine screening (ELITSUR et al. 1997).

In humans salivary antibodies are secreted as part of the humoral immune response. Salivary concentrations of *H. pylori* specific IgG antibodies have been compared to serum IgG levels and found to be strongly correlated (LUZZA et al. 1995a). This has led to the development of salivary antibody test kits for *H. pylori*. The major advantage of a saliva test is that it is minimally invasive. This can be particularly useful in pediatric patients where it is desirable to avoid needle sticks. However, the sensitivity and specificity of the saliva tests are still lower than those of serum ELISAs (LUZZA et al. 1995b, 1997; LOEB et al. 1997; REILLY et al. 1997; CHRISTIE et al. 1996). At present they can be recommended as a noninvasive test in children, but assessment of their usefulness in adult populations must await further studies.

Used in the correct population, antibody tests such as the serum ELISAs can be accurate and relatively inexpensive diagnostic tools. However, their use is limited to initial diagnosis. Once a patient has been treated, a different test, such as the urea breath test, should be used to confirm eradication of *H. pylori*. This is because antibody levels decline very slowly after eradication, leading to false-positive results. A 50% decline in antibody levels can be expected after 6–12 months (CUTLER and PRASAD 1996; KOSUNEN et al. 1992; SHIMOYAMA et al. 1996), but a majority of patients still have positive serology after more than 1 year (CUTLER and PRASAD 1996). Using a qualitative ELISA, and comparing pre- and posttreatment samples side by side, it has been suggested that a 20% drop in titers can identify successful eradication with a sensitivity of 93% (CUTLER and PRASAD 1996). However, since physicians do not want to wait several months for an answer, serology is not a suitable test to confirm eradication of *H. pylori*.

6 Urea Breath Tests

Urea breath tests are simple, noninvasive tests for detection of *H. pylori* infection. When an infected patient ingests the isotope-labeled urea, carbon dioxide is liberated by the bacterial urease. This carbon dioxide is exhaled in the breath and can be measured. Two isotopes commonly used to label urea are ^{13}C (GRAHAM et al. 1987) and ^{14}C (MARSHALL and SURVEYOR 1988). These differ from each other in terms of radioactivity and expense. ^{13}C is a nonradioactive isotope and therefore can be used in children and pregnant women. On the other hand, it requires an isotope ratio mass spectrometer which makes it considerably expensive. In contrast, ^{14}C uses a regular scintillation counter for analysis. Such equipment is available in most laboratories and makes the test more affordable. The drawback is that ^{14}C is a radioactive isotope. Even though the doses of radioactivity are extremely low, some patients are apprehensive about consuming radioactive substances.

Urea breath tests have high sensitivity and specificity in the 95%–100% range (THIJS et al. 1996b; ROWLAND et al. 1997; EPPLE et al. 1997; DESROCHES et al. 1997; MOWAT et al. 1998; MALATY et al. 1996). When first introduced, the ^{14}C urea breath test used a dose of 10μCi (370kBq) (MARSHALL and SURVEYOR 1988). Since then the dose has steadily decreased, and a microdose test is now offered using only 1 μCi (37kBq). This lower dose still has a sensitivity and specificity between 95%–98% (PEURA et al. 1996; RAJU et al. 1994). The ^{13}C urea breath test has also undergone modifications since its introduction. The isotope dose has been lowered from 250mg to 50–75mg (LABENZ et al. 1996; ELLENRIEDER et al. 1997; ROWLAND et al. 1997; EPPLE et al. 1997). Air sampling has been reduced to a single sample about 30min after ingestion of the ^{13}C urea (LOTTERER et al. 1991; GOOD et al. 1991) and both the prolonged fasting and the test meal have been eliminated (OKSANEN et al. 1997; ROWLAND et al. 1997; MOAYYEDI et al. 1997; BRADEN et al. 1994). Using gas chromatography–mass spectrometer can eliminate the need for an isotope ratio mass spectrometer (TANIGAWA et al. 1996; KASHO et al. 1996). One can also use an infrared spectrometer (OHARA et al. 1995; BRADEN et al. 1996; TANIGUCHI et al. 1996). All these modifications have now made the ^{13}C urea breath test cheaper and more convenient to use.

Although the urea breath test has high sensitivity and specificity, the results can be influenced by several factors. False-positive results can occur if the patient is colonized with other urease-producing organisms. This is rarely a problem except in patients who are achlorhydric (BRESLIN and O'MORAIN 1997). False-negative results can be seen if the patient has recently consumed antibiotics (STEEN et al. 1995; PEREZ GARCIA et al. 1996; PERRI et al. 1995b), bismuth compounds (BELL et al. 1987; RAUWS et al. 1989; PREWETT et al. 1992; PERRI et al. 1995b; REIJERS et al. 1994), antacids (BERSTAD et al. 1990), H_2 blockers (CHING 1992; CHEY et al. 1997), or proton-pump inhibitors (Chey et al. 1996, 1997; PERRI et al. 1995b; MION et al. 1994; WEIL et al. 1991a). Patients scheduled for a urea breath test should therefore not consume any antisecretory drugs for at least 2 weeks prior to the test.

In spite of these potential problems the urea breath test is a valuable diagnostic tool. Compared to other noninvasive tests, it measures current infection and can therefore be used to confirm eradication, provided the testing is delayed at least 4 weeks after the end of treatment (LAINE 1996; WEIL et al. 1988, 1991b; YAMASHIRO et al. 1995). It measures *H. pylori* activity in the whole stomach and thereby avoids any sampling error that can occur with biopsy tests (GENTA and GRAHAM 1994; BAZZOLI et al. 1997; PERRI et al. 1995a; AXON et al. 1997). In patients who are asymptomatic following treatment endoscopic diagnosis can usually not be justified and the urea breath test has rapidly become the "gold standard" for these situations (BAZZOLI et al. 1997; VELDHUYZEN VAN ZANTEN et al. 1990; ROLLAN et al.

1997; CASPARY 1995; BRESLIN and O'MORAIN 1997). It is also very useful in pediatric patients where traumatic invasive procedures or the use of needles often is
not desirable.

7 Molecular Diagnosis

Molecular tests can be used for very precise diagnosis of *H. pylori* infection. The
techniques do not require the bacteria to be alive when tested. This means that
archival material can be used (SCHOLTE et al. 1997), and that clinical samples can be
shipped between institutions without compromising the results of the tests
(WESTBLOM et al. 1993c). Polymerase chain reaction (PCR) is an excellent method
for diagnosing *H. pylori* when the organism is present in low numbers. Theoretically the method can find and identify an organism if only a few single copies of its
DNA is present. The DNA molecule is very stable chemically and can survive in the
environment for long periods of time (DORAN et al. 1986). This makes the method
suitable for both clinical and environmental sampling.

Several PCR protocols for clinical diagnosis of *H. pylori* have been published.
These differ from each other mostly in the choice of primers. The first PCR protocol
to be published used primers from the 16-S rRNA (HOSHINA et al. 1990). This is an
approach that is well established from work with other bacteria, and many other
investigators have followed their lead (Ho et al. 1991; ENGSTRAND et al. 1992;
MAPSTONE et al. 1993a; MORERA-BRENES et al. 1994; WAHLFORS et al. 1995; ICHI-
KAWA et al. 1996; SMITH et al. 1996; THORESON et al. 1995). Other investigators have
decided to use primers from the genes encoding the uniquely powerful urease of
H. pylori (CLAYTON et al. 1991; WESTBLOM et al. 1993c; WANG et al. 1993; BICKLEY
et al. 1993; LIN et al. 1995, 1996; ASHTON-KEY et al. 1996; KAWAMATA et al. 1996;
SCHWARZ et al. 1997). An alternative approach was chosen by HAMMAR et al. (1992)
who used sequences from a protein antigen that appears to be species specific for
H. pylori (O'TOOLE et al. 1991) and VALENTINE et al. (1991) who picked primers from a
cloned fragment randomly selected from an *H. pylori* library (VALENTINE et al. 1991).

All of these PCR protocols are very accurate in diagnosing *H. pylori* from
clinical biopsy material. However, this may not be the optimal usage for this
technique. PCR usually does not add much to other techniques when used on
biopsy material (EL-ZAATARI et al. 1995; LAGE et al. 1995; ASHTON-KEY et al. 1996).
The combination of culture and histology detects *H. pylori* in almost as many cases
as PCR (SCHWARZ et al. 1997; LAGE et al. 1995; LIN et al. 1996). The exception is in
patients in whom the organism is present in very low numbers following antibiotic
treatment (SHIMADA et al. 1995; THIJS et al. 1996a). The main advantage of PCR,
on the other hand, is in situations requiring a clinical diagnosis but without access
to biopsy material.

Westblom et al. (1993c) studied the use of PCR on gastric juice which can be
collected through a nasogastric catheter. Using only 5ml gastric juice, they correctly

diagnosed *H. pylori* infection with a sensitivity of 96% and a specificity of 100%. These findings have since been verified in other studies showing similar degrees of sensitivity and specificity (MAPSTONE et al. 1993a; KAWAMATA et al. 1996; YOSHIDA et al. 1998; MATSUKURA et al. 1995). *H. pylori* has also been detected in bile samples using PCR (LIN et al. 1995).

Several investigators have used the technique to identify *H. pylori* from oral secretions and stool samples. Cultures from the oral cavity have almost uniformly been negative for *H. pylori* (DIONISIO et al. 1989; KRAJDEN et al. 1989; FERGUSON et al. 1993), but PCR has been able to find the organism in the oral cavity (NGUYEN et al. 1993; LI et al. 1996, 1995; MAPSTONE et al. 1993a). However, it is still an unanswered question whether *H. pylori* actually colonizes the mouth or is found there only coincidentally after regurgitation of gastric secretions. PCR has also been used to diagnose the presence of *H. pylori* in stool samples (VAN ZWET et al. 1994; ENROTH and ENGSTRAND 1995; MAPSTONE et al. 1993b; LI et al. 1996). This is another area in which PCR offers distinct advantages since *H. pylori* may only be present in low numbers and the multitude of contaminating organisms in the bowel makes it very hard to obtain any positive cultures (DIONISIO et al. 1989; KELLY et al. 1994; THOMAS et al. 1992; SAHAY et al. 1995). Still, PCR of stool samples can be unreliable because of inhibitory components that are present in fecal material, mostly complex polysaccharides originating from vegetable material in the diet (MONTEIRO et al. 1997; VAN ZWET et al. 1994). Similar inhibition has been noticed in oral secretions and may explain why some researchers have only rarely found *H. pylori* in the mouth (MAPSTONE et al. 1993a; HAMMAR et al. 1992; HARDO et al. 1995; T.U. Westblom 1998, personal communication). Recently methods to overcome this inhibition have been described using an immunomagnetic separation technique (ENROTH and ENGSTRAND 1995; OSAKI et al. 1998). This opens up the possibility of more routine usage of PCR from oral or fecal material, but the true clinical significance of the test still needs to be determined in larger prospective studies.

8 Other Diagnostic Tests

Several other diagnostic tests have been reported in smaller studies. Most of these are based on the breakdown of urea by *H. pylori*'s strong urease. A simplified alternative to the urea breath test measures ammonia levels in gastric juice (BORNSCHEIN et al. 1989; KIM et al. 1990; TRIEBLING et al. 1991; NEITHERCUT et al. 1991; GOLDMANN 1987; PEDRIALI et al. 1992; YANG et al. 1995). There is a significant increase in gastric juice ammmonia levels in patients infected with *H. pylori* compared to noninfected individuals. This is true both in patients with renal failure and in individuals with normal renal function (KIM et al. 1990; NEITHERCUT et al. 1991). The ammonia levels can be measured by direct colorimetric methods using an automated analyzer and requires no radioactive material. This method is semi-

Table 1. Advantages and disadvantages of common diagnostic tests for *H. pylori* (adapted from WEST-BLOM 1993; AXON et al. 1997)

Diagnostic test	Advantages	Disadvantages
Histology	Can estimate the extent of *H. pylori* infection simultaneously with inflammatory and degenerative mucosal lesions. Available in most institutions. Allows retrospective evaluation of specimens.	Endoscopy needed to obtain the sample Performance depends on the experience of the pathologist. Cannot study antimicrobial resistance or type bacteria. Delayed result.
Culture	100% specific. Allows testing for antimicrobial susceptibility. Permits typing of the strains. Available in most institutions.	Endoscopy needed to obtain the sample. Results take several days. Sensitivity may be impaired by improper sampling, transportation or processing. Does not give insight into the status of the mucosa.
Rapid urease test	Close to 100% specific. results within 1–2h. Inexpensive. Available in most institutions.	Endoscopy needed to obtain the sample. Does not permit antimicrobial susceptibility testing or strain typing. Does not give insight into the status of the mucosa.
Serology	Noninvasive test. Needs no specific transport conditions. Relatively inexpensive. Available in most institutions.	Cannot be used to confirm eradication after treatment. Does not permit antimicrobial susceptibility testing or strain typing. Does not give insight into the status of the mucosa.
Urea breath test	Noninvasive test. High sensitivity and specificity. Needs no specific transport conditions. Tests the whole stomach.	Does not permit antimicrobial susceptibility testing or strain typing Does not give insight into the status of the mucosa. Not available in all institutions.
PCR	High sensitivity and specificity. Needs no specific transport conditions. Results available in a day. Allows strain typing through molecular fingerprinting. Retrospective analysis possible.	Does not permit antimicrobial susceptibility testing. Does not give insight into the status of the mucosa. Not generally available. Risk of contamination of samples if protocols are not strictly followed.

invasive since it requires the collection of gastric juice, but it can be "the poor man's" alternative to the urea breath test. However, it is not as accurate as the breath test. In patients with normal renal function the sensitivity is only 82% and the specificity 93% (KIM et al. 1990). Some improvement can be achieved if urea/ ammonia ratios are calculated (NEITHERCUT et al. 1991, 1993; MOKUOLU et al. 1997), but the method still has not achieved the same accuracy as the urea breath test.

Another variation on the same theme looks at serum levels of ^{13}C bicarbonate (^{13}C-HCO_3) after ingestion of ^{13}C urea. This method has a sensitivity of 91% and a specificity of 86% (KIM et al. 1997). One can also consider urinary levels of the isotopes. When patients are given ^{14}C urea, some of the radioactive carbon can be retrieved from the urine (MUNSTER et al. 1993). The same is true for ^{13}C-labeled urea (TANIGAWA et al. 1996). This has been used as an alternative way to measure *H. pylori* urease activity. PATHAK et al. (1994) measured ^{14}C in 24-h urine and in a

15-min breath sample and found both to be highly sensitive, specific, and cross-confirmatory tests. In the urinary test significantly lower amounts of ^{14}C urea is found in the urine of infected patients as most of the isotope has been exhaled in the form of ^{14}C CO_2. A similar variation on the test uses ^{15}N urea instead and measures the excretion of $^{15}NH_4$ in the urine (Wu et al. 1992). Since ^{15}N is not a radioactive isotope, it can be safely used in women and children. In a small study of 36 patients this test was 96% sensitive and 100% specific (Wu et al. 1992).

There are also single reports of other diagnostic tests. HpSA is a stool assay that uses captured antibodies to *H. pylori*. This test has been used to detect *H. pylori* infection in an 1800-year-old Chilean mummy (Correa et al. 1998), but no prospective studies have been published yet. In a study of 54 patients the urinary interleukin-8/creatinine ratio was measured and found to be correlated with activity of gastritis and presence of *H. pylori* (Taha et al. 1996). The urine has also been used to detect IgG antibodies to *H. pylori*. Using ELISA and western blot, *H. pylori* can be diagnosed in urine with a sensitivity of 96% and a specificity of 90% (Alemohammad et al. 1993). Lactoferrin levels in the stomach are reported to be correlated well with presence of *H. pylori* (Nakao et al. 1997), but no prospective diagnostic study has been reported so far. All these new tests have in common that they have not yet been extensively evaluated in major studies, and assessment of their usefulness must await future research data.

9 Conclusions

There are a wide variety of tests available for diagnosing *H. pylori* infection. They all have their individual advantages and disadvantages as outlined in Table 1. In choosing the proper test it is important to consider its accuracy, the cost of the test, and the experience of the local laboratory. However, the most important consideration is whether the patient will be undergoing endoscopy.

If endoscopy is performed, multiple biopsies from both antrum and body should be taken and submitted for histology, culture, and rapid urease testing. Histology helps both in the diagnosis and by giving important information about the presence of inflammation or metaplasia. Giemsa, H&E, and Genta are the most commonly used stains. Of these, Giemsa is the simplest and least expensive while Genta gives more information about surrounding tissues. Culture helps in selecting the proper therapy if antibiotic resistance is present. The choice of culture method depends on laboratory preferences. A rapid urease test gives a presumptive diagnosis within 1–2h. The CLO test is the most widely used rapid urease test, but the PyloriTek test promises to be as accurate as the CLO test and somewhat faster.

In patients whose symptoms do not warrant endoscopy one of the noninvasive tests should be used. For screening of patients with typical symptoms or with history of peptic ulcer disease a serum antibody test can be used. Of these, the ELISAs outperform the many office-based rapid antibody kits available. There are several commercial ELISAs on the market with sensitivity and specificity of 90% or higher. The antibody tests can be used to make a diagnosis only prior to antibiotic therapy. Since antibody levels take a long time to decline, these tests are not reliable in verifying eradication following treatment.

If a urea breath test is available, it is recommended over the antibody tests. It is a more sensitive and specific test, but it is also more expensive. Following treatment the urea breath test is the only noninvasive test that can accurately determine whether the infection has been eradicated. Although other noninvasive tests have been reported in recent years, the urea breath test remains the gold standard if endoscopy is not performed.

Molecular methods such as PCR can be a complement to the other diagnostic tests but rarely replaces any of them. On fresh biopsy material PCR has no distinct advantage over the combination of histology, culture, and rapid urease testing. However, it can be very useful on archival tissue, environmental samples, gastric juice, oral secretions, and stool samples where the traditional diagnostic tests perform poorly. Still, PCR is an expensive diagnostic tool, and it is used mostly as a component of research protocols.

References

Alemohammad MM, Foley TJ, Cohen H (1993) Detection of immunoglobulin G antibodies to *Helicobacter pylori* in urine by an enzyme immunoassay method. J Clin Microbiol 31:2174–2177

Anderson JC, Cheng E, Roeske M, Marchildon P, Peacock J, Shaw RD (1997) Detection of serum antibodies to *Helicobacter pylori* by an immunochromatographic method. Am J Gastroenterol 92:1135–1139

Andreica V, Dumitrascu D, Sasca N, Toganel E, Suciu A, Draghici A, Pascu O, Sasca C, Suciu M, Andreica M et al (1990) Helicobacter-like organisms in gastroduodenal diseases. Gastroenterol Clin Biol 14:437–441

Ansorg R, von Recklinghausen G, Pomarius R, Schmid EN (1991) Evaluation of techniques for isolation, subcultivation, and preservation of *Helicobacter pylori*. J Clin Microbiol 29:51–53

Ashton-Key M, Diss TC, Isaacson PG (1996) Detection of *Helicobacter pylori* in gastric biopsy and resection specimens. J Clin Pathol 49:107–111

Axon A, Deltenre M, Eriksson S, Fiocca R, Glupczynski Y, Hirschl AM, Hunt R, Kimura K, Logan R, Malfertheiner P, Megraud F, O'Morain C, Pajares Garcia JM, Rauws E, Rune S, Shimoyama T, Unge P, Walan A, Westblom TU (1997) Technical annex: tests used to assess *Helicobacter pylori* infection. Working Party of the European *Helicobacter pylori* Study Group. Gut 41 [Suppl 2]:S10–S18

Aymard B, Labouyrie E, Patris A, de Korwin JD, Foliguet B, Floquet J, Duprez A (1988) Detection of *Campylobacter pylori* in gastric biopsies: a comparative study of 4 histopathologic methods and scanning electron microscopy. [in French]. Arch Anat Cytol Pathol 36:193–199

Bazzoli F, Zagari M, Fossi S, Pozzato P, Ricciardiello L, Mwangemi C, Roda A, Roda E (1997) Urea breath tests for the detection of *Helicobacter pylori* infection. Helicobacter 2 [Suppl 1]:S34-S37

Bell GD, Weil J, Harrison G, Morden A, Jones PH, Gant PW, Trowell JE, Yoong AK, Daneshmend TK, Logan RF (1987) 14C-urea breath analysis, a non-invasive test for *Campylobacter pylori* in the stomach. Lancet 1:1367–1368

Berstad K, Weberg R, Berstad A (1990) Suppression of gastric urease activity by antacids. Scand J Gastroenterol 25:496–500

Bickley J, Owen RJ, Fraser AG, Pounder RE (1993) Evaluation of the polymerase chain reaction for detecting the urease C gene of *Helicobacter pylori* in gastric biopsy samples and dental plaque. J Med Microbiol 39:338–344

Bornschein W, Heilmann KL, Bauernfeind A (1989) Intragastric formation of ammonia in *Campylobacter pylori* associated gastritis. Diagnostic and pathogenetic significance [in German]. Med Klin 84:329–332, 368

Boyanova L, Stancheva I, Todorov D, Kumanova R, Petrov S, Vladimirov B, Pehlivanov N, Mitova R, Chakarski I, Churchev I (1996) Comparison of three urease tests for detection of *Helicobacter pylori* in gastric biopsy specimens. Eur J Gastroenterol Hepatol 8:911–914

Braden B, Duan LP, Caspary WF, Lembcke B (1994) More convenient 13C-urea breath test modifications still meet the criteria for valid diagnosis of *Helicobacter pylori* infection. Z Gastroenterol 32:198–202

Braden B, Schafer F, Caspary WF, Lembcke B (1996) Nondispersive isotope-selective infrared spectroscopy: a new analytical method for 13C-urea breath tests. Scand J Gastroenterol 31:442–445

Breslin NP, O'Morain CA (1997) Noninvasive diagnosis of *Helicobacter pylori* infection: a review. Helicobacter 2:111–117

Burnett RA, Brown IL, Findlay J (1987) Cresyl fast violet staining method for campylobacter like organisms. J Clin Pathol 40:353

Butler GD (1994) Butler modified Wright stain for demonstration of *Campylobacter pylori*. J Histotechnol 13:109–111

Carmona T, Munoz E, Abad MM, Paz JI, Gomez F, Alonso MJ, Sanchez A, Bullon A (1995) Usefulness of antral brushing samples stained with Diff-Quik in the cytologic diagnosis of *Helicobacter pylori*. A comparative methodologic study. Acta Cytol 39:669–672

Caspary WF (1995) 13C-urea breath test. Patient-friendly gold standard in the diagnosis of *Helicobacter pylori* infection with long term cost control potential. Dtsch Med Wochenschr 120:976–978

Chen TS, Chang FY, Lee SD (1997) Serodiagnosis of *Helicobacter pylori* infection: comparison and correlation between enzyme-linked immunosorbent assay and rapid serological test results. J Clin Microbiol 35:184–186

Chey WD, Spybrook M, Carpenter S, Nostrant TT, Elta GH, Scheiman JM (1996) Prolonged effect of omeprazole on the 14C-urea breath test. Am J Gastroenterol 91:89–92

Chey WD, Woods M, Scheiman JM, Nostrant TT, DelValle J (1997) Lansoprazole and ranitidine affect the accuracy of the 14C-urea breath test by a pH-dependent mechanism. Am J Gastroenterol 92:446–450

Chey WD, Murthy UK, Linscheer W, Barish C, Riff D, Rubin H, Safdi M, Schwartz H, Shah U, Wruble L, el-Zimaity HM (1998) The ChemTrak Hp Chek fingerstick whole blood serology test for the detection of *Helicobacter pylori* infection. Am J Gastroenterol 93:16–19

Ching CK (1992) Impaired *Helicobacter pylori* urease enzyme activity by histamine 2 receptor antagonist (letter). Am J Gastroenterol 87:257–258

Christie JM, McNulty CA, Shepherd NA, Valori RM (1996) Is saliva serology useful for the diagnosis of *Helicobacter pylori*? Gut 39:27–30

Clayton C, Kleanthous K, Tabaqchali S (1991) Detection and identification of *Helicobacter pylori* by the polymerase chain reaction. J Clin Pathol 44:515–516

Cohen LF, Sayeeduddin M, Phillips C, Shahab I (1997) A new staining method for identification of *Helicobacter pylori* and simultaneous visualization of gastric morphologic features. Mod Pathol 10:1160–1163

Correa P, Willis D, Allison MJ, Gerszten E (1998) *Helicobacter pylori* in pre-Columbian mummies. Proceedings of digestive disease week abstract 3155

Cutler AF, Prasad VM (1996) Long-term follow-up of *Helicobacter pylori* serology after successful eradication. Am J Gastroenterol 91:85–88

Czinn SJ, Carr H (1987) Rapid diagnosis of *Campylobacter pyloridis*-associated gastritis. J Pediatr 110:569–570

Das SS, Bain LA, Karim QN, Coelho LG, Baron JH (1987) Rapid diagnosis of *Campylobacter pyloridis* infection (letter). J Clin Pathol 40:701–702

Daw MA, Deegan P, Leen E, O'Morain C (1991) Short report: the effect of omeprazole on *Helicobacter pylori* and associated gastritis. Aliment Pharmacol Ther 5:435–439

Deltenre M, Glupczynski Y, De Prez C, Nyst JF, Burette A, Labbe M, Jonas C, DeKoster E (1989) The reliability of urease tests, histology and culture in the diagnosis of *Campylobacter pylori* infection. Scand J Gastroenterol [Suppl] 160:19–24

Desroches JJ, Lahaie RG, Picard M, Morais J, Dumont A, Gaudreau C, Picard D, Chartrand R (1997) Methodological validation and clinical usefulness of carbon-14-urea breath test for documentation of presence and eradication of *Helicobacter pylori* infection. J Nucl Med 38:1141–1145

Dionisio D, Buonamici C, Mazzotta D, Ricciarelli L, Pecile P, Gabbrielli M, Poggiali G, Zanchi R (1989) *Campylobacter pylori* absence in extragastric human intestinal sites and animal stomachs. Boll Ist Sieroter Milan 68:197–198

Doenges JL (1939) Spirochetes in the gastric glands of macacus rhesus and of man without related disease. Arch Pathol 27:469–477

Doglioni C, Turrin M, Macri E, Chiarelli C, Germana B, Barbareschi M (1997) HpSS: a new silver staining method for *Helicobacter pylori*. J Clin Pathol 50:461–464

Doran GH, Dickel DN, Ballinger WE, Agee OF, Laipis PJ, Hauswirth NN (1986) Anatomical, cellular and molecular analysis of 8,000-yr-old human brain tissue from the Windower archeological site. Nature 323:803–806

el-Zaatari FA, Nguyen AM, Genta RM, Klein PD, Graham DY (1995) Determination of *Helicobacter pylori* status by reverse transcription-polymerase chain reaction. Comparison with urea breath test. Dig Dis Sci 40:109–113

Elitsur Y, Neace C, Triest WE (1997) Comparison between a rapid office-based and ELISA serologic test in screening for *Helicobacter pylori* in children. Helicobacter 2:180–184

Elitsur Y, Hill I, Lichtman SN, Rosenberg AJ (1998) Prospective comparison of rapid urease tests (PyloriTek, CLO test) for the diagnosis of *Helicobacter pylori* infection in symptomatic children: a pediatric multicenter study. Am J Gastroenterol 93:217–219

Ellenrieder V, Glasbrenner B, Stoffels C, Weiler S, Bode G, Moller P, Adler G (1997) Qualitative and semi-quantitative value of a modified 13C-urea breath test for identification of *Helicobacter pylori* infection. Eur J Gastroenterol Hepatol 9:1085–1089

Engstrand L, Nguyen AM, Graham DY, el-Zaatari FA (1992) Reverse transcription and polymerase chain reaction amplification of rRNA for detection of Helicobacter species. J Clin Microbiol 30:2295–2301

Enroth H, Engstrand L (1995) Immunomagnetic separation and PCR for detection of *Helicobacter pylori* in water and stool specimens. J Clin Microbiol 33:2162–2165

Epple HJ, Kirstein FW, Bojarski C, Frege J, Fromm M, Riecken EO, Schulzke JD (1997) 13C-urea breath test in *Helicobacter pylori* diagnosis and eradication. Correlation to histology, origin of 'false' results, and influence of food intake. Scand J Gastroenterol 32:308–314

Fallone CA, Mitchell A, Paterson WG (1995) Determination of the test performance of less costly methods of *Helicobacter pylori* detection. Clin Invest Med 18:177–185

Fallone CA, Loo VG, Lough J, Barkun AN (1997) Hematoxylin and eosin staining of gastric tissue for the detection of *Helicobacter pylori*. Helicobacter 2:32–35

Feldman RA, Deeks JJ, Evans SJ (1995) Multi-laboratory comparison of eight commercially available *Helicobacter pylori* serology kits. *Helicobacter pylori* Serology Study Group. Eur J Clin Microbiol Infect Dis 14:428–433

Ferguson DA Jr, Li C, Patel NR, Mayberry WR, Chi DS, Thomas E (1993) Isolation of *Helicobacter pylori* from saliva. J Clin Microbiol 31:2802–2804

Freedberg AS, Barron LE (1940) The Presence of Spirochetes in Human Gastric Mucosa. Am J Dig Dis 7:443–445

Genta RM, Robason GO, Graham DY (1994) Simultaneous visualization of *Helicobacter pylori* and gastric morphology: a new stain. Hum Pathol 25:221–226

Genta RM, Graham DY (1994) Comparison of biopsy sites for the histopathologic diagnosis of *Helicobacter pylori*: a topographic study of H pylori density and distribution. Gastrointest Endosc 40:342–345

Goldmann FL (1987) Ammonia determination in gastric juice. A new simple rapid test for *Campylobacter pylori* (in German). Dtsch Med Wochenschr 112:1643–1644

Good DJ, Dill S, Mossi S, Frey R, Beglinger C, Stalder GA, Meyer-Wyss B (1991) Sensitivity and specificity of a simplified, standardized 13C-urea breath test for the demonstration of *Helicobacter pylori* (in German). Schweiz Med Wochenschr 121:764–766

Goossens H, Glupczynski Y, Burette A, Van den Borre C, Butzler JP (1992) Evaluation of a commercially available second-generation immunoglobulin G enzyme immunoassay for detection of *Helicobacter pylori* infection. J Clin Microbiol 30:176–180

Graham DY, Klein PD, Evans DJ Jr, Evans DG, Alpert LC, Opekun AR, Boutton TW (1987) *Campylobacter pylori* detected noninvasively by the 13C-urea breath test. Lancet 1:1174–1177

Graham DY, Evans DJ Jr, Peacock J, Baker JT, Schrier WH (1996) Comparison of rapid serological tests (FlexSure HP and QuickVue) with conventional ELISA for detection of *Helicobacter pylori* infection. Am J Gastroenterol 91:942–948

Gray SF, Wyatt JI, Rathbone BJ (1986) Simplified techniques for identifying *Campylobacter pyloridis*. J Clin Pathol 39:1279

Grouls V (1988) Detection of *Campylobacter pylori* in gastric mucosa biopsies (letter; in German). Dtsch Med Wochenschr 113:1256

Hammar M, Tyszkiewicz T, Wadström T, O'Toole PW (1992) Rapid detection of *Helicobacter pylori* in gastric biopsy material by polymerase chain reaction. J Clin Microbiol 30:54–58

Hardo PG, Tugnait A, Hassan F, Lynch DA, West AP, Mapstone NP, Quirke P, Chalmers DM, Kowolik MJ, Axon AT (1995) *Helicobacter pylori* infection and dental care. Gut 37:44–46

Hazell SL, Borody TJ, Gal A, Lee A (1987a) *Campylobacter pyloridis* gastritis I: Detection of urease as a marker of bacterial colonization and gastritis. Am J Gastroenterol 82:292–296

Hazell SL, Hennessy WB, Borody TJ, Carrick J, Ralston M, Brady L, Lee A (1987b) *Campylobacter pyloridis* gastritis II: Distribution of bacteria and associated inflammation in the gastroduodenal environment. Am J Gastroenterol 82:297–301

Ho SA, Hoyle JA, Lewis FA, Secker AD, Cross D, Mapstone NP, Dixon MF, Wyatt JI, Tompkins DS, Taylor GR et al (1991) Direct polymerase chain reaction test for detection of *Helicobacter pylori* in humans and animals. J Clin Microbiol 29:2543–2549

Holton J (1997) Clinical relevance of culture: why, how, and when. Helicobacter 2 [Suppl 1]:S25–S33

Hoshina S, Kahn SM, Jiang W, Green PH, Neu HC, Chin N, Morotomi M, LoGerfo P, Weinstein IB (1990) Direct detection and amplification of *Helicobacter pylori* ribosomal 16 S gene segments from gastric endoscopic biopsies. Diagn Microbiol Infect Dis 13:473–479

Huelin J, Sanchez-Galdon S, Cardenas A, Ibanez J, Espana P, de la Cruz J, Jimenez M, Ferreiro B, Lozano JM, Maldonado G (1996) Comparative study of Helisal TM rapid blood and Elisa, Jatrox and pathologic anatomy in the diagnosis of *Helicobacter pylori* infection (in Spanish). Rev Esp Enferm Dig 88:825–827

Ichikawa Y, Mitsuhashi M, Ishikawa T, Wyle F, Chang K, Fujiwara Y, Arakawa T, Shimada H, Tarnawski A (1996) Laboratory diagnosis of *Helicobacter pylori* infection by polymerase chain reaction. Res Commun Mol Pathol Pharmacol 91:117–128

Jones DM, Lessells AM, Eldridge J (1984) Campylobacter like organisms on the gastric mucosa: culture, histological, and serological studies. J Clin Pathol 37:1002–1006

Jones R, Phillips I, Felix G, Tait C (1997) An evaluation of near-patient testing for *Helicobacter pylori* in general practice. Aliment Pharmacol Ther 11:101–105

Kasho VN, Cheng S, Jensen DM, Ajie H, Lee WN, Faller LD (1996) Feasibility of analysing [^{13}C]urea breath tests for *Helicobacter pylori* by gas chromatography-mass spectrometry in the selected ion monitoring mode. Aliment Pharmacol Ther 10:985–995

Kawamata O, Yoshida H, Hirota K, Yoshida A, Kawaguchi R, Shiratori Y, Omata M (1996) Nested-polymerase chain reaction for the detection of *Helicobacter pylori* infection with novel primers designed by sequence analysis of urease A gene in clinically isolated bacterial strains. Biochem Biophys Res Commun 219:266–272

Kehler EG, Midkiff BR, Westblom TU (1994) Evaluation of three commercially available blood culture systems for cultivation of *Helicobacter pylori*. J Clin Microbiol 32:1597–1598

Kelly SM, Pitcher MC, Farmery SM, Gibson GR (1994) Isolation of *Helicobacter pylori* from feces of patients with dyspepsia in the United Kingdom. Gastroenterology 107:1671–1674

Khanna MU, Kochar N, Nair NG, Bhatia SJ, Abraham P (1990) Evaluation of a modified medium for the one hour urease test for *Helicobacter pylori* infection. Indian J Gastroenterol 9:219–220

Kim H, Park C, Jang WI, Lee KH, Kwon SO, Robey-Cafferty SS, Ro JY, Lee YB (1990) The gastric juice urea and ammonia levels in patients with *Campylobacter pylori*. Am J Clin Pathol 94:187–191

Kim MJ, Michener R, Triadafilopoulos G (1997) Serum 13C-bicarbonate assay for the diagnosis of gastric *Helicobacter pylori* infection and response to treatment. Gastroenterology 113:31–37

Kolts BE, Joseph B, Achem SR, Bianchi T, Monteiro C (1993) *Helicobacter pylori* detection: a quality and cost analysis. Am J Gastroenterol 88:650–655

Kosunen TU, Seppala K, Sarna S, Sipponen P (1992) Diagnostic value of decreasing IgG, IgA, and IgM antibody titres after eradication of *Helicobacter pylori*. Lancet 339:893–895

Krajden S, Fuksa M, Anderson J, Kempston J, Boccia A, Petrea C, Babida C, Karmali M, Penner JL (1989) Examination of human stomach biopsies, saliva, and dental plaque for *Campylobacter pylori*. J Clin Microbiol 27:1397–1398

Krienitz W (1906) Über das Auftreten von Spirochäten verschiedener Form im Mageninhalt bei Carcinoma ventriculi. Dtsch Med Wochenschr 28:872

Kroser JA, Faigel DO, Furth EE, Metz DC (1998) Comparison of rapid office-based serology with formal laboratory-based ELISA testing for diagnosis of *Helicobacter pylori* gastritis. Dig Dis Sci 43:103–108

Labenz J, Barsch G, Peitz U, Aygen S, Hennemann O, Tillenburg B, Becker T, Stolte M (1996) Validity of a novel biopsy urease test (HUT) and a simplified 13C-urea breath test for diagnosis of *Helicobacter pylori* infection and estimation of the severity of gastritis. Digestion 57:391–397

Lage AP, Godfroid E, Fauconnier A, Burette A, Butzler JP, Bollen A, Glupczynski Y (1995) Diagnosis of *Helicobacter pylori* infection by PCR: comparison with other invasive techniques and detection of cagA gene in gastric biopsy specimens. J Clin Microbiol 33:2752–2756

Laine L, Estrada R, Lewin DN, Cohen H (1996a) The influence of warming on rapid urease test results: a prospective evaluation. Gastrointest Endosc 44:429–432

Laine L, Lewin D, Naritoku W, Estrada R, Cohen H (1996b) Prospective comparison of commercially available rapid urease tests for the diagnosis of *Helicobacter pylori*. Gastrointest Endosc 44:523–526

Laine L, Lewin DN, Naritoku W, Cohen H (1997) Prospective comparison of H&E, Giemsa, and Genta stains for the diagnosis of *Helicobacter pylori*. Gastrointest Endosc 45:463–467

Laine LA (1996) *Helicobacter pylori* and complicated ulcer disease. Am J Med 100:52S–57S; discussion

Li C, Musich PR, Ha T, Ferguson DA Jr, Patel NR, Chi DS, Thomas E (1995) High prevalence of *Helicobacter pylori* in saliva demonstrated by a novel PCR assay. J Clin Pathol 48:662–666

Li C, Ha T, Ferguson DA Jr, Chi DS, Zhao R, Patel NR, Krishnaswamy G, Thomas E (1996) A newly developed PCR assay of H. pylori in gastric biopsy, saliva, and feces. Evidence of high prevalence of H. pylori in saliva supports oral transmission. Dig Dis Sci 41:2142–2149

Lin SY, Jeng YS, Wang CK, Ko FT, Lin KY, Wang CS, Liu JD, Chen PH, Chang JG (1996) Polymerase chain reaction diagnosis of *Helicobacter pylori* in gastroduodenal diseases: comparison with culture and histopathological examinations. J Gastroenterol Hepatol 11:286–289

Lin TT, Yeh CT, Wu CS, Liaw YF (1995) Detection and partial sequence analysis of *Helicobacter pylori* DNA in the bile samples. Dig Dis Sci 40:2214–2219

Loeb MB, Riddell RH, James C, Hunt R, Smaill FM (1997) Evaluation of salivary antibodies to detect infection with *Helicobacter pylori*. Can J Gastroenterol 11:437–440

Lotterer E, Ramaker J, Ludtke FE, Tegeler R, Geletneky JV, Bauer FE (1991) The simplified 13C-urea breath test – one point analysis for detection of *Helicobacter pylori* infection. Z Gastroenterol 29:590–594

Luger A, Neuberger H (1921) Über Spirochätenbefunde im Magensaft und deren diagnostische Bedeutung für das Carcinoma ventriculi. Z Klin Med 92:54–75

Luzza F, Maletta M, Imeneo M, Doldo P, Marasco R, Biancone L, Pallone F (1995a) Salivary specific IgG is a sensitive indicator of the humoral immune response to *Helicobacter pylori*. FEMS Immunol Med Microbiol 10:281–283

Luzza F, Maletta M, Imeneo M, Marcheggiano A, Iannoni C, Biancone L, Pallone F (1995b) Salivary-specific immunoglobulin G in the diagnosis of *Helicobacter pylori* infection in dyspeptic patients. Am J Gastroenterol 90:1820–1823

Luzza F, Oderda G, Maletta M, Imeneo M, Mesuraca L, Chioboli E, Lerro P, Guandalini S, Pallone F (1997) Salivary immunoglobulin G assay to diagnose *Helicobacter pylori* infection in children. J Clin Microbiol 35:3358–3360

Madan E, Kemp J, Westblom TU, Subik M, Sexton S, Cook J (1988) Evaluation of staining methods for identifying *Campylobacter pylori*. Am J Clin Pathol 90:450–453

Malaty HM, el-Zimaity HM, Genta RM, Klein PD, Graham DY (1996) Twenty-minute fasting version of the US 13C-urea breath test for the diagnosis of H pylori infection. Helicobacter 1:165–167

Malfertheiner P, Enrique Dominguez-Munoz J, Heckenmuller H, Neubrand M, Fischer HP, Sauerbruch T (1996) Modified rapid urease test for detection of *Helicobacter pylori* infection. Eur J Gastroenterol Hepatol 8:53–56

Mapstone NP, Lynch DA, Lewis FA, Axon AT, Tompkins DS, Dixon MF, Quirke P (1993a) Identification of *Helicobacter pylori* DNA in the mouths and stomachs of patients with gastritis using PCR. J Clin Pathol 46:540–543

Mapstone NP, Lynch DA, Lewis FA, Axon AT, Tompkins DS, Dixon MF, Quirke P (1993b) PCR identification of *Helicobacter pylori* in faeces from gastritis patients (letter). Lancet 341:447

Marshall BJ, Royce H, Annear DI, Goodwin CS, Pearman JW, Warren JR, Armstrong JA (1984) Original Isolation of *Campylobacter pyloridis* from human gastric mucosa. Microbios Lett 25:83–88

Marshall BJ, Warren JR, Francis GJ, Langton SR, Goodwin CS, Blincow ED (1987) Rapid urease test in the management of *Campylobacter pyloridis*-associated gastritis. Am J Gastroenterol 82:200–210

Marshall BJ (1989) History of the discovery of C pylori. In: Blaser MJ (ed) *Campylobacter pylori* in gastritis and peptic ulcer disease. Igaku-Shoin, New York, pp 7–23

Marshall BJ, Surveyor I (1988) Carbon-14 urea breath test for the diagnosis of *Campylobacter pylori* associated gastritis. J Nucl Med 29:11–16

Matsukura N, Onda M, Tokunaga A, Kato S, Yamashita K, Ohbayashi M (1995) Detection of *Helicobacter pylori* DNA in gastric juice by the polymerase chain reaction: comparison with findings in bacterial culture and the detection of tissue IgA and serum IgG antibodies against *Helicobacter pylori*. J Gastroenterol 30:689–695

McMullen L, Walker MM, Bain LA, Karim QN, Baron JH (1987) Histological identification of Campylobacter using Gimenez technique in gastric antral mucosa. J Clin Pathol 40:464–465

McNulty CA, Wise R (1985) Rapid diagnosis of Campylobacter-associated gastritis (letter). Lancet 1:1443–1444

Mendoza ML, Martin-Rabadan P, Carrion I, Morillas JD, Lopez-Alonso G, Diaz-Rubio M (1993) *Helicobacter pylori* infection. Rapid diagnosis with brush cytology. Acta Cytol 37:181–185

Mion F, Delecluse HJ, Rousseau M, Berger F, Brazier JL, Minaire Y (1994) 13C-urea breath test for the diagnosis of *Helicobacter pylori* infection. Comparison with histology (in French). Gastroenterol Clin Biol 18:1106–1111

Moayyedi P, Braunholtz D, Heminbrough E, Clough M, Tompkins DS, Mapstone NP, Mason S, Dowell AC, Richards ID, Chalmers DM, Axon AT (1997) Do patients need to fast for a 13C-urea breath test? Eur J Gastroenterol Hepatol 9:275–277

Mokuolu AO, Sigal SH, Lieber CS (1997) Gastric juice urease activity as a diagnostic test for *Helicobacter pylori* infection. Am J Gastroenterol 92:644–648

Monteiro L, Bonnemaison D, Vekris A, Petry KG, Bonnet J, Vidal R, Cabrita J, Megraud F (1997) Complex polysaccharides as PCR inhibitors in feces: *Helicobacter pylori* model. J Clin Microbiol 35:995–998

Montgomery EA, Martin DF, Peura DA (1988) Rapid diagnosis of *Campylobacter pylori* by Gram's stain. Am J Clin Pathol 90:606–609

Morera-Brenes B, Sierra R, Barrantes R, Jonasson J, Nord CE (1994) *Helicobacter pylori* in a Costa Rican dyspeptic patient population. Eur J Clin Microbiol Infect Dis 13:253–257

Morris A, Ali MR, Brown P, Lane M, Patton K (1989) *Campylobacter pylori* infection in biopsy specimens of gastric antrum: laboratory diagnosis and estimation of sampling error. J Clin Pathol 42:727–732

Mowat C, Murray L, Hilditch TE, Kelman A, Oien K, McColl KE (1998) Comparison of helisal rapid blood test and 14C-urea breath test in determining *Helicobacter pylori* status and predicting ulcer disease in dyspeptic patients. Am J Gastroenterol 93:20–25

Munster DJ, Chapman BA, Burt MJ, Dobbs BR, Allardyce RA, Bagshaw PF, Troughton WD, Cook HB (1993) The fate of ingested 14C-urea in the urea breath test for *Helicobacter pylori* infection. Scand J Gastroenterol 28:661–666

Nakao K, Imoto I, Gabazza EC, Yamauchi K, Yamazaki N, Taguchi Y, Shibata T, Takaji S, Ikemura N, Misaki M (1997) Gastric juice levels of lactoferrin and *Helicobacter pylori* infection. Scand J Gastroenterol 32:530–534

Narvaez Rodriguez I, Saez de Santamaria J, Alcalde Rubio MM, Pascasio Acevedo JM, Pabon Jaen M, Campos de Orellana AM, Soria Monge A (1995) Cytologic brushing as a simple and rapid method in the diagnosis of *Helicobacter pylori* infection. Acta Cytol 39:916–919

Neithercut WD, Milne A, Chittajallu RS, el Nujumi AM, McColl KE (1991) Detection of *Helicobacter pylori* infection of the gastric mucosa by measurement of gastric aspirate ammonium and urea concentrations. Gut 32:973–976

Neithercut WD, Rowe PA, el Nujumi AM, Dahill S, McColl KE (1993) Effect of *Helicobacter pylori* infection on intragastric urea and ammonium concentrations in patients with chronic renal failure. J Clin Pathol 46:544–547

Nguyen AM, Engstrand L, Genta RM, Graham DY, el-Zaatari FA (1993) Detection of *Helicobacter pylori* in dental plaque by reverse transcription-polymerase chain reaction. J Clin Microbiol 31:783–787

Nichols L, Sughayer M, DeGirolami PC, Balogh K, Pleskow D, Eichelberger K, Santos M (1991) Evaluation of diagnostic methods for *Helicobacter pylori* gastritis. Am J Clin Pathol 95:769–773

O'Toole PW, Logan SM, Kostrzynska M, Wadström T, Trust TJ (1991) Isolation and biochemical and molecular analyses of a species-specific protein antigen from the gastric pathogen *Helicobacter pylori*. J Bacteriol 173:505–513

Ohara H, Suzuki T, Nakagawa T, Yoneshima M, Yamamoto M, Tsujino D, Murai S, Saito N, Kokubun N, Kajiwara M (1995) 13C-UBT using an infrared spectrometer for detection of *Helicobacter pylori* and for monitoring the effects of lansoprazole. J Clin Gastroenterol 20 [Suppl 2]:S115–S117

Oksanen A, Bergstrom M, Sjostedt S, Gad A, Hammarlund B, Seensalu R (1997) Accurate detection of *Helicobacter pylori* infection with a simplified 13C urea breath test. Scand J Clin Lab Invest 57:689–694

Osaki T, Taguchi H, Yamaguchi H, Kamiya S (1998) Detection of *Helicobacter pylori* in fecal samples of gnotobiotic mice infected with H pylori by an immunomagnetic-bead separation technique. J Clin Microbiol 36:321–323

Owen RJ, Martin SR, Borman P (1985) Rapid urea hydrolysis by gastric Campylobacters. Lancet 1:111

Palmer ED (1954) Investigation of the Gastric Mucosa Spirochetes of the Human. Gastroenterology 27:218–220

Pathak CM, Bhasin DK, Panigrahi D, Goel RC (1994) Evaluation of 14C-urinary excretion and its comparison with 14CO2 in breath after 14C-urea administration in *Helicobacter pylori* infection. Am J Gastroenterol 89:734–738

Pedriali R, Cantarini D, Gullini S (1992) The importance of determining both urea and ammonium levels in gastric juice for rapid diagnosis of *Helicobacter pylori* infection. Endoscopy 24:292

Perez Garcia JI, Pajares Garcia JM, Jimenez Alonso I (1996) C13 urea breath test in the diagnosis of *Helicobacter pylori* infection in the gastric mucosa. Validation of the method (in Spanish. Rev Esp Enferm Dig 88:202–208

Perri F, Ghoos Y, Hiele M, Andriulli A, Rutgeerts P (1995a) The urea breath test: a non-invasive clinical tool for detecting *Helicobacter pylori* infection. Ital J Gastroenterol 27:55–63

Perri F, Maes B, Geypens B, Ghoos Y, Hiele M, Rutgeerts P (1995b) The influence of isolated doses of drugs, feeding and colonic bacterial ureolysis on urea breath test results. Aliment Pharmacol Ther 9:705–709

Peura DA (1995) *Helicobacter pylori*: a diagnostic dilemma and a dilemma of diagnosis. Gastroenterology 109:313–315

Peura DA, Pambianco DJ, Dye KR, Lind C, Frierson HF, Hoffman SR, Combs MJ, Guilfoyle E, Marshall BJ (1996) Microdose 14C-urea breath test offers diagnosis of *Helicobacter pylori* in 10 min. Am J Gastroenterol 91:233–238

Pinto MM, Meriano FV, Afridi S, Taubin HL (1991) Cytodiagnosis of *Campylobacter pylori* in Papanicolaou-stained imprints of gastric biopsy specimens. Acta Cytol 35:204–206

Prewett EJ, Luk YW, Fraser AG, Lam WM, Pounder RE (1992) Comparison of one-day oral dosing with three bismuth compounds for the suppression of *Helicobacter pylori* assessed by the 13C-urea breath test. Aliment Pharmacol Ther 6:97–102

Puetz T, Vakil N, Phadnis S, Dunn B, Robinson J (1997) The Pyloritek test and the CLO test: accuracy and incremental cost analysis. Am J Gastroenterol 92:254–257

Raju GS, Smith MJ, Morton D, Bardhan KD (1994) Mini-dose (1-microCi) 14C-urea breath test for the detection of *Helicobacter pylori*. Am J Gastroenterol 89:1027–1031

Rauws EA, Royen EA, Langenberg W, Woensel JV, Vrij AA, Tytgat GN (1989) 14C-urea breath test in C pylori gastritis. Gut 30:798–803

Reijers MH, Noach LA, Tytgat GN (1994) Short report: evaluation of *Helicobacter pylori* eradication with bismuth sucralfate. Aliment Pharmacol Ther 8:351–352

Reilly TG, Poxon V, Sanders DS, Elliott TS, Walt RP (1997) Comparison of serum, salivary, and rapid whole blood diagnostic tests for *Helicobacter pylori* and their validation against endoscopy based tests. Gut 40:454–458

Riard P, Hostein J, Croize J, Bourguignon G, Le Marc'Hadour F, Faure H, Fournet J (1989) *Campylobacter pylori*: diagnostic value of the urease test during endoscopy (in French). Gastroenterol Clin Biol 13:8–13

Robey-Cafferty SS, Ro JY, Cleary KR (1989) The prevalence of *Campylobacter pylori* in gastric biopsies from cancer patients. Mod Pathol 2:473–476

Rocha GA, Queiroz DM, Mendes EN, Lage AP, Barbosa AJ (1989) Simple carbolfuchsin staining for showing C pylori and other spiral bacteria in gastric mucosa. J Clin Pathol 42:1004–1005

Rollan A, Giancaspero R, Arrese M, Figueroa C, Vollrath V, Schultz M, Duarte I, Vial P (1997) Accuracy of invasive and noninvasive tests to diagnose *Helicobacter pylori* infection after antibiotic treatment. Am J Gastroenterol 92:1268–1274

Rowland M, Lambert I, Gormally S, Daly LE, Thomas JE, Hetherington C, Durnin M, Drumm B (1997) Carbon 13-labeled urea breath test for the diagnosis of *Helicobacter pylori* infection in children. J Pediatr 131:815–820

Sahay P, West AP, Hawkey PM, Axon AT (1995) Isolation of *Helicobacter pylori* from faeces. J Infect 30:262–263

Salmenkyla S, Hyvarinen H, Halonen K, Sipponen P (1997) Frozen-section biopsy in perendoscopic diagnosis of *Helicobacter pylori*. Helicobacter 2:123–126

Sang FC, Lule GN, Ogutu EO (1991) Evaluation of culture media and antimicrobial susceptibility of *Helicobacter pylori*. East Afr Med J 68:865–868

Schnadig VJ, Bigio EH, Gourley WK, Stewart GD, Newton GA, Shabot JM (1990) Identification of *Campylobacter pylori* by endoscopic brush cytology. Diagn Cytopathol 6:227–234

Scholte GH, van Doorn LJ, Quint WG, Lindeman J (1997) Polymerase chain reaction for the detection of *Helicobacter pylori* in formaldehyde-sublimate fixed, paraffin-embedded gastric biopsies. Diagn Mol Pathol 6:238–243

Schrier WH, Schoengold RJ, Baker JT, Norell JL, Jaseph CL, Okin Y, Doe JY, Chandler H (1998) Development of FlexSure HP – an immunochromatographic method to detect antibodies against *Helicobacter pylori*. Clin Chem 44:293–298

Schwarz E, Plum G, Mauff G, Hasbach H, Eidt S, Schrappe M, Kruis W (1997) Molecular biology in diagnosis and epidemiology of *Helicobacter pylori*: PCR for the detection and AP-PCR for characterization of patient isolates. Zentralbl Bakteriol 285:368–378

Sharma TK, Young EL, Miller S, Cutler AF (1997) Evaluation of a rapid, new method for detecting serum IgG antibodies to *Helicobacter pylori*. Clin Chem 43:832–836

Shimada T, Ogura K, Ota S, Terano A (1995) Clinical efficacy of lansoprazole-amoxicillin treatment in eradicating *Helicobacter pylori*: evaluation by the polymerase chain reaction method. J Clin Gastroenterol 20 [Suppl 2]:S100–S103

Shimoyama T, Fukuda Y, Fukuda S, Munakata A, Yoshida Y (1996) Validity of various diagnostic tests to evaluate cure of *Helicobacter pylori* infection. J Gastroenterol 31:171–174

Sjöstrom JE, Kuhler T, Larsson H (1997) Basis for the selective antibacterial activity in vitro of proton pump inhibitors against Helicobacter spp. Antimicrob Agents Chemother 41:1797–1801

Slater B (1990) Superior stain for *Helicobacter pylori* using toluidine O. J Clin Pathol 43:961

Smith JG, Kong L, Abruzzo GK, Gill CJ, Flattery AM, Scott PM, Bramhill D, Cioffe C, Thompson CM, Bartizal K (1996) PCR detection of colonization by *Helicobacter pylori* in conventional, euthymic mice based on the 16 S ribosomal gene sequence. Clin Diagn Lab Immunol 3:66–72

Steen T, Berstad K, Meling T, Berstad A (1995) Reproducibility of the 14C urea breath test repeated after 1 week. Am J Gastroenterol 90:2103–2105

Stone MA, Mayberry JF, Wicks AC, Livsey SA, Stevens M, Swann RA, Robinson RJ (1997) Near patient testing for *Helicobacter pylori*: a detailed evaluation of the Cortecs Helisal Rapid Blood test. Eur J Gastroenterol Hepatol 9:257–260

Taha AS, Kelly RW, Carr G, Stiemer B, Morton R, Park RH, Beattie AD (1996) Altered urinary interleukin-8/creatinine ratio in peptic ulcer disease: pathological and diagnostic implications. Am J Gastroenterol 91:2528–2531

Tanigawa T, Mizo-Oku Y, Moriguchi K, Suzuki T, Osumi T, Odomi M (1996) Simple and rapid quantitative assay of 13C-labelled urea in human serum using liquid chromatography-atmospheric pressure chemical ionization mass spectrometry. J Chromatogr B Biomed Appl 683:135–142

Taniguchi Y, Kimura K, Sohara H, Shirasaki A, Kawada H, Satoh K, Kihira K, Wang XM, Takimoto T, Goto Y, Takatori K, Iida K, Kajiwara M (1996) Simple 13C-urea breath test with infra-red spectrophotometer. J Gastroenterol 31 [Suppl 9]:37–40

Tee W, Fairley S, Smallwood R, Dwyer B (1991) Comparative evaluation of three selective media and a nonselective medium for the culture of *Helicobacter pylori* from gastric biopsies. J Clin Microbiol 29:2587–2589

Thijs JC, van Zwet AA, Moolenaar W, Wolfhagen MJ, ten Bokkel Huinink J (1996a) Triple therapy vs. amoxicillin plus omeprazole for treatment of *Helicobacter pylori* infection: a multicenter, prospective, randomized, controlled study of efficacy and side effects. Am J Gastroenterol 91:93–97

Thijs JC, van Zwet AA, Thijs WJ, Oey HB, Karrenbeld A, Stellaard F, Luijt DS, Meyer BC, Kleibeuker JH (1996b) Diagnostic tests for *Helicobacter pylori*: a prospective evaluation of their accuracy, without selecting a single test as the gold standard. Am J Gastroenterol 91:2125–2129

Thillainayagam AV, Arvind AS, Cook RS, Harrison IG, Tabaqchali S, Farthing MJ (1991) Diagnostic efficiency of an ultrarapid endoscopy room test for *Helicobacter pylori*. Gut 32:467–469

Thomas JE, Gibson GR, Darboe MK, Dale A, Weaver LT (1992) Isolation of *Helicobacter pylori* from human faeces. Lancet 340:1194–1195

Thoreson AC, Borre MB, Andersen LP, Elsborg L, Holck S, Conway P, Henrichsen J, Vuust J, Krogfelt KA (1995) Development of a PCR-based technique for detection of *Helicobacter pylori*. FEMS Immunol Med Microbiol 10:325–333

Trevisani L, Sartori S, Ruina M, Caselli M, Abbasciano V, Grandi E, Forini E (1997) Touch cytology. A reliable and cost-effective method for diagnosis of *Helicobacter pylori* infection. Dig Dis Sci 42: 2299–2303

Triebling AT, Korsten MA, Dlugosz JW, Paronetto F, Lieber CS (1991) Severity of Helicobacter-induced gastric injury correlates with gastric juice ammonia. Dig Dis Sci 36:1089–1096

Vaira D, Holton J, Cairns S, Polydorou A, Falzon M, Dowsett J, Salmon PR (1988) Urease tests for *Campylobacter pylori*: care in interpretation. J Clin Pathol 41:812–813

Valentine JL, Arthur RR, Mobley HL, Dick JD (1991) Detection of *Helicobacter pylori* by using the polymerase chain reaction. J Clin Microbiol 29:689–695

van de Wouw BA, de Boer WA, Jansz AR, Roymans RT, Staals AP (1996) Comparison of three commercially available enzyme-linked immunosorbent assays and biopsy-dependent diagnosis for detecting *Helicobacter pylori* infection. J Clin Microbiol 34:94–97

van der Hulst RW, Verheul SB, Weel JF, Gerrits Y, ten Kate FJ, Dankert J, Tytgat GN (1996) Effect of specimen collection techniques, transport media, and incubation of cultures on the detection rate of *Helicobacter pylori*. Eur J Clin Microbiol Infect Dis 15:211–215

Van Horn KG, Dworkin BM (1990) Direct gram stain and urease test to detect *Helicobacter pylori*. Diagn Microbiol Infect Dis 13:449–452

van Zwet AA, Thijs JC, Kooistra-Smid AM, Schirm J, Snijder JA (1994) Use of PCR with feces for detection of *Helicobacter pylori* infections in patients. J Clin Microbiol 32:1346–1348

Veenendaal RA, Lichtendahl-Bernards AT, Pena AS, Endtz HP, van Boven CP, Lamers CB (1993) Effect of transport medium and transportation time on culture of *Helicobacter pylori* from gastric biopsy specimens. J Clin Pathol 46:561–563

Veldhuyzen van Zanten SJ, Tytgat KM, Hollingsworth J, Jalali S, Rshid FA, Bowen BM, Goldie J, Goodacre RL, Riddell RH, Hunt RH (1990) 14C-urea breath test for the detection of *Helicobacter pylori*. Am J Gastroenterol 85:399–403

Wahlfors J, Meurman JH, Toskala J, Korhonen A, Alakuijala P, Janatuinen E, Karkkkainen UM, Nuutinen P, Janne J (1995) Development of a rapid PCR method for identification of *Helicobacter pylori* in dental plaque and gastric biopsy specimens. Eur J Clin Microbiol Infect Dis 14:780–786

Walters LL, Budin RE, Paull G (1986) Acridine-orange to identify *Campylobacter pylori*dis in formalin fixed, paraffin-embedded gastric biopsies. Lancet 1:42

Wang JT, Lin JT, Sheu JC, Yang JC, Chen DS, Wang TH (1993) Detection of *Helicobacter pylori* in gastric biopsy tissue by polymerase chain reaction. Eur J Clin Microbiol Infect Dis 12:367–371

Warren JR, Marshall B (1983) Unidentified curved bacilli on gastric epithelium in active chronic gastritis. Lancet 1:1273–1275

Weil J, Bell GD, Jones PH, Gant P, Trowell JE, Harrison G (1988) "Eradication" of *Campylobacter pylori*: are we being misled? Lancet 2:1245

Weil J, Bell GD, Powell K, Morden A, Harrison G, Gant PW, Jones PH, Trowell JE (1991a) Omeprazole and *Helicobacter pylori*: temporary suppression rather than true eradication. Aliment Pharmacol Ther 5:309–313

Weil J, Bell GD, Powell K, Morden A, Harrison G, Gant PW, Trowell JE, Burridge S (1991b) *Helicobacter pylori*: treatment with combinations of pivampicillin and tripotassium dicitrato bismuthate. Aliment Pharmacol Ther 5:543–547

Westblom TU, Madan E, Kemp J, Subik MA (1988a) Evaluation of a rapid urease test to detect *Campylobacter pylori* infection. J Clin Microbiol 26:1393–1394

Westblom TU, Madan E, Kemp J, Subik MA, Tseng J (1988b) Improved visualisation of mucus penetration by *Campylobacter pylori* using a Brown-Hopps stain (letter). J Clin Pathol 41:232

Westblom TU (1991) Laboratory diagnosis and handling of *Helicobacter pylori*. In: Marshall BJ, McCallum RW, Guerrant RL (eds) *Helicobacter pylori* in peptic ulceration and gastritis. Blackwell Scientific, Boston, pp 81–91

Westblom TU, Gudipati S, Madan E, Midkiff BR (1991a) Improved growth of *Helicobacter pylori* using a liquid medium supplemented with human serum. Ital J Gastroenterol 23 [Suppl 2]:48

Westblom TU, Madan E, Midkiff BR (1991b) Egg yolk emulsion agar, a new medium for the cultivation of *Helicobacter pylori*. J Clin Microbiol 29:819–821

Westblom TU, Madan E, Gudipati S, Midkiff BR, Czinn SJ (1992) Diagnosis of *Helicobacter pylori* infection in adult and pediatric patients by using Pyloriset, a rapid latex agglutination test. J Clin Microbiol 30:96–98

Westblom TU (1993) The comparative value of different diagnostic tests for *Helicobacter pylori*. In: Goodwin CS, Worsley BW (eds) *Helicobacter pylori*: biology and clinical practice. CRC Press, Boca Raton, pp 329–342

Westblom TU, Lagging LM, Midkiff BR, Czinn SJ (1993a) Evaluation of QuickVue, a rapid enzyme immunoassay test for the detection of serum antibodies to *Helicobacter pylori*. Diagn Microbiol Infect Dis 16:317–320

Westblom TU, Lagging LM, Milligan TW, Midkiff BR, Czinn SJ (1993b) Differences in antigenic recognition between adult and pediatric patients infected with *Helicobacter pylori*: analysis using Western blot technique. Acta Gastroenterol Belg 56 [Suppl]:84

Westblom TU, Phadnis S, Yang P, Czinn SJ (1993c) Diagnosis of *Helicobacter pylori* infection by means of a polymerase chain reaction assay for gastric juice aspirates. Clin Infect Dis 16:367–371

Wilcox MH, Dent TH, Hunter JO, Gray JJ, Brown DF, Wight DG, Wraight EP (1996) Accuracy of serology for the diagnosis of *Helicobacter pylori* infection – a comparison of eight kits. J Clin Pathol 49:373–376

Woo JS, el-Zimaity HM, Genta RM, Yousfi MM, Graham DY (1996) The best gastric site for obtaining a positive rapid urease test. Helicobacter 1:256–259

Wu JC, Liu GL, Zhang ZH, Mou YL, Chen QA, Yang SL (1992) 15NH4+ excretion test: a new method for detection of *Helicobacter pylori* infection. J Clin Microbiol 30:181–184

Xia HX, Keane CT, O'Morain CA (1993) Determination of the optimal transport system for *Helicobacter pylori* cultures. J Med Microbiol 39:334–337

Yamashiro Y, Oguchi S, Otsuka Y, Nagata S, Shioya T, Shimizu T (1995) *Helicobacter pylori* colonization in children with peptic ulcer disease. III. Diagnostic value of the 13C-urea breath test to detect gastric H. pylori colonization. Acta Paediatr Jpn 37:12–16

Yang DH, Bom HS, Joo YE, Choi SK, Rew JS, Yoon CM (1995) Gastric juice ammonia vs CLO test for diagnosis of *Helicobacter pylori* infection. Dig Dis Sci 40:1083–1086

Yeung CK, Yuen KY, Fu KH, Tsang TM, Seto WH, Saing H (1990) Rapid endoscopy room diagnosis of *Campylobacter pylori*-associated gastritis in children. J Pediatr Gastroenterol Nutr 10:357–360

Yoshida H, Hirota K, Shiratori Y, Nihei T, Amano S, Yoshida A, Kawamata O, Omata M (1998) Use of a gastric juice-based PCR assay to detect *Helicobacter pylori* infection in culture-negative patients. J Clin Microbiol 36:317–320

Yousfi MM, el-Zimaity HM, Genta RM, Graham DY (1996) Evaluation of a new reagent strip rapid urease test for detection of *Helicobacter pylori* infection. Gastrointest Endosc 44:519–522

Yousfi MM, el-Zimaity HM, Cole RA, Genta RM, Graham DY (1997) Comparison of agar gel (CLOtest) or reagent strip (PyloriTek) rapid urease tests for detection of *Helicobacter pylori* infection. Am J Gastroenterol 92:997–999

Economic Perspectives in the Management of *Helicobacter pylori* Infections

A. SONNENBERG and J.M. INADOMI

1 Introduction

The infection with *Helicobacter pylori* contributes to the occurrence of at least four diseases, that is, gastric ulcer, duodenal ulcer, gastric cancer and gastric mucosa-associated lymphoma tissue lymphoma. Many gastroenterologists believe that infection with *H. pylori* can also result in epigastric symptoms and nonulcer dyspepsia. The health economics of *H. pylori* infection relates to the cost-benefit relationship of preventing, treating or curing these various conditions through

Gastroenterology Section, Department of Veterans Affairs, Medical Center 111F, 2100 Ridgecrest Drive SE, Albuquerque, NM 87108, USA medical measures directed against the infectious organism. In addition, economic analyses have addressed various other aspects of diagnosis and management of patients infected with *H. pylori*. A minority of analyses were based on real data generated from prospective clinical trials or retrospective analysis of utilization of health care resources, while the majority of studies used economic modeling to predict the influence of various medical measures. The models used mostly decision trees, Markov chains, the declining exponential approximation of life expectancy (DEALE), and the accounting technique of net present value. The following three sections of the present chapter are focused towards the management of the three most common conditions associated with *H. pylori*, that is, peptic ulcer, gastric cancer, and nonulcer dyspepsia. In a subsequent section we discuss the workup of patients with upper abdominal symptoms and a few other economic issues related to the management of patients infected with *H. pylori*.

2 Peptic Ulcer

Most studies that test the influence of *H. pylori* treatment on peptic ulcer deal with duodenal ulcer or duodenal plus gastric ulcer. All studies show similarly that antibiotic therapy to eradicate *H. pylori* is cheaper and far more cost-effective than any previous conventional therapy to inhibit gastric acid secretion. Four different types of economic studies have analyzed the economics of peptic ulcer with respect to *H. pylori*, that is (a) prospective randomized clinical trial, (b) Markov chain, (c) decision tree, and (d) DEALE.

2.1 Clinical Trial in Peptic Ulcer

In a large multicenter study in the United States, adult patients infected with *H. pylori* in the presence of active duodenal ulcer were randomized to double-blind treatment with clarithromycin 500mg t.i.d. plus omeprazole 40mg q.d. for 14 days followed by omeprazole alone 20mg q.d. for 14 days, omeprazole 20mg q.d. for 28 days, or ranitidine 150mg b.i.d. for 28 days (SONNENBERG 1996c, 1977a; SONNENBERG et al. 1998). After the initial therapy, all patients were followed for 1 year. During this period, investigators accumulated all ulcer-related utilization of health care resources, such as gastrointestinal endoscopies, clinic visits, visits to the emergency room, medications, and hospital admissions. In addition, work days lost secondary to ulcer disease were recorded. Average cost data for the United States from the Health Care Financing Administration, the Bureau of the Census, and the Average Wholesale Price List for drugs were used to convert resource utilization into dollar amounts.

Of the 819 patients enrolled 727 completed the study, that is, 243 on omeprazole plus clarithromycin, 248 on omeprazole alone, and 236 on ranitidine alone. Based on the results of a 13C-urea breath tests 6 weeks after completion of treatment, *H. pylori* was eradicated in 68% of patients on omeprazole plus clarithromycin, 7% on omeprazole, and 4% on ranitidine. Patients in the clarithromycin plus omeprazole treatment group utilized fewer ulcer-related health care resources during the 1 year after therapy, compared with the omeprazole or ranitidine treatment groups: the difference between the omeprazole plus clarithromycin group and the two conventional groups was significant with respect to the number of endoscopies, number of patients receiving medications for upper gastrointestinal symptoms, clinic visits, and hospital days. The costs of the initial antibiotic drug therapy were more expensive than either of the two antisecretory therapies, while the total ulcer-related costs during the 1-year follow-up were higher in the two antisecretory therapies than the antibiotic therapy (Fig. 1). The incremental cost-savings correspond to the difference in total costs between each two therapies, divided by the difference between their drug costs. Although it was initially more expensive, antibiotic therapy resulted in less utilization of health care resources than conventional antisecretory therapy. For every dollar spent on short-term antibiotic therapy, $1.94 and $2.96 were saved within the first year after completion of therapy by a reduced utilization of care resources compared with omeprazole or ranitidine, respectively.

For three reasons the results the study might have been biased against a stronger economic benefit associated with antibiotic eradication. First, when the study was initiated in 1994, clarithromycin plus omeprazole was a state of the art regimen. Since then other treatment modalities based on triple therapy with omeprazole 20mg b.i.d., clarithromycin 500mg b.i.d., and amoxicillin 1g b.i.d. or metronidazole 500mg b.i.d. have consistently provided higher eradication rates of 90%–95%. Second, after the initial double-blind treatment phase, the participating

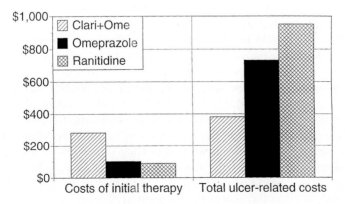

Fig. 1. Cost of initial ulcer therapy and subsequent ulcer-related costs per patient treated with clarithromycin and omeprazole, omeprazole alone, or ranitidine alone. Data accumulated during a prospective randomized clinical trial following 727 duodenal ulcer patients over a time period of 1 year after the initial ulcer therapy

trial centers could use any type of treatment regimen to manage recurrent ulcer symptoms. A large number of patients randomized initially into the omeprazole or ranitidine arm were subsequently given antibiotic therapy for recurrent ulcer symptoms. Third, all analyses are based on the intention to treat rather than a successful completion of the antibiotic course. For financial reasons a study of this size could be carried on for only 1 year. Much larger savings are likely to accumulate if the observation period is extended beyond 1 year, as little additional cost should accrue in the patients with successfully eradicated *H. pylori* while further maintenance therapy is needed and breakthrough ulcers are to be expected in conventionally treated patients.

2.2 Markov Chain in Peptic Ulcer

Intermittent or maintenance therapy with histamine-2 receptor antagonists, highly selective vagotomy, or antibiotic therapy to eradicate *H. pylori* represent four options to manage duodenal ulcer disease. A Markov chain was used to compare their efficacy and cost over a time period of 15 years (SONNENBERG and TOWNSEND 1995). The direct costs were calculated from the average wholesale prices of drugs and from charges for medical services submitted to the Health Care Financing Administration in 1993. The average annual income in the United States in 1993 was used to estimate the indirect costs.

The concept of a Markov chain is relatively simple and straightforward. It can be easily analyzed on a computerized spreadsheet, such as Excel from Microsoft. Any patient with duodenal ulcer disease can be considered to be in one of the six states shown in Fig. 2. The transitions between the states are governed by the probability of infection with *H. pylori*, ulcer relapse, ulcer healing, eradication of *H. pylori*, and the occurrence of ulcer complications. Duodenal ulcers accompanied by bleeding but without need for surgery are treated as ordinary ulcers. However, duodenal ulcers associated with severe hemorrhage, perforation, or any other severe complication would require surgical intervention with either a favorable or lethal outcome. Using the scoring system suggested by Visick, the favorable postoperative state is further separated into grades 1–3, representing satisfactory outcomes, and grade 4, representing an unsatisfactory outcome of surgery. The analysis is started with 1000 hypothetical patients with an active ulcer, i.e., 1000 patients in the state of "duodenal ulcer without complication." Every month the patients are newly distributed among the various states of the Markov chain according to the transition probabilities taken from the literature. The fraction of subjects in each state and the costs which arise from drugs, hospitalization, surgery, and income losses due to absenteeism, disability, and premature death are then accumulated on a monthly basis for a duration of 15 years.

The model predicts that after antibiotic therapy, 99.7% of patient time is spent free of duodenal ulcer. The corresponding percentages for maintenance therapy are 96.6%, for vagotomy 94.4%, for intermittent therapy 89.4%, and without therapy

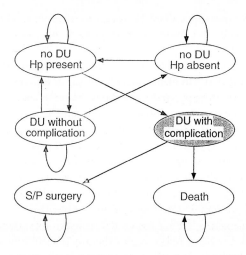

Fig. 2. A Markov state model of duodenal ulcer. *Ovals,* different states in the natural history of the disease; *straight arrows,* transitions between various states, the probabilities of which were taken from the literature; *curved arrows,* patients who stay in the same state. The transition probabilities associated with *straight and curved arrows* that leave a single state add up to 100%. The model was run on a monthly cycle for 1 year with patients being distributed among the various states according to the transition probabilities associated with *each arrow.* The model was started with 1000 patients in the state of "DU without complication"

82.8%. For an individual patient after 15 years, the expected total costs of a treatment approach involving antibiotics are \$978, compared with \$10,350 for intermittent therapy with H_2 antagonists, \$11,186 for maintenance therapy with H_2 antagonists, and \$17,661 after vagotomy. Compared with other options, antibiotics to eradicate *H. pylori* appear to be the cheapest therapy of duodenal ulcer and provide the least time spent with an active ulcer. From an economic perspective, antibiotics represent the treatment of choice. The striking difference between antibiotic and other types of therapy proved quite insensitive to a wide range of variations regarding antibiotic efficacy, reinfection rates, and various means to assess successful eradication. Even with the changes in health care market from fee-for-service to a capitated system and a marked drop in the cost of most endoscopic procedures, the difference between the various therapeutic treatment options would remain largely unaffected.

BRIGGS et al. (1996) used a slightly different Markov chain than shown in Fig. 2 to assess the long-term benefit of eradicating *H. pylori*. The results of their study also suggested the antibiotic regimen to be the preferred treatment strategy.

2.3 Decision Trees in Peptic Ulcer

O'BRIEN et al. (1995) used a decision tree to compare the direct costs accumulating during 1 year with three treatment strategies of duodenal ulcer: [1] immediate *H. pylori* eradication. [2] *H. pylori* eradication only after the first ulcer recurrence, and [3] maintenance therapy with an H_2 receptor antagonist. The first strategy was found to be less costly and result in fewer ulcer recurrences than the other two options.

IMPERIALE et al. (1995) used a decision tree to compare the direct costs per symptomatic treatment of duodenal ulcer with (a) a H_2 receptor antagonist for 8 weeks, (b) antibiotic therapy, and (c) a choice between the two former therapies based on the outcome of a urease breath test. Patients were followed for 1 year. If the infection rate with *H. pylori* in duodenal ulcer exceeded 66%, the second strategy was the least expensive. Initial testing for *H. pylori* by breath tests in all duodenal ulcer patients (as suggested by the third treatment option) was the preferred strategy if *H. pylori* infection rates in duodenal ulcer ranged between 3 and 66%. Antisecretory therapy was only cost-effective with extremely low *H. pylori* infection rates of less than 3% in duodenal ulcer patients.

VAKIL and FENNERTY (1995) compared antisecretory therapy of the initial duodenal ulcer with 6 weeks of H_2 receptor therapy to antibiotic therapy. The costs of potential complications and ulcer recurrences were accumulated over a time period of 2 years. As in the previous two studies, antibiotic therapy was found to be the least expensive treatment option.

2.4 DEALE in Peptic Ulcer

The DEALE allows one to estimate the influence of a particular disease or a medical measure on life expectancy. The technique of DEALE has been utilized to estimate how eradication of *H. pylori* would affect life expectancy by preventing peptic ulcer disease (INADOMI and SONNENBERG 1998). The DEALE assumes that survival in human populations follows an exponential decline (BECK et al. 1982a,b):

$$S = S_0 \cdot e^{-\mu_{age} \cdot time} \tag{1}$$

S_0 and S represent the number of survivors at time $= 0$ and some other given time, respectively (Fig. 3). If no other diseases are present, μ_{age} corresponds to the age-dependent mortality force of each age group. It can be shown that in each age group the average life expectancy (LE) equals (DRAKE 1967; GROSS and CLARK 1975)

$$LE = \frac{1}{\mu_{age}}. \tag{2}$$

The age-specific life expectancy (LE) is readily available through various publications of the Vital Statistics of the United States and the NATIONAL CENTER FOR HEALTH STATISTICS (1995, 1996). If a disease such as peptic ulcer (PUD) is present, the overall mortality force becomes a composite of the age-specific mortality force plus the disease-specific mortality force:

$$LE = \frac{1}{\mu} = \frac{1}{\mu_{age} + \mu_{pud}}. \tag{3}$$

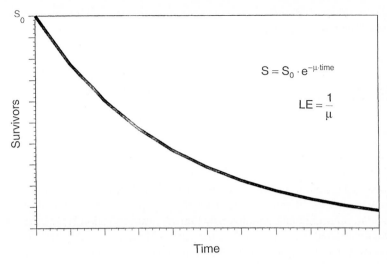

Fig. 3. The model of declining exponential approximation of life expectancy (DEALE) assumes that over time the number of survivors in each age group drops according to an exponential law

These approximations hold true as long as the disease-specific mortality is small compared with the overall mortality of a particular age group. The disease-specific mortality force is assumed to act independently of age. The age-specific increase in mortality is postulated to stem solely from the age-dependent μ_{age}. The ulcer-specific mortality force can be calculated from the number of deaths listed in the Vital Statistics or obtained through the internet from the Centers for Disease Control (http://www.wonder.cdc.gov/). In 1992, 6058 Americans aged over 35 years died from peptic ulcer, that is, ICD codes 531 through 533. The total United States population over 35 years was 120,522,342 persons. For the contribution of peptic ulcer alone to survival, Eq. 1 can be rewritten as:

$$S = S_0 \cdot e^{-\mu_{pud} \cdot time}. \tag{4}$$

The number of survivors after 1 year corresponds to the original population S_0 minus the annual number of deaths D secondary to peptic ulcer, that is, $S = S_0 - D$. After solving Eq. 4 for μ_{pud}, Eq. 3 yields the life expectancy modified by the presence of peptic ulcer disease. The difference between the life expectancies of Eqs. 2 and 3 represents the reduction in life expectancy of the general population secondary to peptic ulcer.

In the general population, cure of PUD increases life expectancy by 34 days in persons aged 35–39 years and by 4 days in persons aged 70–74 years. In subjects with a previous PUD history the increases in life expectancy are 322 and 36 days, respectively. Patients with active PUD may expect gains ranging between 2.4 years and 101 days. The most substantial impact occurs in persons with complicated PUD, with increases in life expectancy ranging between 28.5 and 5.6 years after curing the disease. The benefit of PUD cure diminishes as age advances. In young patients with active ulcers or ulcer complications, cure of PUD results in an appreciable increase in life expectancy.

3 Gastric Cancer

The economics of *H. pylori* in gastric cancer center around two related questions. [1] Are childhood vaccination against *H. pylori* or its eradication among adults worthwhile medical pursuits to prevent the future development of gastric cancer? [2] Could the prevention of *H. pylori* infection be made less costly than treatment of the actual diseases, that is gastric cancer and peptic ulcer? Although epidemiological data indicate quite unanimously that *H. pylori* infection represents a strong risk factor for the occurrence of gastric cancer (FORMAN et al. 1994), no experimental data exist to show that eradication of *H. pylori* actually prevents the occurrence of gastric cancer. It is also presently unknown at what point in the natural history of an *H. pylori*-induced gastritis one can prevent the future development of gastric cancer and what features characterize the earliest point of no return when gastritis becomes irreversible. Antibiotic eradication of *H. pylori* does not appear to reverse intestinal metaplasia (VAN DER HULST et al. 1997), although several pathophysiological changes still separate intestinal metaplasia from cancer. Appreciable efforts have been spent in the development of a vaccine, however, a functional vaccine does not yet exist nor is it foreseeable for the near future (CORTHÉSY-THEULAZ et al. 1995; LEE 1996; SELLMAN et al. 1995). Since many of the crucial clinical, as well as pathophysiological data, are still missing, economic analyses of *H. pylori* therapy to prevent gastric cancer are based on a mixture of guesswork and modeling, using estimated rates of efficacy and utilization of health care resources. Three types of modeling techniques have been used: decision trees, DEALE, and the concept of the net present value.

3.1 Decision Trees in Gastric Cancer

As with most other preventive programs in medicine, the decision in favor of or against screening for *H. pylori* and its subsequent therapy can be reduced to a simple question of balance. On one side of the scale is the large benefit experienced by a small group of subjects in whom gastric cancer becomes prevented through screening and therapy. On the other side are the relatively low costs associated with screening and therapy to whom a large group of subjects needs to be exposed in order to prevent a few cancers. Rather than phrase the problem as a cost-benefit issue, one can also compare the current costs invested in screening and therapy to save the future costs associated with gastric cancer. Figure 4 illustrates such a decision tree.

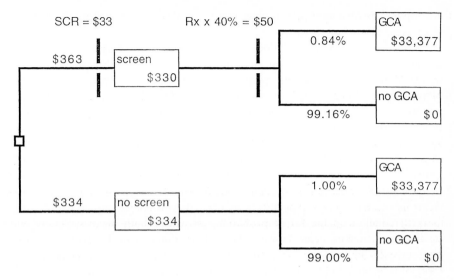

Fig. 4. The decision tree of screening (*SCR*) and therapy (*Rx*) for *H. pylori* to prevent gastric cancer (*GCA*). *Numbers inside the boxes, above toll bars,* costs associated with various outcomes and transitions

The lower branch represents the decision against screening. The cumulative life time probability of gastric cancer has been estimated to be 1% (WELLER et al. 1993). The costs of managing gastric cancer have been estimated to amount to $52,000 (PARSONNET et al. 1996). If the screening program is aimed at preventing a gastric cancer that would possibly occur in 15 years, the net present value of a future gastric cancer equals:

$$\$33,377 = \$52,000/1.03^{15years} \tag{5}$$

The denominator $1.03^{15\ years}$ represents the adjustment of future cost to its present value, assuming a discount rate of 3% over 15 years. In a decision tree, all probabilities at a chance fork need to add up to 100%. The weighted average cost of all branches emanating from a chance fork are calculated as the sum of all costs multiplied by their associated probability of occurrence. Hence, $334 = 1% × $33,377 + 99% · $0. The upper branch represents the decision in favor of screening. Screening and therapy are represented by two toll bars. Screening is assumed to $33. Since only 40% of the population are assumed to test positive for *H. pylori* and require the subsequent expenditure of $125 for antibiotic therapy, therapy costs $50 = 40% · $125. The toll blocking each branch is added to the weighted average cost of the branches emanating from it. Under baseline conditions, the cumulative risk of gastric cancer is assumed to drop from 1% to 0.84% after successful eradication of *H. pylori*. This reduced cancer risk after *H. pylori* eradication represents the most crucial and least understood probability of the present decision tree. It reflects the separate influences of (at least) two factors on cancer development: (a) the actual contribution of *H. pylori* to the overall risk of developing gastric cancer, and (b) the efficacy of *H. pylori* eradication in reducing this risk of future gastric cancer.

Under the baseline conditions shown in Fig. 4 the decision in favor of screening and treating costs more than the decision against it. Figure 5 shows the results of two one-way sensitivity analyses. The y-axis represents the difference between the outcome of the lower minus the upper branch. Positive values indicate cost savings associated with screening and therapy, as the upper branch becomes cheaper than the lower branch. Varying the future cost of gastric cancer between $0 and $320,000 on the upper x-axis changes the combination of screening and treating for *H. pylori* from a cost-incurring to a cost-saving strategy. Varying the probability of gastric cancer after *H. pylori* eradication between 0.0% and 1.0% changes the combination of screening and treating from a cost-saving to a cost-incurring strategy. High expenditure associated with future gastric cancer or a marked reduction in the future probability of cancer both make screening and treating a worthwhile medical option. Time affects outcome of the analysis through Eq. 5 by reducing the net present value of gastric cancer and making the decision in favor of screening and treating less costly than the decision against it.

More refined decision trees than shown in Fig. 4 can be designed (SONNENBERG and INADOMI 1998). For instance, one could include additional branches that consider the positive and negative predictive values of screening tests or the success and failure rates of antibiotic therapy. In a small fraction of subjects, antibiotic

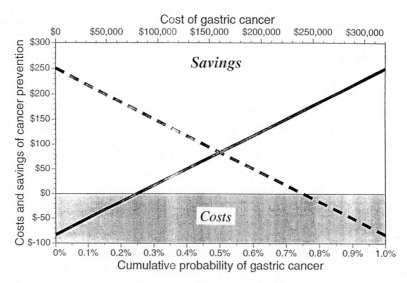

Fig. 5. One-way sensitivity analysis of the decision analysis from Fig. 4. *Broken line* and *lower a-axis*, effect of the reduced cumulative probability of gastric cancer after eradication of *H. pylori*; *unbroken line* and *upper axis*, effect of varying the future cost of gastric cancer between $0 and $320,000. *Negative values on y-axis* (and *shaded area*), values for which screening and therapy for *H. pylori* to prevent gastric cancer are more expensive than not doing it; *positive values on y-axis* (and *white area*) values for which screening and therapy for *H. pylori* to prevent gastric cancer would save money

eradication of *H. pylori* may lead to costs from side effects, the worst being pseudomembraneous colitis or long-term development of antibiotic resistance in the population. Such refinements change little in the overall outcome of the analysis. In addition to considering the future cost of gastric cancer and the immediate cost of screening and antibiotic treatment, PARSONNET et al. (1996) considered the benefit of life time gained by preventing gastric cancer. Their decision analysis reported the outcome as a ratio of dollars spent per life year gained. None of these more detailed decision analyses can bypass the principal problem of not knowing how *H. pylori* eradication will actually affect mortality from gastric cancer. Simultaneous changes of multiple variables within a clinically reasonable range can change the outcome of the economic analysis tenfold (SONNENBERG and INADOMI 1998).

3.2 The Concept of Present Value in Gastric Cancer

In principle, a cheap vaccination today is supposed to prevent a costly gastric cancer in the future. One may try to simplify the analyses from above even further and ask how much a gastric cancer in the future is worth in present dollars. Does its present value justify the cost of the means to prevent its occurrence? In general, the present value (PV) of future costs is given by the economic equation:

$$PV = \frac{future.costs}{(1 + discount.rate)^{years}}. \tag{6}$$

The discount rate reflects the depreciation of money and all material values over time. It accounts for the lost opportunity of future earnings through present investment (WEINSTEIN and STASON 1977). For instance, if one assumes an annual discount rate of 3%, the present value of a gastric cancer that will cost \$52,000 in 65 years from now amounts to:

$$PV = \frac{\$52,000}{(1 + 3\%)^{65years}} = \$7,613. \tag{6a}$$

About 40% of the general population are infected with *H. pylori*, and the cumulative chance of developing gastric cancer over lifetime in the general population is 1%. Infection with *H. pylori* leads to a fourfold increased risk of gastric cancer (FORMAN et al. 1994). These data can be used to calculate a 1.81% cumulative probability of developing gastric cancer in subjects infected with *H. pylori* (SONNENBERG and INADOMI 1998). It has been estimated that the cure or the prevention of an *H. pylori* infection will be 30% efficacious in preventing future gastric cancer (PARSONNET et al. 1996). Therefore, the present value of gastric cancer prevention is:

$$PE = \frac{future.costs}{(1 + discount.rate)^{years}} \times Hp.prevalence.rate \times lifetime.cancer.rate \\ \times Rx.efficacy.rate. \tag{7}$$

Using the values from above, Eq. 7 yields:

$$\$17 = \$7,613 \times 40\% \times 1.81\% \times 30\% \tag{7b}$$

According to this calculation, a childhood vaccination must not cost more than \$17 to be cost advantageous in preventing *H. pylori*-related gastric cancer. A need to establish the *H. pylori* status prior to the vaccination would increase the cost of vaccination in each individual subject. Any side effects of vaccination would increase the overall costs in the total population of all vaccinated subjects and, hence, the expected cost of vaccination per individual subject. With these constraints in mind, it seems doubtful that in the United States childhood vaccination for the sole purpose of preventing gastric cancer in adults will ever become a feasible option.

It is conceivable that vaccination could be effective in infected adults to help their immune system clear *H. pylori*. Even if vaccination failed or never materialized, we would still have the means of antibiotic therapy to eradicate the organism and heal the gastroduodenal inflammation. Compared with childhood conditions, vaccination or antibiotic therapy of adults would be directed towards prevention of gastric cancer that is expected to occur in closer temporal proximity to the preventive measure. For instance, one could imagine a prevention directed against cancer 15 years from now. Assuming cancer cost of \$52,000, discount rate of 3%, infection rate of 40%, and efficacy rate of 30%, the present value of such a strategy amounts to \$73. In general, the shorter the time period between the preventive measure and the potential occurrence of cancer, the greater the impact of future cancer and the more important its prevention. However, even without temporal discounting of future costs, the present value does not exceed \$113, since the cancer cost still applies to only a relatively small fraction of the population.

3.3 DEALE in Gastric Cancer

In 1992, 12,862 Americans aged over 35 years died from cancer of the gastric corpus and antrum, that is, ICD codes 151.1 through 151.9. This number excludes the 24 deaths before the age of 35 years or the few deaths from cancer of the gastric cardia (ICD code 151.0). The total US population over 40 years was 120,522,342 persons. Using the same equations as outlined above for peptic ulcer, one can calculate the impact of gastric cancer on life expectancy (SONNENBERG and INADOMI 1998). If prevention or cure of *H. pylori* infection were able to prevent all gastric cancers, life expectancy would increase by 71 days in persons aged 35–39 years and by 8 days in persons aged 70–74 years. The small changes in life expectancy associated with gastric cancer are a direct result of its small mortality force μ_{gca}. A small mortality force is calculated from Eq. 4, because the large United States population S_0 is affected by a very small number of cancer deaths ($D = S_0 - S$). A better knowledge of all risk factors involved in the development of gastric cancer may provide the opportunity to concentrate the preventive efforts on a high risk population. Such a concentration would be achievable, for instance, if we were able to diagnose cancerogenic strains of *H. pylori*, test an underlying genetic susceptibility for cancer, or reliably pinpoint other environmental risk factors in addition to

H. pylori. Mathematically, such knowledge would leave the value of D unchanged, but the size of the population at risk S_0 would shrink considerably, thus increasing the mortality force μ_{gca} associated with gastric cancer and increase its impact on life expectancy in the high risk population.

One can also use Eq. 3 to assess the joint influence of both peptic ulcer and gastric cancer on life expectancy of the general population (INADOMI and SONNENBERG 1998). Life expectancy would be prolonged by 105 days in subjects 35–39 years old and by 12 days in subjects 70–74 years old, if all mortality from peptic ulcer and gastric cancer were preventable through eradication of *H. pylori*. If preventive measures could be restricted to only 40% of the general population infected with *H. pylori*, their respective life expectancies would increase by 259 and 29 days. These numbers are overly optimistic, because they are based on the assumptions that, first, all cancers and ulcers are attributable to an underlying *H. pylori* infection and, second, eradication of *H. pylori* through vaccination or antibiotic therapy would be 100% efficacious.

A larger increase in life expectancy is seen in the younger than in the older age groups. The increase in life expectancy that could be achieved by prevention of gastric cancer (and peptic ulcer) decreases with advancing age, despite the age-independent nature of the mortality force of gastric cancer. This phenomenon can be explained mathematically by the structure of Eq. 2. Since the age-dependent mortality force (μ_{age}) increases with age, the relative contribution of the constant disease-specific mortality forces (μ_{gca} or μ_{pud}) to the overall mortality force (μ) decreases with advancing age (WELCH et al. 1996). This phenomenon has also a real medical background: as subjects age, their life expectancy decreases and their risk of dying from many different diseases increases. In the elderly, the elimination of a single disease from a large list of potential afflictions contributes little to their overall survival.

4 Nonulcer Dyspepsia

The key issue in the economics of nonulcer dyspepsia (NUD) relates to the question of whether this disorder responds to the eradication of *H. pylori*. Epidemiological studies have yielded similar infection rates among patients with nonulcer dyspepsia as in asymptomatic controls (VELDHUYZEN VAN ZANTEN and SHERMAN 1994). With few noteworthy exceptions, the majority of interventional studies failed to show that eradication of *H. pylori* improves dyspeptic symptoms in patients without peptic ulcer (LAHEIJ et al. 1996; TALLEY 1994). The success of few and the failure of many studies in affecting dyspeptic symptoms through antibiotic therapy have been ascribed to different selections of patients, different amounts of bacterial load or severity of gastritis, and different lengths of follow-up among the various studies. The group of patients with nonulcer dyspepsia presents with a hotchpotch of symptoms and diseases. Although it has remained difficult to separate them into clear-cut entities (TALLEY et al. 1992, 1993), some gastroenterologists feel that there may exist a smaller subgroup of NUD patients whose symptoms reflect primarily *H. pylori*-induced gastritis. The beneficial influence of *H. pylori* eradication in this particular subgroup would become masked by the large number of other NUD patients who fail therapy. Since NUD itself is characterized by waxing and waning of symptoms, longer observation periods than the usual 4–8 weeks of most clinical trials dealing with acid-peptic disorders may be needed to assess the influence of antibiotic therapy. The economic analysis of *H. pylori* eradication will fail to give conclusive answers as long as these key issues remain unresolved.

4.1 Decision Trees in NUD

Figure 6 illustrates the decision tree of testing for *H. pylori* in dyspeptic patients. Similar decision trees with slightly different transition rates and costs have been used in previous publications (SONNENBERG 1996a; SONNENBERG et al. 1997). To be consistent with the analyses outlined above, the decision tree covers an arbitrary time frame of 15 years. If one decides to order a serological test for *H. pylori* in each dyspeptic patient at the estimated cost of −$33, about 60% of the tests will have a negative result, while 40% will return positive (VELDHUYZEN VAN ZANTEN and SHERMAN 1994). Testing is done to subsequently treat the infection with antibiotics. Antibiotic therapy in combination with antisecretory therapy costs about −$125. Additional −$50 are spent on the physician visit. A baseline 80% cure rate and 20% failure rate are assumed. Eradication of *H. pylori* in dyspeptic patients may lead to a resolution of a nonulcer dyspepsia in 10% of all treated patients. In an additional 10% of all treated patients, a peptic ulcer becomes cured or prevented (SONNENBERG and EVERHART 1996). In 0.12% of dyspeptic patients, *H. pylori*

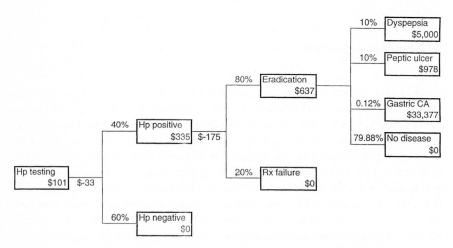

Fig. 6. Decision tree of testing for *H. pylori* in patients with dyspepsia. Costs and benefits are shown as negative and positive dollar amounts, respectively. *CA*, Cancer; *Hp*, *H. pylori*; *Rx*, therapy

eradication may be associated with prevention of gastric cancer. This rate is derived by multiplying the annual incidence rate of gastric cancer in the United States with an expected follow-up period of 15 years (WELLER et al. 1993). However, in the vast majority of patients treated for *H. pylori*, that is almost 80%, little is achieved, as no specific disease is cured or prevented, and the symptoms of dyspepsia do not improve.

In 80% of dyspeptic subjects, the benefit of the approach involving testing and empirical therapy is zero. The prevention of gastric cancer is assumed to be associated with the benefit of $33,337. This amount is taken from the above calculations. It also corresponds to about 1.5 times the Medicare charges for the DRG code 154 of one major gastric surgery (SONNENBERG and TOWNSEND 1995). The benefit of peptic ulcer prevention is assumed to be $978. As shown above, this amount corresponds to the expected cost of a duodenal ulcer over a 15 year period (SONNENBERG and TOWNSEND 1995). As workup of dyspepsia may be associated with a large variety of diagnostic tests and therapeutic trials, it is estimated that successfully treating dyspepsia would save $5,000 in overall diagnostic and therapeutic expenditures. In the sensitivity analysis this value is varied between $1,000 and $5,000.

Costs and benefits are counted as negative and positive dollar amounts, respectively. In calculating the expected costs or benefits of any individual branch of the decision tree, the various cost items must be multiplied with the probability of their occurrence. All in all, averaging out from right to left provides a net benefit of $101 associated with *H. pylori* testing of dyspeptic patients. The prevalence rate of peptic ulcer in dyspeptic subjects and the response rate of nonulcer dyspepsia to treatment of *H. pylori* are both debatable (VELDHUYZEN VAN ZANTEN and SHERMAN 1994; LAHEIJ et al. 1996). Similarly, the benefit of curing dyspepsia is not known. Therefore, in a sensitivity analysis, these three parameters of the decision tree were subjected to variations over a wide range (Fig. 7). The gray area of Fig. 7 denotes combinations of the prevalence rate of PUD and the response rate of NUD to antibiotics for which the strategy to screen and treat for *H. pylori* is beneficial. The prevalence rate of PUD and the response rate of NUD to antibiotics are inversely correlated. If the screened population of dyspeptics is characterized by a high prevalence rate of peptic ulcer, the response rate of NUD to antibiotics becomes largely irrelevant, because most of the benefit is wrought from curing and preventing peptic ulcer. On the other hand, if the PUD prevalence is low, all the benefit of screening and treatment depends of the response rate of NUD to *H. pylori* eradication. In addition, this relationship is influenced by the monetary benefit of curing nonulcer dyspepsia. Changing the benefit from $1,000 to $5,000 shifts the border between the decision in favor and against screening and treatment downwards. The gray area expands and, hence, the combinations of PUD prevalence and NUD response rates, for which screening and treatment are favorable, becomes more numerous as the financial benefit of curing dyspepsia increases.

Rather than spending money on an initial serological test, some physicians may opt for antibiotic therapy in all patients who present initially with symptoms of dyspepsia, irrespective of the outcome of a serological test. In terms of the model

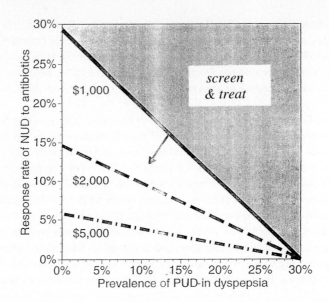

Fig. 7. Three-way sensitivity analysis of the decision analysis from Fig. 6. *Shaded area*, all combinations of PUD prevalence and NUD response rate for which screening and treatment for *H. pylori* is associated with a net benefit. As the benefit of curing dyspepsia through antibiotic therapy increases from $1000–2000 and $5000, the *gray area* expands and the number of combinations of PUD prevalence and NUD response rate increases, for which screening and treatment lead to a net benefit

shown in Fig. 6, the initial branch would be associated with −$175 in all patients, representing the costs of antibiotics therapy rather than the cost of −$33 for the initial serological test. This yields a lower expected benefit, that is $29, than the previous approach of initial serological testing. Since the serological test for *H. pylori* is cheaper than the antibiotic therapy, the initial test helps to save money and increase the expected benefit by restricting the more expensive antibiotic therapy to a subset of patients.

Other authors have modeled similar decision trees to address the issue of empiric therapy in dyspepsia (FENDRICK et al. 1995; OFMAN et al. 1997; SILVER-STEIN et al. 1996). All decision analyses depend on a similar set of assumptions built into the model, although the authors do not always openly address the dependency of their models on the response rate of NUD to eradication of *H. pylori*. It seems that the published models used overly optimistic cure rates of NUD, leading to seemingly robust and unequivocal results of the decision analyses.

4.2 The Concept of Marginal Cost-Benefit Ratio in NUD

It is important to distinguish between the a-priori decision to test (or treat dyspeptic patients empirically) and the a-posteriori decision to respond to a positive test of *H. pylori*. Here, we deal with a patient who has been worked-up for whatever clinical reasons and in whom a positive *H. pylori* status was established. It does not matter in the present context whether the *H. pylori* infection was diagnosed during endoscopy, urea breath test, or simple serology. All that matters is the fact that after already investing in diagnostic procedures, *H. pylori* became intentionally or serendipitously diagnosed. Should such newly diagnosed subjects be treated for their infection? Conceptually and ethically the present decision is rather distinct from the situation discussed in the previous section.

The issue at stake it best analyzed in terms of marginal costs and benefits (SONNENBERG et al. 1997). We will assume that to arrive at knowledge about the *H. pylori* infection we invested in a serological test. Such a test costs −$33, but yields no benefit. Compared with doing nothing, there is no increase in benefit but only an increase in cost. The marginal ratio between the benefit difference and the cost difference amounts to:

$$R = (benefit_2 - benefit_1)/(cost_2 - cost_1) = \$0/\$33 = 0. \tag{8}$$

In the decision tree of NUD, the expected benefit of eradicating *H. pylori* in dyspeptic patients was estimated at $637 (Fig. 6). This benefit can be bought at the expense of −$175 for antibiotic therapy plus physician charges. The marginal ratio between benefit and cost yields:

$$R = (benefit_2 - benefit_1)/(cost_2 - cost_1) = (\$637 - \$0)/(\$175 - \$33) = 4.5$$

If −$2,000 were spent in a patient with vague abdominal pain to find *H. pylori* infection as the only tangible diagnosis, the marginal ratio is:

$$R = (\$637 - \$0)/(\$2,175 - \$2,000) = 3.6$$

The marginal cost of −$175 spent on the additional antibiotic eradication of *H. pylori* pales in comparison with the previous investment of −$2000 spent on the diagnostic workup. In other words, it would seem justified to spend the relatively small amount of money on antibiotic therapy to gain at least some potential benefit.

5 Diagnostic Workup and Related Issues in the Management of Dyspeptic Patients

The discovery of *H. pylori* and its role in peptic ulcer disease has opened a variety of new ways to workup patients with upper abdominal symptoms. Different forms of management have been compared in clinical trials or analyzed by means of medical decision analysis. The present section focuses on the differential diagnosis of epigastric symptoms and the most cost-effective usage of diagnostic procedures in the workup of patients with dyspepsia or acid-peptic disorders.

5.1 Diagnostic Procedures in Dyspepsia

Empiric therapy constitutes a possible option in the initial management of dyspepsia. Therefore, some of the issues discussed in the present section overlap with
those covered in the previous section on NUD therapy. Table 1 lists the articles
that have studied competing strategies in the workup of patients with dyspepsia.
The variety of partly contradictory recommendations given by different authors
suggests that no clearcut answer exists and that professional bias must have
influenced the findings. Gastroenterologists tend to recommend endoscopy as a

Table 1. Management of patients with dyspepsia

Author	Study type	Results/recommendation
READ et al. (1982)	Medical decision analysis	Empiric therapy with antacids least expensive, initial barium swallow reduces mortality, least pain days associated with ulcer therapy
KAHN et al. (1985)	Editorial/meta-analysis	Start with empiric H_2 RA therapy
JONES (1988)	Clinical study	Negative EGD have positive influence on NUD patients
GOODSON et al. (1989)	Randomized clinical trial	Empiric antacid therapy results in similar benefit but less cost
LONGSTRETH (1992)	Randomized clinical trial	EGD cheaper than barium swallow
BYTZER et al. (1994)	Randomized clinical trial	EGD more cost-effective than empiric H_2 RA therapy
SOBALA et al. (1994)	Clinical study	Hp test reduces need for EGD by 23%, but 3% of PUD would be missed
PATEL et al. (1995)	Clinical study	Hp test reduces need for EGD by 36% without negative influence on overall outcome
FENDRICK et al. (1995)	Medical decision analysis	Empiric antibiotic therapy least expensive
SILVERSTEIN et al. (1996)	Medical decision analysis	Start workup with EGD, because empiric antibiotic therapy and EGD are equally expensive
SONNENBERG (1996)	Medical decision analysis	No empiric antibiotic therapy of Hp
OFMAN et al. (1997)	Medical decision analysis	Empiric antibiotic therapy most cost-effective
BRIGNOLI et al. (1997)	Randomized clinical trial	Empiric therapy with prokinetics less expensive than initial EGD at the expense of missing peptic lesions

H_2 RA, Histamine-2 receptor antagonist; *Hp, Helicobacter pylori*; EGD, esophagogastroduodenoscopy.

cost-effective means of workup, radiologists find barium swallow a worthwhile procedure, while general internists appear to favor empiric therapy. In addition, numerous methodological differences seem to have contributed to the discrepancies between the individual studies. Different management strategies underlie both the clinical trials as well as the decision models investigated by different authors. The management strategies variably involved initial endoscopy or barium swallow, empirical therapy with antacids, H_2 receptor antagonists, screening for *H. pylori*, or a combination of such measures. Moreover, different authors have used different methods of accounting by analyzing only direct versus total costs or ignoring costs associated with delayed and missed diagnoses. The transition probabilities built into the decision models were based on fragmented knowledge and were often influenced by the authors' bias. Economic studies, in general, are limited by the fact that many factors relevant to the patients or their physicians do not enter the analysis. Patients' motivations remain unaccounted for, such as hypochondria, fear of disease or diagnostic tests, and pursuits of disability pensions. Economic analyses also tend to ignore the utilities associated with negative diagnoses, the contribution of comorbid conditions and past medical histories, or the varying physician attitude and diagnostic intensity at the beginning versus the end of a diagnostic workup (SONNENBERG 1997b).

While some authors did not assign any benefit to establishing a correct and timely diagnosis (OFMAN et al. 1997), others restricted their spectrum of potential differential diagnoses to four, that is, malignant neoplasm of the stomach, reflux esophagitis, peptic ulcer, and nonulcer dyspepsia (SILVERSTEIN et al. 1996). In the clinical studies, the fraction of patients with positive findings was crucially dependent on the selection criteria and population size. It is amazing that, in spite of the inclusion of retrosternal pain and heartburn into the definition of dyspepsia (COLIN-JONES et al. 1988), none of the studies seemed to have spent large amounts of money on cardiological workups. A large variety of organic diseases can present with symptoms of dyspepsia or upper abdominal pain. These diseases can affect the chest or abdominal wall, heart, lungs, esophagus, stomach, duodenum, liver, pancreas, bile ducts, small and large intestine. The issue of dyspepsia becomes further confounded by the fact that many patients who complain about symptoms of dyspepsia do not present with any organic disease at all, but suffer from somatization or have no disease at all. Since dyspepsia and upper abdominal pain are located at the cross-road of so many heterogeneous diagnoses, it remains doubtful that a single strategy can be developed to accommodate all patients.

The benefits of individual diagnoses increase as we acquire more knowledge and better means of treatment. At a time when H_2 receptor antagonists represented the most efficacious therapy for nonulcer dyspepsia, peptic ulcer, and reflux disease alike, the diagnostic distinction between the three diseases had little if any therapeutic consequence (KAHN et al. 1985). Nowadays, the missed opportunity to cure peptic ulcer is associated with large cumulative costs in the long-run (SONNENBERG and TOWNSEND 1995). The assessment of a short-term benefit associated with empirical H_2 receptor antagonists or antacids in ulcer patients may not reveal this cost difference, however, because ulcer patients would respond symptomatically to antisecretory therapy. In all clinical studies, the study populations were too small to assess the impact of rare but costly side effects of any proposed strategies. Such potential side effects include complications of diagnostic and therapeutic procedures, side effects of drugs, or costs associated with missed diagnoses.

A newly emerging management concept recommends the separation of patients with dyspepsia into those below and above the age of 45 (AXON 1997; STEVENS et al. 1996). Patients over the age of 45 are worked-up by all available endoscopic and radiological means until the cause of their symptoms has been found or a serious diagnosis has been ruled out. Since serious life threatening diagnoses are rare among younger patients, further diagnostic workup of those under the age of 45 is restricted to patients who test positive for *H. pylori* by a urea breath test or a serological antibody test. Others have gone one step further and recommended that testing for *H. pylori* is made the pivotal diagnostic test in every dyspeptic patient and that all decisions about empiric therapy or further diagnostic procedures should be based on the outcome of this test (FENDRICK et al. 1995; OFMAN et al. 1997). For the reasons outlined above, however, we do not think that this concept represents a workable option that would be truly applicable in the routine management of all upper abdominal symptoms/dyspepsia.

5.2 Resistance Testing Before Antibiotic Therapy

BREUER and GRAHAM (1997) used a decision tree to analyze whether testing for antibiotic resistance before initiating therapy would be cost effective. Without resistance testing, the prevalence rate of resistant strains and the response rate of such resistant strains to untested antibiotics determine the rate of patients who fail therapy. The cost of failed therapy must be balanced against the $55 spent on resistance testing. In their model, failed therapy was relatively expensive, because every treatment course was associated with an endoscopy to assess eradication. Failed eradication led to a cumulative increase in the number of endoscopies and, accordingly, cost. The authors concluded that resistance testing in each patient is worthwhile, if 35% or more of *H. pylori* strains are resistant to the commonly used antibiotics and the response rate of such strains to untested antibiotic therapy drops from 90% or more to 75% or less. In addition to the two latter rates, the outcome of the decision analysis depends crucially on the cost associated with failure. Most physicians would probably not test whether the eradication was successful unless the patient developed symptoms of recurrent ulcers. Lower costs associated with failure of antibiotic therapy diminish the cost saving effect of resistance testing.

5.3 Confirmation of Eradication

RABENECK et al. (1997) assessed the cost-effectiveness of the urea breath test to assess infection status after antibiotic therapy. The authors concluded that in asymptomatic patients the use of the urea breath test to confirm eradication resulted in less symptomatic recurrences in the long run at a cost equal to that of the urea breath test. In symptomatic patients a repeat antibiotic regimen represented the least costly approach.

5.4 Threshold Analysis of Antibiotic Therapy

In addition to *H. pylori* induced gastritis and duodenitis, other mechanisms can underlie the occurrence of an ulcer in the upper gastrointestinal tract. For instance, consumption of nonsteroidal anti-inflammatory drugs (NSAIDs), gastric hyperse-cretion (in Zollinger-Ellison syndrome, in G-cell hyperplasia or secondary to other disorders), and portal hypertension can all result in peptic ulcers. Occasionally, such patients also test positive for *H. pylori* and the exact mechanism contributing to the occurrence of their ulcer is difficult to disentangle. SONNENBERG (1996b) used a threshold analysis to calculate the probability of an *H. pylori*-induced ulcer that would render antibiotics the cheapest therapy. In essence, his analysis compares the costs of an erroneous antibiotic regimen in patients without *H. pylori*-induced ulcers to the foregone opportunity of an inexpensive antibiotic cure of most ulcers. The threshold for using antibiotics is less than 20%. In other words, if the likeli-hood for an *H. pylori*-induced ulceration exceeds 20%, antibiotic eradication represents the cheapest treatment option. The results suggest that the vast majority of ulcer patients infected with *H. pylori* should undergo antibiotic therapy, even if other etiologies are considered possible.

6 Conclusions

A prospective randomized clinical trial and several types of economic modeling studies alike showed that eradication of *H. pylori* is the least expensive and most cost-effective means of treating peptic ulcer disease. The advantage of antibiotic cure of peptic ulcer disease becomes evident even within a time frame of 1 year after eradication of *H. pylori*. All other issues related to the treatment of *H. pylori* infection, unfortunately, are less clear, because important clinical information is missing and economic modeling is not able to overcome this dearth of crucial data. In gastric cancer, the outcome of a strategy of *H. pylori* eradication to prevent gastric cancer depends on the risk reduction achieved by antibiotic therapy and the costs of future gastric cancer. Cancer prevention could save cost, if the cancer risk can be reduced by more than 20%. As the cost of future gastric cancer depreciates over time, cancer prevention becomes a feasible option, if the time period between the preventive measures and the occurrence of gastric cancer can be made relatively short. In nonulcer dyspepsia, the economics of treatment of *H. pylori* infection depend heavily on the prevalence rate of peptic ulcer and the response rate of nonulcer dyspepsia to antibiotics, as well as the monetary benefit associated with curing both diseases. None of these values is known with certainty. The discovery of *H. pylori* has changed the workup of patients with dyspepsia. In dyspeptic patients without serious symptoms, such as severe pain, weight loss or hematemesis, it would be important to establish that no disease outside the upper gastrointestinal tract is missed. Once the cause of dyspepsia can be associated relatively confidently with the gastroduodenal area, patients could be grouped into those below and above the age of 45 years. Patients over the age of 45 are worked-up by the available endoscopic and radiological means until the cause of their symptoms has been found. Since serious life threatening diagnoses are rare among patients younger than 45, they would be first subjected to empiric therapy with antibiotics or H_2 receptor antagonists depending on the outcome of a urea breath test or a serological antibody test. Only if such means fail would they undergo further diagnostic workup.

Acknowledgement. Supported by a grant from the Centers for Disease Control and Prevention, Atlanta, GA.

References

Axon AT (1997) Chronic dyspepsia: who needs endoscopy? Gastroenterology 112:1376–1380

Beck JR, Kassirer JP, Pauker SG (1982a) A convenient approximation of life expectancy (the "DEALE"). Validation of the method. Am J Med 73:883–888

Beck JR, Pauker SG, Gottlieb JE, Klein K, Kassirer JP (1982b) A convenient approximation of life expectancy (the "DEALE"). Use in medical decision-making. Am J Med 73:889–896

Breuer T, Graham DY (1997) When does choosing the treatment regimen based on sensitivity testing become cost effective? Gastroenterology 112:A7

Briggs AH, Sculpher MJ, Logan RPH, Aldous J, Ramsay ME, Baron JH (1996) Cost effectiveness of screening for and eradication of *Helicobacter pylori* in management of dyspeptic patients under 45 years of age. Br Med J 312:1321–1325

Brignoli R, Watkins P, Halter F (1997) The Omega-Project – a comparison of two diagnostic strategies for risk and cost oriented management of dyspepsia. Eur J Gastroenterol Hepatol 9:337–343

Bytzer P, Møller Hansen J, Schaffalitzky de Muckadell OB (1994) Empirical H2-blocker therapy or prompt endoscopy in management of dyspepsia. Lancet 343:811–816

Colin-Jones DG, Bloom B, Bodemar G, Crean G, Freston J, Gugler R, Malagelada J, Nyrén O, Petersen H, Piper D (1988) Management of dyspepsia: report of a working party. Lancet 1:576–579

Corthésy-Theulaz I, Porta N, Glauser M, Saraga E, Vaney AC, Haas R, Kraehenbuhl JP, Blum AL, Michetti P (1995) Oral immunization with *Helicobacter pylori* urease B subunit as a treatment against Helicobacter infection in mice. Gastroenterology 109:115–121

Drake AW (1967) Fundamentals of applied probability theory. McGraw-Hill, New York, p 273

Fendrick AM, Chernew ME, Hirth RA, Bloom AS (1995) Alternative management strategies for patients with suspected peptic ulcer disease. Ann Intern Med 123:260–268

Forman D, Webb P, Parsonnet J (1994) H pylori and gastric cancer. Lancet 343:243–244

Goodson JD, Lehman JW, Richter JM, Read JL, Atamian S, Colditz GA (1989) Is upper gastrointestinal radiography necessary in the initial management of uncomplicated dyspepsia? A randomized controlled trial comparing empiric antacid therapy plus patient reassurance with traditional care. J Gen Intern Med 4:367–374

Gross AJ, Clark VA (1975) Survival distributions: reliability applications in the biomedical sciences. Wiley, New York, pp 49–94

Imperiale TF, Speroff T, Cebul RD, McCullough AJ (1995) A cost analysis of alternative treatments for duodenal ulcer. Ann Intern Med 123:665–672

Inadomi JM, Sonnenberg A (1998) The impact of peptic ulcer disease and *Helicobacter pylori* infection on life expectancy. Am J Gastroenterol 93:1286–1290

Jones R (1988) What happens to patients with non-ulcer dyspepsia after endoscopy? Practitioner 232: 75–78

Kahn KL, Health and Public Policy Committee, American College of Physicians (1985) Endoscopy in the evaluation of dyspepsia. Ann Intern Med 102:266–269

Laheij RJF, Jansen JBMJ, van de Lisdonk EH, Severens JL, Verbeek ALM (1996) Symptom improvement through eradication of *Helicobacter pylori* in patients with non-ulcer dyspepsia. Aliment Pharmacol Ther 10:843–850

Lee A (1996) Vaccination against *Helicobacter pylori*. J Gastroenterol 31 [Suppl 9]:69–74

Longstreth GF (1992) Long-term costs after gastroenterology consultation with endoscopy versus radiography in dyspepsia. Gastrointest Endosc 38:23–26

National Center for Health Statistics (1995) Vital statistics of the United States, 1990, vol 2, Mortality, Part A. Public Health Service, Washington DC

National Center for Health Statistics (1996) Vital statistics of the United States, 1992, Vol 2, section 6. DHHS Publication No. (PHS) 96–1104. US Department of Health and Human Services, Washington DC

O'Brien B, Goeree R, Mohamed HA, Hunt R (1995) Cost-effectiveness of *Helicobacter pylori* eradication for the long-term management of duodenal ulcer in Canada. Arch Intern Med 155:1958–1964

Ofman JJ, Etchason J, Fullerton S, Kahn KL, Soll AH (1997) Management strategies for *Helicobacter pylori*-seropositive patients with dyspepsia: Clinical and economic consequences. Ann Intern Med 126:280–291

Parsonnet J, Harris RA, Hack HM, Owens DK (1996) Modelling cost-effectiveness of *Helicobacter pylori* screening to prevent gastric cancer: a mandate for clinical trials. Lancet 348:150–154

Patel P, Khulusi S, Mendall MA, Llyod R, Jazrawi R, Maxwell JD, Northfield TC (1995) Prospective screening of dyspeptic patients by Helicobacter serology. Lancet 346:1315–1318

Rabeneck L, Griffiths RI, Guzman G, Cromwell DM, Strauss MJ, Robinson JW, Winston B, Li T, Graham DY (1997) Management of H pylori-infected ulcer patients following initial therapy: costs and outcomes of alternative approaches. Gastroenterology 112:A37

Read L, Pass TM, Komaroff AL (1982) Diagnosis and treatment of dyspepsia. A cost-effectiveness analysis. Med Decis Making 2:415–438

Sellman S, Blanchard TG, Nedrud JG, Czinn SJ (1995) Vaccine strategies for prevention of *Helicobacter pylori* infection. Eur J Gastroenterol Hepatol 7 [Suppl 1]:S1–S6

Silverstein MD, Petterson T, Talley N (1996) Initial endoscopy or empirical therapy with or without testing for *Helicobacter pylori* for dyspepsia: a decision analysis. Gastroenterology 110:72–83

Sobala GM, Crabtreee JE, Pentith JA, Rathbone BJ, Shallcross TM, Wyatt JI, Dixon MF, Heatley RV, Axon ATR (1991) Screening dyspepsia by serology to *Helicobacter pylori* Lancet 338:94–96

Sonnenberg A (1996a) Cost-benefit analysis of testing for *Helicobacter pylori* in dyspeptic subjects. Am J Gastroenterol 91:1773–1777

Sonnenberg A (1996b) Model of *Helicobacter pylori* treatment and disease outcome: a threshold analysis. In: Hunt RH, Tytgat GM (eds) *Helicobacter pylori*: basic mechanisms to clinical cure 1996. Kluwer Academic, Dordrecht, pp 398–405

Sonnenberg A (1996c) Cost-impact of clarithromycin plus omeprazole compared to traditional therapies for treatment of H pylori associated duodenal ulcers. Gut 39 [Suppl 2]:A22

Sonnenberg A (1997a) Comparative cost-effectiveness of three ulcer therapies. Gastroenterology 112:A43

Sonnenberg A (1997b) Economic analysis of dyspepsia. Eur J Gastroenterol Hepatol 9:323–326

Sonnenberg A, Everhart JE (1996) The prevalence of self-reported peptic ulcer in the United States. Am J Public Health 86:200–205

Sonnenberg A, Inadomi JM (1998) Medical decision models of *Helicobacter pylori* therapy to prevent gastric cancer. Aliment Pharmacol Ther 12 [Suppl 1]:111–121

Sonnenberg A, Townsend WF (1995) Costs of duodenal ulcer therapy with antibiotics. Arch Intern Med 155:922–928

Sonnenberg A, Delcò FR, Inadomi JM (1997) When to eradicate *Helicobacter pylori*? a decision analytic approach. Gastroenterol Int 10:1–7

Sonnenberg A, Schwartz JS, Cutler AF, Vakil N, Bloom BS (1998) Cost savings in duodenal ulcer treatment through H. pylori eradication compared to conventional therapies: results of a randomized, double blind, multicenter trial. Arch Int Med 158:852–860

Stevens R, Clinical Services and Standards Committee (1996) Dyspepsia management guidelines. British Society of Gastroenterology, London
Talley NJ (1994) A critique of therapeutic trials in *Helicobacter pylori*-positive functional dyspepsia. Gastroenterology 106:1174–1183
Talley NJ, Zinsmeister AR, Schleck CD, Melton LJ III (1992) Dyspepsia and dyspepsia subgroups: a population-based study. Gastroenterology 102:1259–1268
Talley NJ, Weaver AL, Tesmer DL, Zinsmeister AR (1993) Lack of discriminant value of dyspepsia subgroups in patients referred for upper endoscopy. Gastroenterology 105:1378–1386
Vakil N, Fennerty MB (1996) Cost-effectiveness of treatment regimens for the eradication of *Helicobacter pylori* in duodenal ulcer. Am J Gastroenterol 91:239–245
van der Hulst RWM, van der Ende A, Dekker FW, ten Kate FJW, Weel JFL, Keller JJ, Kruizinga SP, Dankert J, Tytgat GNJ (1997) Effect of *Helicobacter pylori* eradication on gastritis in relation to cagA: a prospective 1-year follow-up study. Gastroenterology 113:25–30
Veldhuyzen van Zanten SJO, Sherman PM (1994) *Helicobacter pylori* infection as a cause of gastritis, duodenal ulcer, gastric cancer and nonulcer dyspepsia: a systematic overview. Can Med Assoc J 150:177–185
Weinstein MC, Stason WB (1977) Foundations of cost-effectiveness analysis for health and medical practice. N Engl J Med 296:716–721
Welch HG, Albertsen PC, Nease RF, Bubolz TA, Wasson JH (1996) Estimating treatment benefits for the elderly: the effect of competing risks. Ann Intern Med 124:577–584
Weller EA, Blot WJ, Kaplan R (1993) Stomach cancer. In: Miller BA, Ries LAG, Hankey BF, Kosary CL, Harras A, Devesa SS, Edwards BK (eds) SEER cancer statistics review: 1973–1990. NIH Publication No 93–2789. National Cancer Institute, Bethesda, MD, XXIII.1–15

Antibiotic Treatment of *Helicobacter pylori* Infection

P. UNGE

1 Introduction

1.1 The Organism as a Target for Therapy

The most common infection in the world is caused by *Helicobacter pylori*, a very specific organism which cannot be treated conventionally. Animal models, mouse, ferret etc., are so far not reliable screening models for evaluation of *H. pylori* as a pathogen or efficacy of treatment regimens. Old-fashioned trial-and-error research of infected humans is still the gold standard for evaluation of *H. pylori* infection. The bacterium has found a unique niche in the gastric mucosa with a neutral environment, but is also present in the gastric lumen in an extremely acidic milieu.

Department of Medicine, Budst 126, Länssjukhuset Gävle Sandviken, S-80187 Gävle, Sweden

Its tremendous urease activity, which converts urea in the stomach to carbon dioxide and ammonia, neutralizes the gastric acid. All infected stomachs present with significant inflammation, which is histologically classified as chronic active gastritis, based on the infiltration of both mononuclear and polynuclear cells. The immune reaction causes an increased and easily detected level of IgG antibodies directed towards *H. pylori*. It is notable that, until recently, the infection per se, was not regarded as an infectious disease that should be treated. Treatment of the infection was recommended only when complications such as peptic ulcer disease appeared, according to the NIH meeting 1994. A number of diseases possibly associated with *H. pylori* infection are currently under investigation. IARC, the WHO organization, classified *H. pylori* as a group I carcinogen in 1994, causing gastric cancer, the link being comparable to that of smoking and lung cancer. Mucosa-associated lymphoma tissue lymphoma is closely associated with *H. pylori* infection and eradication of the infection can reverse the lymphoma completely in early stages. Gastric bleed and development of peptic ulcer due to NSAID use seem to be more frequent in infected patients.

The bacterium seems fragile in an in vitro environment and its sensitivity to a large number of antibiotics suggests an "easy scenario" when it comes to in vivo therapy. In vivo experiences, however, clearly show that *H. pylori* is not an easy target to hit. Most antimicrobials are either not effective or only partly effective in vivo.

The evaluation of therapeutic efficacy in vivo has been controversial. Differences exist in assessment methods and their sensitivity, specificity and predictive value. Authorities have continuously changed the approved combination of tests necessary for regulatory purposes and very few studies in the literature have used the required tests. Data must therefore be scrutinized carefully.

2 Antimicrobial Therapy: General Aspects on Mechanisms, Drug Delivery and Local Activity

*The Target for the Most Frequently Used Anti-*H. pylori *Antimicrobials.* H. pylori is sensitive to a number of antimicrobials in vitro (Loo et al. 1992; MILLAR et al. 1992; RUBINSTEIN et al. 1994), but only a few of them are active enough against the organism in vivo to cure the infection. Nitroimidazoles, for example, metronidazole and tinidazole, are metabolized in the bacterium to an active form destroying the bacterial DNA. Macrolides, such as clarithromycin, erythromycin, roxithromycin, and azithromycin, block the RNA synthesis in the bacterium. Penicillins such as amoxicillin are active against the cell wall.

Intraluminal Acidity as a Destroyer of the Antimicrobials and Their Efficacy. The acidic gastric environment has been blamed for drug delivery deficiency. Oral formulations of antibiotics or antimicrobials with medium or low acid stability might be expected to be less effective as monotherapy. A pronounced altered secretion of gastric acid might open an opportunity for acid labile drugs. Intravenous administration of antimicrobials is, at least theoretically, a suitable method to improve drug delivery to the bacterium but has not been confirmed effectively in large controlled trials.

Local Activity in the Gastric Lumen. Bismuth containing compounds are usually only partially absorbed and have a local inhibitory effect on the organism. Intraluminal concentrations of antibiotics have been claimed to be a key factor and local therapy, as performed by KIMURA et al. (1994), is effective. However, amoxicillin in a formulation that stayed in the gastric lumen for 4–8 h has not shown a clear beneficial advantage over the immediate release formulation (UNGE et al. 1994). Frequent and irregular gastric emptying may affect local antibacterial potential. Gastric Secretion. Gastric secretion of the antimicrobial is suggested as a favorable property facilitating the transportation of the drug to the target, *H. pylori.* Macrolides such as clarithromycin and azithromycin are concentrated in the gastric mucosa and secreted into the gastric lumen and they have a detectable effect on the organism. Amoxicillin is concentrated in the gastric mucosa, but without significant secretion into the gastric lumen. Hence the relatively low cure rate by amoxicillin monotherapy may suggest that this mucosal concentration is a less important factor for treatment success.

Antimicrobial Resistance. Resistance development towards nitroimidazoles and/or macrolides varies in grade and frequency, and the clinical impact is not yet defined. Data to date are relatively weak but suggest that resistance to nitroimidazoles is a predictor of failure which increases according to degree of resistance (MEGRAUD et al. 1997). Resistance to macrolides and its importance as a negative predictive factor for failure is little documented. No plasmid-transferred resistance has been reported for *H. pylori.*

Summary. It is not possible to eradicate *H. pylori* infection effectively, using only one drug and the ideal therapy for cure is lacking. No mechanism(s) has been postulated that truly explains the lack of efficacy of antimicrobial activity in vivo. *H. pylori* seems to be an extremely well adapted organism quite capable of defending itself when attacked in a traditional way, i.e., with monotherapy.

3 Pooled Analysis of the Clinical Efficacy of Regimens Directed Towards *H. pylori*

Identifying the important key factors that predict treatment success, has proved difficult, and we base our efficacy evaluation of drugs and drug combinations on clinical trial data. Large numbers of drug combinations have been investigated worldwide in studies of varying quality and results. Both formal meta-analyses and pooled analyses have been published. Efficacy and safety data, however, are often weak and results vary according to the methods used for analysis. Following is an attempt to transfer available data from the literature to one analysis model, the ITT analysis, in order to increase the reliability of this pooled analysis.

3.1 Criteria for the Pooled Analysis

The quality of the included studies was ranked according to blindness, i.e., blind (single or double), open-randomized or open without the use of randomization procedure. Whenever a random allocation of the patient to a treatment was stated, it was accepted even if the methodology could be questioned. Data on efficacy were pooled in the drug combination groups. Only patients who were *H. pylori*-negative or who had an unknown *H. pylori* status preentry were excluded from the efficacy analysis. A worst case analysis was performed, i.e., intention to treat analysis, which probably reflects the clinical setting as closely as possible since all patients intended to treat are included in the evaluation. Only patients with confirmed conversion from infected to negative *H. pylori* status were regarded as cured. If data in an abstract were extended or changed in a poster presentation, the poster data were regarded as more reliable, after discussion with the authors.

Confidence intervals were calculated as if pooled data were from one study only. To compensate for the weakness of the variations in study design, timing etc. confidence intervals were enlarged arbitrarily by 1.5 and called credibility values (CV). The efficacy, i.e., eradication rates, were calculated on pooled data from all studies on the specified drug combination, on data from each of the three quality levels, as well as on data from larger studies with 50 patients or more in the treatment arms. Dose interval, duration of therapy etc. are most likely to affect compliance which is an important factor for success. However, the ITT analysis comprised all patients including treatment failures as a result of bad drug compliance. Data on the total number of doses, total number of tablets or capsules, and duration of therapy are given for each treatment group. Side effects were rarely reported in a form that was possible to evaluate and pool in an acceptable way. No pooled evaluation of the predictive value of bacterial resistance was performed. Med-Line search in combination with scrutiny of available posters and abstracts from the American Gastroenterology Association meetings of 1988–1996 and the European *Helicobacter* pylori Study Group meetings of 1988–1996 revealed 1409 treatment arms, evaluating therapies aimed to eradicate *H. pylori*, to be dissected. A number of dual publications were identified and deleted, as were reports which did not present the number of included and cured patients per study arm. This was the most common reason for exclusion of studies from the analysis. The remaining reports included one or more of the stated drug combinations (Table 1) and fulfilled the inclusion criteria. A large number of publications were available as abstracts and posters only. One study could include more than one treatment arm per treatment group. Data from this analysis will be used as efficacy data in this chapter. Table 1 shows the drug combinations evaluated in this analysis.

Table 1. Treatment groups in the pooled analysis. PPI = proton pump inhibitor

---

Bismuth-based therapy
  Bismuth-based triple therapy
    Bismuthdicitrate or bismuthsubsalicylate, nitroimidazole, tetracycline
    Bismuthdicitrate or bismuthsubsalicylate, nitroimidazole, amoxicillin
Therapies based on acid inhibitory drugs
  Dual therapy
    Omeprazole, amoxicillin
    Omeprazole, clarithromycin
    Omeprazole, azithromycin
  Triple therapy
    H$_2$ antagonist based triple, quadruple therapy
    H$_2$ antagonist, nitroimidazole, amoxicillin
    Bismuth-ranitidine, clarithromycin
    Bismuth-ranitidine, clarithromycin, amoxicillin
    Bismuth-ranitidine, clarithromycin, nitroimidazole
    PPI based triple therapy
  PPI plus amoxicillin plus a nitroimidazole
    Omeprazole, amoxicillin, nitroimidazole
    Lansoprazole, amoxicillin, nitroimidazole
    Pantoprazole, amoxicillin, nitroimidazole
  PPI plus amoxicillin plus a macrolide (Bordeaux strategy)
    Omeprazole, amoxicillin, clarithromycin
    Lansoprazole, amoxicillin, clarithromycin
    Pantoprazole, amoxicillin, clarithromycin
  PPI plus nitroimidazole plus a macrolide (Bazzoli strategy)
    Omeprazole, nitroimidazole, clarithromycin
    Omeprazole, nitroimidazole, azithromycin
    Omeprazole, nitroimidazole, roxithromycin
    or
    Lansoprazole, nitroimidazole, clarithromycin
    Pantoprazole, nitroimidazole, clarithromycin
  Mucosa protective agent based combinations)
    sucralfate plus two of either amoxicillin, nitroimidazole or clarithromycin
    Sofalcone, ranitidine, clarithromycin
  Quadruple therapy
  PPI, bismuth based quadruple therapy
    Omeprazole, bismuthdicitrate or bismuthsubsalicylate, nitroimidazole, tetracycline
    Omeprazole, bismuthdicitrate or bismuthsubsalicylate, nitroimidazole, amoxicillin

---

Figures 1–9 show the eradication rates for each combination, and Fig. 10 is a summary of the efficacy of all combinations.

3.2 Results

3.2.1 Bismuth-Based Triple Therapies

There are two major therapeutic options, bismuth plus a nitroimidazole combined with either tetracycline or amoxicillin (ALCALDE et al. 1992; BANCU et al. 1996; BELL et al. 1993; BOR-SHYANG SHEN et al. 1995; BRUNO et al. 1994; BURETTE et al.

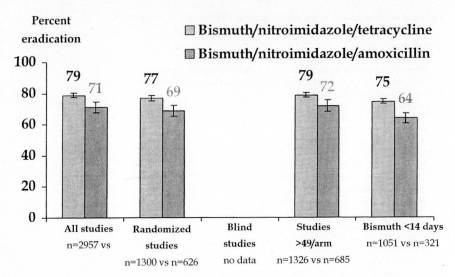

Fig. 1. Pooled efficacy data on two bismuth-based triple therapy; bismuth/nitroimidazole/tetracycline and bismuth/nitroimidazole/amoxicillin

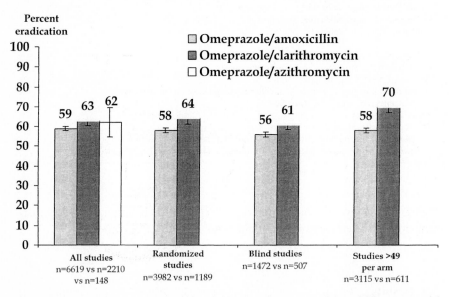

Fig. 2. Pooled efficacy data on omeprazole-based dual therapies; omeprazole/amoxicillin, omeprazole/ clarithromycin and omeprazole/azithromycin

1992; CATALANO et al. 1992, 1994a; DE BONA et al. 1994; DE KOSTER et al. 1992a; DOPPL et al. 1994; EL-OMAR et al. 1995; FIXA et al. 1994; GUPTA et al. 1994; HU et al. 1994; JAN et al. 1994; JAUP et al. 1991; KORDECKI et al. 1996; LIBERTI et al.

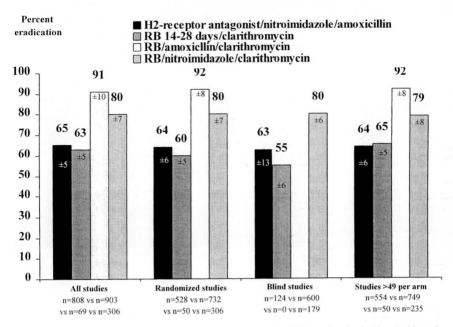

Fig. 3. Pooled efficacy data on H_2 antagonist combined with amoxicillin and a nitroimidazole, bismuth-ranitidine (RB) plus clarithromycin alone or together with one of amoxicillin or nitroimidazole. *Above bars*, eradication rates; *within bars*, confidence interval

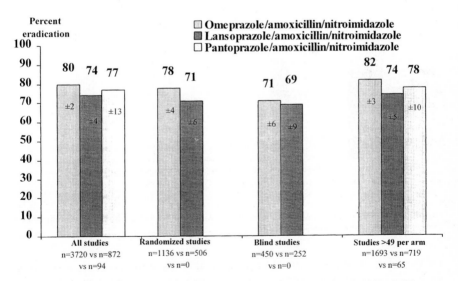

Fig. 4. Pooled efficacy data on PPI (omeprazole, lansoprazole and pantoprazole) combined with amoxicillin and a nitroimidazole. *Above bars*, eradication rates; *within bars*, confidence interval

268   P. Unge

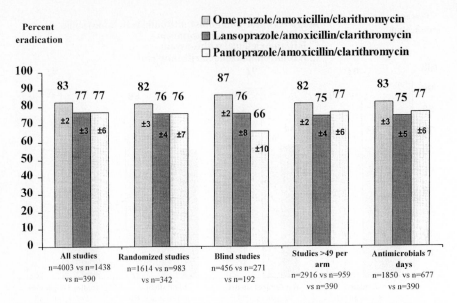

Fig. 5. Pooled efficacy data on PPI (omeprazole, lansoprazole and pantoprazole) combined with amoxicillin and clarithromycin. *Above bars*, eradication rates; *within bars*, confidence interval

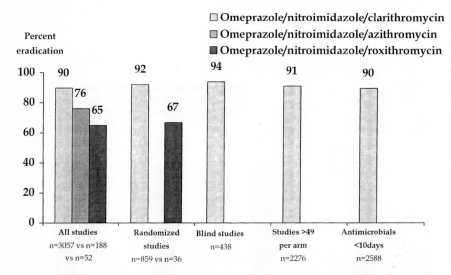

Fig. 6. Pooled efficacy data on omeprazole combined with a nitroimidazole and either clarithromycin, azithromycin or roxithromycin

1995; LOGAN et al. 1991, 1994a; MESSA et al. 1996, MIDOLO et al. 1994, 1996; MOSHKOWITZ et al. 1995; O'RIORDAN et al. 1990; PAJARES et al. 1994; PATCHETT et al. 1991; QURESHI et al. 1995; RAUWS et al. 1990a,b; ROKKAS et al. 1994; ROSSI

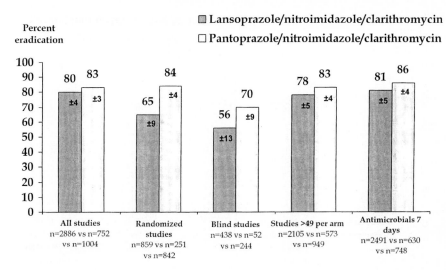

Fig. 7. Pooled efficacy data on omeprazole lansoprazole and pantoprazole combined with a nitroimidazole and clarithromycin. *Above bars*, eradication rates; *within bars*, confidence interval

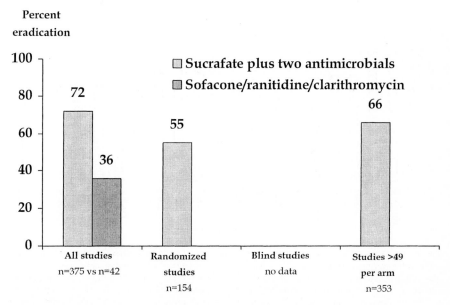

Fig. 8. Pooled efficacy data on sucralfate plus two antimicrobials and sofalcone plus ranitidine and clarithromycin

et al. 1996; SANTANDER et al. 1994, 1995; SCHEIMAN et al. 1996; SEPPÄLÄ et al. 1992; SHEU et al. 1996a; SOBALA et al. 1992; TAKATS et al. 1993; TAN et al. 1995; TUCCI et al. 1994; VALLE et al. 1991; WAGNER et al. 1991, 1992).

270   P. Unge

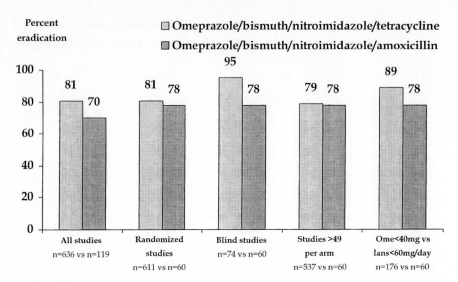

Fig. 9. Pooled efficacy data on omeprazole and bismuth combined with a nitroimidazole and tetracycline or amoxicillin

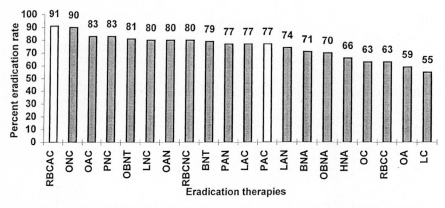

Fig. 10. Eradication therapies ranked by efficacy based on all available studies. *Light-shaded bars*, therapies with fewer than 100 patients. *Above bars*, eradication rates. *RBAC*, ranitidinebismuth, amoxicillin, clarithromycin; *ONC*, omeprazole, nitroimidazole, clarithromycin; *OAC*, omeprazole, amoxicillin, clarithromycin; *PNC*, pantoprazole, nitroimidazole, clarithromycin; *OBNT*, omeprazole, bismuthdicitrate or bismuthsubsalicylate, nitroimidazole, tetracycline; *LNC*, lansoprazole, nitroimidazole, clarithromycin; *OAN*, omeprazole, amoxicillin, nitroimidazole; *RBNC*, ranitidinebismuth, nitroimidazole, clarithromycin; *BNT*, bismuthdicitrate, subsalicylate or nitrate, nitroimidazole, tetracycline; *PAN*, pantoprazole, amoxicillin, nitroimidazole; *LAC*, lansoprazole, amoxicillin, clarithromycin; *PAC*, pantoprazole, amoxicillin, clarithromycin; *LAN*, lansoprazole, amoxicillin, nitroimidazole; *BNA*, bismuthdicitrate, subsalicylate or nitrate, nitroimidazole, amoxicillin; *OBNA*, omeprazole, bismuthdicitrate-bismuthsubsalicylate, nitroimidazole, amoxicillin; *HNA*, H₂ antagonist, nitroimidazole, amoxicillin; *OC*, omeprazole, clarithromycin; *RBC*, ranitidinebismuth, clarithromycin; *OA*, omeprazole, amoxicillin; *LC*, lansoprazole, clarithromycin

The tetracycline triple therapy is about 10% more effective than the amoxicillin one (Fig. 1). Study design, i.e., randomized, blind or uncontrolled, did not significantly influence the outcome in any of the combinations. Duration of bismuth or antimicrobial therapy of less than 14 days was slightly inferior in both groups. Side effects were reported in some studies and were usually in the range of 10%–40% of patients or sometimes higher. Convenience and compliance factors (Table 2) are in the low range, due to the large number of tablets, dosage and long duration of therapy.

– Dose recommendation: depends on approved bismuth formulation
– Mean eradication rate: 71%–79%

3.2.2 Therapies Based on Acid-Inhibitory Drugs

3.2.2.1 Dual Therapies

Amoxicillin, clarithromycin or azithromycin given in combination with the strong acid inhibitory drug, omeprazole (a proton pump inhibitor, PPI), had a synergistic antibacterial effect. This was most likely driven by the altered acid secretion and not the weak antibacterial property of proton pump inhibitors. The additional effect of acid inhibitory drugs on antimicrobials is dose dependent and, for amoxicillin, is also dependent on the dose frequency, i.e., twice daily is more effective than once daily. Clarithromycin interacts with omeprazole and increases the absorption of both clarithromycin and omeprazole. Dose frequency higher than once daily was not more effective. Pretreatment with omeprazole might influence patients' drug compliance but does not change the efficacy of the subsequent eradication therapy. *Omeprazole (PPI), Amoxicillin.* Amoxicillin and omeprazole given twice daily were effective in the range of 55%–60% (Fig. 2) (ADAMEK et al. 1992, 1993a,b, 1994a–c,

Table 2. Evaluation of therapeutic strategies with regards to the convenience of therapy

	Number of tablets	Number of intakes	Duration of therapy (days)	Significant side effects (%)
Bismuth, nitroimidazole, tetracycline or amoxicillin	> 100	> 50	8–14	> 10
Omeprazole, amoxicillin	< 50	15–50	8–14	5–15
Omeprazole, clarithromycin	50–100	15–50	8–14	> 5
H₂ antagonist, nitroimidazole, amoxicillin	50–100	15–50	8–14	5–15
Bismuth-ranitidine, clarithromycin	50–100	15–50	8–14	> 5
PPI, amoxicillin, nitroimidazole	< 50	15–50	8–14	> 5%
PPI, amoxicillin, macrolide	< 50	< 15	1–7	< 10%
PPI, nitroimidazole, macrolide	< 50	< 15	1–7	< 10%
Sucralfate, two antibiotics	50–100	> 50	> 14	> 5%
Sofalcone, ranitidine, clarithromycin	50–100	> 50	> 14	> 5%
PPI, bismuth, nitroimidazole, tetracycline or amoxicillin	> 100	> 50	8–14	> 10%

1995a,b; AL-ASSI et al. 1994; ATHERTON et al. 1993, 1994; AVUNDUK et al. 1995; BACK et al. 1995; BANK et al. 1995; BAYERDÖRFFER et al. 1992, 1993, 1995a–c; BELL et al. 1991, 1992, 1993; BERTONI et al. 1996; BIANCHI PORRO et al. 1996a; BUCKLEY et al. 1994; BURES et al. 1994a,b; BURETTE et al. 1994; CAROLI et al. 1995a,b; CARPINTERO et al. 1995; CATALANO et al. 1994a,b, 1995; CIRILLO et al. 1994; COLLINS et al. 1992, 1993b; DE KOSTER et al. 1992a; DE MEDICI et al. 1994; DELCHIER et al. 1995; DELTENDRE et al. 1994, 1995a,b; FERULANO et al. 1994; GOH et al. 1993; GOVOSDIS et al. 1994a,b; GRAHAM et al. 1995; HACKELSBERGER et al. 1996; HU et al. 1995; HUBER 1993; JASPERSEN et al. 1994; KATELARIS et al. 1995; KATICIC et al. 1996; KOELZ et al. 1995; KRAUSSE et al. 1994; LABENZ et al. 1992b,c; 1993a–e, 1994a,b; LAHAIE et al. 1995; LAINE et al. 1995; LAMBERT et al. 1994; LAMOULIATTE et al. 1989, 1990, 1994a; LIBERTI et al. 1995; LIDTK et al. 1994; LOGAN et al. 1992b, 1993b; LONDONG et al. 1995; MACONI et al. 1996; MAIER et al. 1994; MANES et al. 1996; MASSARRAT et al. 1995; MEINING et al. 1996; MELONI et al. 1995; MOSCA et al. 1995a,b; NAIR et al. 1995; NEBIKI et al. 1994; NERI et al. 1995; OTERO et al. 1995; PATCHETT et al. 1994; PIERAMICO et al. 1996; POMMERLEN et al. 1995; POPOVIC et al. 1996; REINAUER et al. 1994; REJCHRT et al. 1994; RIZZO et al. 1993; ROKKAS et al. 1993a,b, 1994; SABERI-FIROOZI et al. 1995; SANTANDER et al. 1994, 1995; SCHEIMAN et al. 1996; SPADACCINI et al. 1995a; SPINZI et al. 1993, 1996; SUNG et al. 1995c; TAN et al. 1995a,b; TREIBER et al. 1994; TYSZKIEWICZ et al. 1994; UNGE et al. 1989, 1993, 1994; VA et al. 1995; WAGNER et al. 1992; YANG et al. 1996; ZALA et al. 1993a,b, 1994, 1995). The results were similar in blinded studies and open studies. Blind studies showed no differences in cure rate whether or not patients were pretreated with omeprazole. Side effects such as skin reactions were reported in about 5% and gastrointestinal symptoms, mostly loose stool, in about 10%. Convenience factors were in the medium range (Table 2). Data on lansoprazole plus amoxicillin were similar but slightly lower. Resistance to amoxicillin is not yet defined.

– Dose recommendation: omeprazole 20–40 mg plus amoxicillin 1000 mg b.i.d. 14 days
– Mean eradication rate: 59%

Omeprazole (PPI), Clarithromycin. Clarithromycin plus omeprazole was the most effective dual therapy with an overall efficacy of 60%–70% eradication (Fig. 2) (BAZZOLI et al. 1996a,b; BERTRAMS et al. 1994; BURETTE et al. 1993b, BURETTE et al. 1997b; CATALANO et al. 1995; CAYLA et al. 1993; CHIBA et al. 1994, 1996; DELTENDRE et al. 1994, 1995a,b; FERRINI et al. 1994; FORNE et al. 1995; GOH et al. 1993; GOVOSDIS et al. 1994a,b; GRAHAM et al. 1995; GREAVES et al. 1994; GREENBERG et al. 1996; GURBUZ et al. 1994; HABU et al. 1996; HUNT et al. 1995; KALANTZIS et al. 1994, 1995; LABENZ et al. 1993e, 1995a; LAMOULIATTE et al. 1994a; LOGAN et al. 1992a, 1993a,b, 1994b, 1995a; MATTLE 1994; MEGRAUD et al. 1997b; MELONI et al. 1995; MENDELSON et al. 1992; NERI et al. 1994a,b, 1995; PARASAKTHI et al. 1995; PATCHETT et al. 1994; PEURA et al. 1996; PIERAMICO et al. 1996; PILOTTO et al. 1994a,c,d, 1995; SPADACCINI et al. 1995a; SPINZI et al. 1996; TAN et al. 1995a; THAM et al. 1995; VAN DER HULST et al. 1996; VEENENDAAL et al. 1996a,b; WURZER et al.

1996). The antibiotic was given three times daily and omeprazole once daily. Side effects were common but mild. Taste disturbances were prevalent in 20%–80%. Gastrointestinal side effects were reported in about 5%–10%. Resistance to clarithromycin varied in different areas from 0.5%–10%. Posttherapy resistance was usually a negative predictive factor.

– Dose recommendation: omeprazole 40 mg o.m. plus clarithromycin 500mg t.i.d. 14 days
– Mean eradication rate: 64%

Omeprazole (PPI), Azithromycin. This combination is not well studied (Caselli et al. 1996; Pilotto et al. 1994a,c,d, 1995). Azithromycin has a long half-life in plasma and there have been some worries about its accumulation. A three day antibiotic regimen was the most common. The limited data on azithromycin are similar to the clarithromycin combination (Fig. 2)

– Dose recommendation: no consistent data
– Mean eradication rate: 62%

3.2.3 Triple Therapies

Two antimicrobials combined with one acid inhibitory drug have been carefully studied since the first report was published on an H_2 antagonist plus two antibiotics (Hentschel et al. 1993). This specific combination has been less successful in some centers, but highlighted the awareness and acceptance of combining three drugs. A more effective acid inhibition using PPIs has optimized the antibacterial efficacy of this triple therapy principle. In this group of drug combinations we can find the most effective and well tolerated options available today.

3.2.3.1 H_2 Receptor Antagonist Based Triple Therapy

H_2 Antagonist, Nitroimidazole, Amoxicillin. The most commonly used H_2 antagonist in this combination was ranitidine, but there are a few studies on cimetidine and a few data on famotidine and roxatidine triples (Alcalde et al. 1992; Bardhan et al. 1996a; Chen et al. 1995; De Koster et al. 1992a, 1993, 1994; Ferrini et al. 1995a; Hentschel et al. 1993; Hirschl et al. 1991; Lahaie et al. 1995; Lamouliatte et al. 1991, 1992, 1996a; Lee et al. 1995; Pajares et al. 1994; Popovic et al. 1997; Powell et al. 1994; Savarino et al. 1997; Sobhani et al. 1995; Spadaccini et al. 1995a; Tham et al. 1995) (Fig. 3). Study design and size did not significantly affect the result. Treatment duration of less than ten days was slightly inferior to longer treatment periods. Side effects were in the range of 10%–20%. Convenience factor was in the medium range (Table 2).

– Dose recommendation: ranitidine 300mg o.d. plus amoxicillin 750mg t.i.d. plus metronidazole 400mg t.i.d. for 12 days
– Mean eradication rate: 65%

Bismuth-Ranitidine Plus One or Two Antimicrobials. Bismuth-ranitidine is a salt and can therefore, be regarded as dual therapy. However, bismuth is released in an early phase after digestion, which is why this therapeutic strategy is classified as a triple combination in this analysis. Available efficacy and safety data on the bismuth-ranitidine, -clarithromycin combination come from studies which were designed to show an ulcer preventive effect of eradication and not primarily the eradication rate (CARDELLI et al. 1997; GUDJONSSON et al. 1997; MARCHI et al. 1997; MEGRAUD et al. 1997b; PETERSON et al. 1995, 1996a–d; WYETH et al. 1994) (Fig. 3). The use of the ITT analysis may be too conservative, but any other analysis approach could also be criticised. A large number of patients were not followed up and consequently were regarded as treatment failures. Duration of therapy was 2–4 weeks and dose frequency varied from two to four times daily (Table 2). When bismuth-ranitidine is combined with clarithromycin plus amoxicillin (LAINE et al. 1997; SAVARINO et al. 1997b; WYETH et al. 1994; Fig. 3) or clarithromycin plus nitroimidazole (GUD-JONSSON et al. 1997; SAVARINO et al. 1997a; Fig. 3), there is a marked increase in efficacy to 91% and 80%, respectively. However, data are limited.

– Mean eradication rate: 63%
– Mean eradication rate bismuth-ranitidine, -clarithromycin, -amoxicillin: 90%
– Mean eradication rate bismuth-ranitidine, -clarithromycin, -nitroimidazole: 80%

3.2.3.2 PPI-Based Triple Therapy

PPI, Amoxicillin, Nitroimidazole. The triple combinations omeprazole plus amox-icillin and metronidazole or tinidazole (ANGELETTI et al. 1995; AVELLINI et al. 1994; BELL et al. 1993, 1995; BIANCHI PORRO et al. 1996b; CAMMAROTA et al. 1994; CAVIGLIA et al. 1995, 1996; CHOW et al. 1996; DE MEDICI et al. 1995; FERULANO et al. 1994; FIOCCA et al. 1992; GISBERT et al. 1997; GOH et al. 1993; HUDSON et al. 1995; JAUP 1991; KADAYIFCI et al. 1997; KATICIC et al. 1996, 1997; KORDECKI et al. 1996; LABENZ et al. 1995c; LAMOULIATTE et al. 1991, 1992, 1993a, 1994a; LAZZA-RONI et al. 1995; LERANG et al. 1994a,b, 1995a; LIND et al. 1995; MASSARRAT et al. 1995; MISIEWICZ et al. 1996; MORGANDO et al. 1995; PIERAMICO et al. 1996; POPOVIC et al. 1997; ROSSI et al. 1996; SABERI-FIROOZI et al. 1995; SAVARINO et al. 1997b; SIGNORELLI et al. 1994; SPADACCINI et al. 1995a; THAM et al. 1995; TREIBER et al. 1997; VAN DER HULST et al. 1996; VELDHUYZEN VAN ZANTEN et al. 1994; VIGNERI et al. 1996; YANG et al. 1996; ZHOU et al. 1991) or lansoprazole plus amoxicillin and metronidazole or tinidazole, (AKAMATSU et al. 1997; BOUCHARD et al. 1996; DE KORWIN et al. 1993; KALACH et al. 1995; KATICIC et al. 1996; KORDECKI et al. 1996; LABENZ et al. 1995c; LAMOULIATTE et al. 1993a, 1996d; MISIEWICZ et al. 1996; MIYAJI et al. 1997; MOAYYEDI et al. 1997; PILOTTO et al. 1997; SAGGJORO et al. 1997; TACHIBANA et al. 1997; VAN OIJEN et al. 1997; Fig. 4) have been studied frequently and are effective in about 80% (omeprazole) and 70% (lansoprazole). Data on pantoprazole, amoxicillin, nitroimidazole are limited (ADAMEK et al. 1997d; STÖLZLE et al. 1997; Fig. 4). A dose of omeprazole lower than 40mg daily was a negative predictive factor. Increased study quality gave lower efficacy. However, short treatment periods using a b.i.d. regimen might explain the inferior results in the blind studies. The lansoprazole dose was usually comparable to less than 40 mg omeprazole, which may explain the lower efficacy in the lansoprazole studies. Resistance to metronidazole seemed to be a weak but negative predictive factor. Significant side effects were in the range of 5%–20%. The convenience factor was in the high-medium range (Table 2).

- Dose recommendation: omeprazole 20mg b.i.d. plus amoxicillin 1000mg b.i.d. plus metronidazole 400mg b.i.d. for 10 days
- Mean eradication rate: 81%
- Dose recommendation: lansoprazole 30mg b.i.d. plus amoxicillin 1000mg b.i.d. plus metronidazole 400mg b.i.d. for 10 days
- Mean eradication rate: 74%

or

- Dose recommendation: not established for pantoprazole
- Mean eradication rate: 77%

PPI, Amoxicillin, Clarithromycin. There are three important combinations: omeprazole, amoxicillin, clarithromycin, named the Bordeaux regimen since it was first studied in France (BERTONI et al. 1996; BUDA et al. 1997; BURETTE et al. 1995, 1997a,b; CATALANO et al. 1996, 1997; CHEN et al. 1997; CHING et al. 1997; COLOMBO et al. 1997; DELCHIER et al. 1995; FERRINI et al. 1995b; FIOCCA et al. 1995; GEORGOPOULOS et al. 1997; GISBERT et al. 1997; HABU et al. 1996; HERMIDA et al. 1996, 1997; HUELIN-BENITEZ et al. 1997; KADAYIFCI et al. 1997; KATICIC et al. 1996, 1997; LABENZ et al. 1995c; LAINE et al. 1995; LAMOULIATTE et al. 1993a,c, 1994a,b, 1996c; LERANG et al. 1996, 1997; LIND et al. 1995; MALFERTHEINER et al. 1997; MANTZARIS et al. 1997; MIWA et al. 1997; MOAYYEDEI et al. 1995; MONES et al. 1996; PEITZ et al. 1996c, 1997; PIERAMICO et al. 1996; REILLY et al. 1995; SAINZ et al. 1997; SAVARINO et al. 1997b; VA et al. 1995; VELDHUYZEN VAN ZANTEN et al. 1997; WURZER et al. 1996; YOUSFI et al. 1996), the lansoprazole, amoxicillin, clarithromycin (BUDA et al. 1997; BURETTE et al. 1996; COLOMBO et al. 1997; CATALANO et al. 1996; COSTA et al. 1997; HO et al. 1996; KRAUSE et al. 1997; LAMOULIATTE et al. 1995a, 1996b,e; LAMY et al. 1996; MISIEWICZ et al. 1996; MIYAJI et al. 1997; MOAYYEDI et al. 1997; NAKATA et al. 1996; PILOTTO et al. 1997; SCHüTZE et al. 1995; TURSI et al. 1996b) and the pantoprazole, amoxicillin, clarithromycin (FREVEL et al. 1997; LAMOULIATTE et al. 1997; LUNA et al. 1997). The most frequently used PPI was omeprazole and the overall mean efficacy was 83% (Fig. 5). Study quality was a major positive predictor probably because of the high drug compliance and the low number of patients lost to follow-up in the blind studies. Resistance to clarithromycin was a negative predictive factor for success. The lansoprazole combination was effective in 77%, and study quality did not change the mean cure rate substantially. The pantoprazole combination was equally effective in the overall evaluation. Significant side effects were in the range 5%–20% and convenience level is high (Table 2).

– Dose recommendation: omeprazole 20mg b.i.d. plus amoxicillin 1000mg b.i.d. plus clarithromycin 500mg b.i.d. for 7 days
– Mean eradication rate: 83%

or

– Dose recommendation: lansoprazole 30mg b.i.d. plus amoxicillin 1000mg b.i.d. plus clarithromycin 500mg b.i.d. for 7 days
– Mean eradication rate: 77%

or

– Dose recommendation: not established for pantoprazole
– Mean eradication rate: 77%

PPI, Nitroimidazole, Macrolide. Data from BAZZOLI and coworkers in Italy, using omeprazole as the PPI, showed 100% efficacy in the very first study of the combination: omeprazole, nitroimidazole, clarithromycin (BAZZOLI et al. 1993, 1994a–c, 1995a, 1996a,b; BERTRAMS et al. 1994; BUCKLEY et al. 1995; CHIBA et al. 1994; DAL BO et al. 1994a,b; DELTENDRE et al. 1994, 1995a,b; GEORGOPOULOS et al. 1996; GODDARD et al. 1996; HO et al. 1996; JAUP et al. 1994, 1995a; KALANTZIS et al. 1994; KAMBEROGLOU et al. 1995; LABENZ et al. 1994c, 1995a,b; LIND et al. 1995; MEINING et al. 1996; MELONI et al. 1995; MOAYYEDI et al. 1994a,b, 1996; MÖLLHAUPT et al. 1996; O'CONNOR et al. 1996; PEITZ et al. 1996a,b; PILOTTO et al. 1995; PRZYTULSKI et al. 1996; ROSSI et al. 1995; SACCA et al. 1996; SALADIN et al. 1995; SOLIMAN et al. 1996; SPADACCINI et al. 1995b,c; VEENENDAAL et al. 1996a,b; WU et al. 1996; YOUSFI et al. 1995; Fig. 6). The overall pooled result today is 90% efficacy and again a higher mean cure rate, 92%–94%, in controlled studies. Resistance to clarithromycin was a negative predictive factor for success. Metronidazole was the most commonly used nitroimidazole and the twice daily dosing during seven days therapy was dominated. The use of roxithromycin was less effective (65% cure rate) than clarithromycin when combined with omeprazole (BURETTE et al. 1993c; GLUPCZYNSKI et al. 1993; VAN GANSE et al. 1993; Fig. 6). Data on azithromycin instead of clarithromycin are limited indicating an efficacy of 76% (DI MARIO et al. 1994a,b, 1996; GASPERONI et al. 1994; TURSI et al. 1996a; Fig. 6). The combination lansoprazole, nitroimidazole, clarithromycin was effective in 80% (CHEN et al. 1996; CHEY et al. 1997; JAUP et al. 1995b; KIHIRA et al. 1996a; LAMOULIATTE et al. 1995c, 1996b,e; MOAYYEDI et al. 1997; MÖLLHAUPT et al. 1996; OZMEN et al. 1995; PILOTTO et al. 1997; PRYCE et al. 1996; SEBESTA et al. 1996; SPADACCINI et al. 1997; TAKIMOTO et al. 1996; Fig. 7) and pantoprazole, nitroimidazole, clarithromycin in 83% (ADAMEK et al. 1996a,b, 1997a–c; BARDHAN et al. 1996b; DAMMANN et al. 1997; FREVEL et al. 1997; KIST et al. 1997; LABENZ et al. 1995d; WITZEL et al. 1997; Fig. 7). Side effects were in the range of 5%–20% and the convenience level is high (Table 2).

– Dose recommendation: omeprazole 20mg b.i.d. plus metronidazole 400mg (or tinidazole 250–500mg) b.i.d. plus clarithromycin 250–500mg b.i.d. for 7 days
– Mean eradication rate: 90%

or

– Dose recommendation: lansoprazole 30mg b.i.d. plus metronidazole 400mg (or tinidazole 250–500mg) b.i.d. plus clarithromycin 250–500mg b.i.d. for 7 days
– Mean eradication rate: 80%

or

– Dose recommendation: pantoprazole 40mg b.i.d. plus metronidazole 400mg (or tinidazole 250–500mg) b.i.d. plus clarithromycin 250–500mg b.i.d. for 7 days
– Mean eradication rate: 83%

3.2.3.3 Mucosal Protective Agent Based Triple Combinations

Sucralfate and sofalcone are mucosal protective agents. Both drugs have an inhibitory effect on *H. pylori*, clearing, but not eradicating the bacterium, according to data from Japan. Data on sucralfate plus two of either amoxicillin, nitroimidazole, tetracycline or clarithromycin are limited and the efficacy did not confirm sucralfate's significant additive effect in the eradication of *H. pylori* (PEDRAZZOLI et al. 1994; STUPNICKI et al. 1994a,b, 1995; SUNG et al. 1994, 1995b; Fig. 8). The mean overall cure rate was 72%. Sofalcone in combination with ranitidine and clarithromycin, was less effective and the overall success rate was 36% (KODAMA et al. 1994; Fig. 8). The convenience factor is medium to low (Table 2; Fig. 8) (KODAMA et al. 1994; PEDRAZZOLI et al. 1994; STUPNICKI et al. 1994a,b, 1995; SUNG et al. 1995b).

– Dose recommendation: no consistent data
– Mean eradication rates: 72% and 36% for Sucralfate and sofalcone, respectively

3.2.4 Quadruple Therapy

3.2.4.1 PPI-, Bismuth-Based Quadruple Therapies

The so-called quadruple therapies has been reported to be extremely effective. However, pooled data shows only 81% efficacy for the omeprazole, bismuthdicitrate or bismuthsubsalicylate, nitroimidazole, tetracycline combination (BORODY et al. 1992a, 1994, 1995; HOSKING et al. 1992, 1994; KUNG et al. 1996; Fig. 9), and 70% efficacy for the omeprazole, bismuthdicitrate or bismuthsubsalicylate, nitroimidazole, amoxicillin combination (DE MEDICI et al. 1995; DOBRUCALI et al. 1995; FIGUEROA et al. 1996; MACRI et al. 1995; TAKATS et al. 1994; TUCCI et al. 1991, 1993; Fig. 9). It is suggested that this combination might be more likely to overcome metronidazole resistance, but further studies are needed. The convenience factor is low (Table 2).

– Dose recommendation: no consistent data
– Mean eradication rate: 81% and 70% for PPI- and bismuth-based therapies, respectively

3.3 Comments to Efficacy Data

When pooling efficacy data from various studies, there are a number of limitations to consider when interpreting the results. How many dual publications are there? Is the study design correctly stated? Was the statistical analysis adequately performed? Have the methods used for assessments been validated? Had the patients been regular participants in previous studies? The weakness of any pooled analysis is that the material will probably consist of a mixture of studies of varying statistical standards, but on the other hand the strength of such an analysis is that it mimics the clinical setting at a practical level.

The worst case approach used in this analysis might be too conservative and might explain why hardly any of the therapies reached the 90% success level in the overall analysis. However, the mixture of several patient groups, variations in the total daily dose, duration of therapy and dose frequency, different physician-patient relations are the realities of daily medical care. The most effective anti-*H. pylori* treatment strategies according to this analysis are a PPI plus clarithromycin plus nitroimidazole or a PPI plus clarithromycin plus amoxicillin. Bismuth triple combinations are frequently used, but were less efficacious in some reports and highly effective in others. The dose frequency and duration of therapy were repeatedly shown to be important factors for treatment success in general. Short treatment courses with twice daily dosing are likely to be key features for the PPI-based triple combinations. More frequent dosing over a longer period might explain the variable results with bismuth triple combinations. Dual therapies are inferior in efficacy and need a longer duration of therapy. Omeprazole plus amoxicillin has a low success rate and is influenced by compliance, smoking habits, etc.

Bearing that in mind, there are some trends in the results (Fig. 10). One antimicrobial is not effective, two antimicrobials plus either a proton pump inhibitor or bismuth increase the efficacy significantly, while four drugs given as quadruple therapy seem equally or less efficacious than triple combinations. PPI-based triple therapies are equally effective when given for 7 days or longer. Bismuth-based regimens should be given for at least fourteen days. Theoretically there are no major indications of significant differences in efficacy between the three PPIs as part of triple therapy against *H. pylori*. However, lansoprazole data show consistently lower success rates despite comparable dosing and daily dosage. This may be due to patient characteristics, drug compliance, resistance prevalence and other prognostic factors and the fact that the total number of patients studied is limited. Small differences in interaction profiles, the dose response curve of acid inhibition etc. do not provide an adequate explanation for this discrepancy in the cure of *H. pylori* infection.

3.4 Resistance Development

H. pylori easily develops resistance towards nitroimidazoles and also to macrolides and tetracycline. Resistance is usually defined as "reduced sensitivity of the bacterium to a given concentration of the antimicrobial." Whether this definition allows resistance data to predict the clinical outcome is controversial. Metronidazole resistance is probably of minor importance when using PPI triple regimens, while bismuth based triples appear more vulnerable. Clarithromycin resistance is regarded as more likely to predict treatment failure, although recent data show a minor clinical impact of in vitro resistance to clarithromycin (MEGRAUD et al. 1997a). However, data are far too limited to draw any conclusions. A cutoff level for a potential amoxicillin resistance has yet to be defined.

3.5 Cost-Effectiveness

The cost-effectiveness of anti-*H. pylori* therapy in duodenal ulcer patients is closely associated with efficacy based on Intention to treat analyses (UNGE et al. 1995). Compared to maintenance strategy, eradication of *H. pylori* pays off within 1 year. It is also cost-effective to check for eradication and the pay off period is less than 3 years. Thus it is cost-effective to use eradication therapy in almost all patients with peptic ulcer disease.

4 Current Research

Therapy. Combination therapy is efficacious but an extended use of antimicrobials is probably increasing the risk for resistance development and also the risk for severe adverse events. New chemical entities are under development as well as vaccines. The aim of the vaccine projects is to develop a protective and therapeutic vaccine. *Who to Treat?* Should all infected objectives be found by a screening procedure and treated or shall we select the group based on certain diagnosis or symptom complex? The cancer link is still under debate also in high risk areas in which the benefit of eradication of *H. pylori* is obvious. There are a number of studies ongoing aimed to clarify the link between *H. pylori* and gastric cancer.

5 Conclusions

In the treatment of *H. pylori* infection it is necessary to use well defined and validated drug combinations. Efficacy is the major determining factor for therapeutic success both regarding clinical cure of the disease and cost efficacy. The ideal therapy directed towards *Helicobacter pylori* eradication is still lacking. Bismuth-based triple therapy is effective, but influenced by compliance factors and bacterial resistance. Bismuth-ranitidine combinations awaits further development. Based on this analysis the best current drug combination is a PPI based triple therapy regimen. Of the eleven different drug combinations ($n > 100$) in this category (See Table 1) the highest eradication rate (90%) was achieved using Omeprazole 20mg b.i.d. plus metronidazole 400mg (or tinidazole 250–500mg) b.i.d. plus clarithromycin 250–500mg b.i.d. for 7 days. Studies searching for even better eradication rates are ongoing and may modify treatment strategies in the future as new compounds and preventive modalities such as vaccines are developed.

References

Adamek RJ, Wegener M, Birkholz S, Opferkuch W, Rühl GH, Ricken D (1992) Modifizierte kombinierte omeprazole/amoxicillin-therapie zur Helicobacter pylori-eradication: eine pilotstudie. Leber Magen Darm 6:222–224

Adamek RJ, Wegener M, Opferkuch W, Freitag M, Birkholz S, Rühl GH, Ricken D (1993a) Long-term and short-term intravenous antibiotic therapy of Helicobacter pylori-associated peptic ulcer disease. UEGW A 102:

Adamek RJ, Wegener M, Ricken D, Opferkuch W, Birkholz S, Freitag M, Rühl GH (1993b) Successful Helicobacter pylori eradication: a systemic or a topic effect of antibiotics? Gastroenterology 104(4):A29

Adamek RJ, Freitag M, Opferkuch W, Rühl GH, Wegener M (1994a) Duration of therapy plays a decisive role in H. pylori eradication using omeprazole and amoxicillin. Am J Gastroenterol 89:A301

Adamek RJ, Freitag M, Opferkuch W, Rühl GH, Wegener M (1994b) Intravenous omeprazole/amoxicillin and omeprazole pretreatment in Helicobacter pylori-positive acute peptic ulcer bleeding. Scand J Gastroenterol 29:880–883

Adamek RJ, Wegener M, Freitag M, Opferkuch W, Rühl GH (1994c) Combined intravenous and oral omeprazole/amoxicillin therapy in patients with H. pylori positive acute peptic ulcer bleeding. Gastroenterology 106:A15

Adamek RJ, Labenz J, Opferkuch W, Stolte M, Wegener M (1995a) Ranitidine/amoxicillin vs omeprazole/amoxicillin for cure of H. pylori positive gastric ulcer – role of acid suppression. Gastroenterology 108:A2599

Adamek RJ, Plaffenbach B, Opferkuch W, Freitag M, Szymaski CH, Wegener M (1995b) Role of duration of treatment in cure of H. pylori infection. Gastroenterology 108:A2096

Adamek, Bethke T, IPHPSG (1996a) One-week triple vs two-weeks dual therapy with pantoprazole for cure of H. pylori infection. Gut 39 [Suppl 2]:4A:32

Adamek RJ, Bethke T (1996b) Pantoprazole, clarithromycin and metronidazole vs pantoprazole and clarithromycin for cure of H. pylori infection in duodenal ulcer patients. Gastroenterology 112:A1235

Adamek RJ, Pfaffenbach B, Szymanski C (1997a) Does pre-treatment with pantoprazole affect the efficacy of a modern triple therapy in Hp cure? Gastroenterology 112:A2192

Adamek RJ, Pfaffenbach B, Szymanski C (1997b) Does pre-treatment with pantoprazole affect the efficacy of a modern triple therapy in Hp cure? Gut 41 [Suppl 1]:A348

Adamek RJ, Szymanski C, Pfaffenbach B (1997c) Pantoprazole vs omeprazole in one-week low-dose triple therapy for cure of H. pylori infection. Gastroenterology 112:A 2193

Adamek RJ, Pfaffenbach B, Suerbaum S, Philippou S, Opferkuch W (1997d) Pantoprazole plus amoxicillin and metronidazole: a safe, cost-effective therapy for Helicobacter pylori infection. Gastroenterology 112:A2194

Akamatsu T, Gotoh A, Shimizu T, Maeyama H, Fujimori K, Shimodaira K, Kiyosawa K, Kawakami Y, Ota H, Katsuyama T (1997) Combination effect of pronase for eradication therapy against Helicobacter pylori. Gastroenterology 112:A2229

AL-Assi MT, Karttunen T, Genta RM, Graham DY (1994) Which is important for omeprazole antimicrobial therapies: pH or antimicrobial activity? Comparison of amoxicillin and omeprazole and high dose ranitidine plus sodium bicarbonate. Am J Gastroenterol 89:A310

Alcalde M, Blanco M, Pajares JM (1992) Relationship between eradication of *Helicobacter pylori* and duodenal ulcer relapse after three different therapies: long term follow up. Gastroenterology 102:A43

Angeletti S, Caviglia R, Marcheggiano A, D'Ambra G, Marignani M, Paoletti M, Iannoni C, Annibale C, Delle Fave G (1995) Evidence that *H. pylori* eradication is not always associated with peptic ulcer healing. Gastroenterology 108:A2069

Atherton JC, Hudson N, Kirk GE, Hawkey CJ, Spiller RC (1993) Should amoxycillin be taken before or after meals when prescribed omeprazole for the eradication of *Helicobacter pylori*? A randomized controlled trial. Gastroenterology 104(4):A36

Atherton JC, Cullen DJE, Hawkey CJ, Spiller RC (1994) Enhanced eradication of *Helicobacter pylori* by pre- versus post-prandial amoxicillin suspension with omeprazole: implications for mode of action. Gastroenterology 106:A3203

Avellini C, Maieron R, Bardus P, Scott CA, Zoratti L, Da Broi GL, Beltrami CA (1994) Helicobacter (Hp) eradication and gastric mucosal changes. Am J Gastroenterol 89:249

Avsar E, Kalayci C, Tözön N, Göltekin O, Kiziltas S (1994) Refractory duodenal ulcer healing and relapse: comparison of omeprazole versus *Helicobacter pylori* eradication. World congress LA A 17P

Avunduk C, Navab F, Hampf F, Coughlin B (1995) Prevalence of *Helicobacter pylori* infection in patients with large gastric folds: evaluation and follow-up with endoscopic ultrasound before and after antimicrobial therapy. Am J Gastroenterol 90:1969–1973

Back S, Carling L, Ekström P, Glise H, Idström JP, Hellblom M, Ström M, Unge P, Weywadt L, Wrangstadh M (1995) Eradication of *Helicobacter pylori* with either phenoxymethylpenicillin, benzylpenicillin or amoxicillin in combination with omeprazole: a swedish multicentre study. Gastroenterology 108:A2125

Balatsos V, Delis V, Skandalis N, Archimandritis A (1993) Triple therapy after duodenal ulcer healing with omeprazole or ranitidine eradicates h pylori and prevents ulcer relapses: preliminary results of a year follow-up study. Gastoenterology 104(4):A37

Bancu L, Marian D, Bancu S, Marina M (1996) The role of nizatidine in *Helicobacter pylori* treatment. Helicobacter 1:274

Bank S, Blumstein M, Greenberg R, Kops R, Magier D, Twersky Y, Brigante L (1995) Amoxicillin 1g tid when combined with omeprazole gives high Hp eradication rates – preliminary report. Gastroenterology 108:A2123

Bardhan KD, Wurzer H, Marcelino M, Jahnsen J, Lotay N (1996a) High cure rates with ranitidine bismuth citrate (pylorid) plus clarithromycin given twice daily. Gut 39 [Suppl 2]4A:24

Bardhan KD, Slater DN, Morton D, Perry MJ, Cherian P, Jones RB, Brooks A, Thompson M, Morris P, Heinzerling H (1996b) Pantoprazole (panto)-based 10-days triple therapy is effective for *H. pylori* eradication. Gastroenterology 112:A2581

Bayerdörffer E, Mannes G A, Sommer A, Höchter W, Wiengardt J, Hatz R, Lehn N, Ruckdeschel G, Dirschedl P, Stolte M (1992) High dose omeprazole treatment combined with amoxicillin eradicates *Helicobacter pylori*. Eur J Gastroenterol Hepatol 4:697–702

Bayerdörffer E, Mannes GA, Miehlke S, Sommer A, Höchter W, Weingart J, Hatz R, Lehn N, Ruckdeschel G, Dirschedl P, Stolte M (1993) Two-year follow-up of duodenal ulcer patients after combined high dose omeprazole + amoxicillin treatment. UEGW A99

Bayerdörffer E, Meining A, Höchter W, Weingart J, Sommer A, Klann H, Simon T, Bästlein E, Huber F, Bolle KH, Schmitt W, Hatz R, Schulz H, Heldwein W, Zoller WG, Heidt H, Lehn N, Stolte M (1995a) Double-blind trial of 80 mg omeprazole and 2250 mg amoxicillin for cure of *Helicobacter pylori* infection in gastric ulcer patients. Gut 37 [Suppl 1]:A175

Bayerdörffer E, Miehlke S, Mannes GA, Sommer A, Höchter W, Weingart J, Heldwein W, Klann H, Simon T, Schmitt W, Bästlein E, Eimiller A, Hatz R, Lehn N, Dirschedl P, Stolte M (1995b) Double-blind trial of omeprazole and amoxicillin to cure *Helicobacter pylori* infection in patients with duodenal ulcers. Gastroenterology 108:1412–1417

Bayerdörffer E, Neubauer A, Rudolph B, Thiede C, Lehn N, Eidt S, Stolte M (1995c) Regression of primary gastric lymphoma of mucosa-associated lymphoid tissue type after cure of *Helicobacter pylori* infection. Lancet 345:1591–1594

Bazzoli F, Zagari RM, Fossi F, Pozzato P, Simoni P, Roda A, Roda E (1993) Efficacy and tolerability of a short term, low dose triple therapy for eradication of *Helicobacter pylori*. UEGW A101

Bazzoli F, Gullini S, Zagari RM, Pazzi P, Libera M, Pozzato P, Sottili S, Fossi S, Carli G, Scagliarini R, Simoni P, Roda E (1994a) Am J Gastroenterol 89:A316

Bazzoli F, Zagari RM, Fossi S, Pozzato P, Alampi G, Simoni P, Sottili S, Roda A, Roda E (1994b) Short-term low-dose triple therapy for the eradication of *Helicobacter pylori*. Eur J Gastroenterol Hepatol 6:773–777

Bazzoli F, Zagari RM, Fossi S, Pozzato P, Simoni P, Roda A, Roda E (1994c) Efficacy and tolerability of a short term, low dose triple therapy for eradication of *Helicobacter pylori*. Am J Gastroenterol 89:A317

Bazzoli F, Gullini S, Zagari RM, Pazzi P, Dalla Libera M, Pozzato P, Sottili S, Fossi S, Carli G, Scagliarini R, Simoni P, Roda E (1995a) Effect of omeprazole and clarithromycin plus tinidazole on the eradication of *Helicobacter pylori* and the recurrence of duodenal ulcer UEGW A2066

Bazzoli F, Gullini S, Zagari RM, Pazzi P, Dalla Libera M, Sottili S, Fossi S, Carli G, Scagliarini R, Simoni P, Roda E (1995b) Effect of omeprazole and clarithromycin plus tinidazole on the eradication of *Helicobacter pylori* and the recurrence. Gastroenterology 108:A2066

Bazzoli F, Zagari RM, Fossi S, Pozzato P, Alampi G, Sottili S, Simoni P, Mwangemi C, Ricciardiello L, Roda A, Roda E (1996a) Short-term low-dose triple therapy for the eradication of *Helicobacter pylori*: a randomized double-blind controlled study. Gastroenterology 112:A1244

Bazzoli F, Zagari RM, Fossi S, Pozzato P, Alampi G, Sottili S, Simoni P, Mwangemi C, Ricciardiello L, Roda A, Roda E (1996b) Short-term low-dose triple therapy for the eradication of *Helicobacter pylori*: a randomized, double blind, controlled study. Gut 39 [Suppl 2]4A:12

Bell DG, Powell K, Weil J, Burridge S M, Morden A, Harrison G, Gant PW, Jones PH, Trowell JE (1991) Experience with omeprazole in combination with either amoxycillin or colloidal bismuth subcitrate in patients with metronidazole-resistant *Helicobacter pylori*. Eur J Gastroenterol Hepatol 3:923–926

Bell GD, Powell KU, Burridge SM, Spencer G, Bolton G, Purser K, Brooks S, Prosser S, Harrison G, Gant PW, Jones PH, Trowell JE (1992) Short report: omeprazole plus antibiotic combinations for the eradication of metronidazole-resistant *Helicobacter pylori*. Aliment Pharmacol Ther 6:751–758

Bell GD, Powell KU, Burridge SM, Bowden AN, Rameh B, Bolton G, Purser K, Harrison G, Brown C, Gant PW, Jones PH, Trowell JE (1993) *Helicobacter pylori* eradication: efficacy and side-effect profile of a combination of omeprazole, amoxycillin and metronidazole compared with four alternative regimens. Q J Med 86:743–750

Bell GD, Powell KU, Burridge SM, Bowden AF, Atoyebi W, Bolton GH, Jones PH, Brown C (1995) Rapid eradication of *Helicobacter pylori* infection. Aliment Pharmacol Ther 9:41–46

Bertoni G, Sassatelli R, Nigrisoli GE, Tansini P, Bianchi G, Della Casa G, Bagni A, Bedogni G (1996) Triple therapy with azithromycin, omeprazole and amoxicillin is highly effective in the eradication of *Helicobacter pylori*: a controlled trial versus omeprazole plus amoxicillin. Am J Gastroenterol 91: 258–263

Bertrams J, Börsch G (1994) Efficacy of low-dose one-week triple therapy to cure *H. pylori* infection. Am J Gastroenterol 89:A364

Bertschinger Ph, Brunner J, Flury R, Lammer F, Jost R, Häcki WH (1992) Vergleich der Wirksamheit von omeprazole/bismuthsubcitrate oder tripleterapie bei Helicobacter-pylori-gastritis. Schweiz Med Wochenschr 122:1446–1451

Bianchi Porro G, Parente F, Imbesi V, Montrone F, Caruso I (1996a) Role of *Helicobacter pylori* infection in healing and recurrence of NSAID-associated peptic ulcer. Gastroenterology 112:A1210

Bianchi Porro G, Lazzaroni M, Bargigggia S, Maconi G, Trespi E, Perego M, Villani L, Luinetti O, Fiocca R, Franceschi M, Cesana B, Solcia E (1996b) Omeprazole coupled with two antibiotics for *Helicobacter pylori* eradication and prevention of ulcer recurrence. Am J Gastroenterol 91:695–700

Bor-Shyang Shen, Lin XZ, Lin CY, Shiesh SC (1995) Is triple therapy beneficial to patients with *Helicobacter pylori* related nonulcer dyspepsia. UEGW A0095

Borody TJ, Brandl S, Andrews P, Jankiewicz E, Ostapowicz N (1992a) H pylori eradication failure (EF) – further treatment possibilities. Gastroenterology 102:A43

Borody TJ, George LL, Brandl P, Andrews P, Lenne J, Moore-Jones D, Devine M, Walton M (1992b) *Helicobacter pylori* eradication with doxycycline-metronidazole-bismuth subcitrate triple therapy. Scand J Gastroenterol 27:281–284

Borody T, Andrews P, Shortis NP, Bae H, Brandl S (1994) Optimal H pylori (Hp) therapy-a combination of omeprazole and triple therapy (TT). Gastroenterology 106:A63

Borody T, Andrews P, Fracchia G, Brandl S, Shortis NP, Bae H (1995) Omeprazole enhances efficacy of triple therapy in eradicating *Helicobacter pylori*. Gut 37:477–481

Bouchard S, Birac C, Lamouliatte H, Forestier S, Megraud F (1996) Correlation between the MICs metronidazole on *Helicobacter pylori* strains and the outcome of a lansoprazole-amoxicillin-metronidazole therapy. Gut 39 [Suppl 2]1A:05

Bruno M, Peyre S, Grosso S, Sategna-Guidetti C (1994) Eradication of *Helicobacter pylori* (Hp) in duodenal ulcer disease: comparison between two different treatments. UEGW OSLO III:A1501

Buckley M, Keating S, Xia H, Beattie S, Hamilton H, O'Morain C (1995) Omeprazole plus one or two antibiotics to eradicate *H. pylori*. Gastroenterology 108:A2131

Buda A, Dal Bò N, Kusstatscher S, Grassi SA, Crestani B, Battaglia G, Pilotto A, Franceschi M, De Bona M, Salanadin S, Di Mario F (1997) Different lansoprazole dosages in *H. pylori* eradication therapy: a prospective multicenter randomized study comparing 30 mg b.i.d. vs 15 mg b.i.d. Gut 41 [Suppl 1]:A335

Bures J, Krejsek J, Kolesar J, Rejchrt S, Drahosova M, Horasek J, Pidrman V (1994a) Serum IgG and IgA anti-*Helicobacter pylori* antibodies in duodenal ulcer treated by omeprazole and amoxicillin. UEGW OSLO III:A1428

Bures J, Malirbreveova E?, Krejsek J, Reichrt S, Kolesar J, Drahosova M, Viczbreveda J, Pidrman V (1994b) Serum group I pepsinogens and IgG & IgA anti-*Helicobacter pylori* antibodies in duodenal ulcer treated by omeprazole and amoxicillin. World congress LA A 707P

Burette A, Glupczynski Y, Deprez C (1992) Two weeks triple therapy for *Helicobacter pylori* overcomes metronidazole resistance. Results of a randomized double/triple therapy. Gastroenterology 102:A46

Burette A, Glupczynski Y, DePrez C, Ramdani B (1993a) Two-week combination therapies with tetracycline are less effective than similar regimens with amoxicillin. Acta Gastroentrol Belg 56 [Suppl]:A131

Burette A, Glupczynski Y, DePrez C, DeKoster E, Urbain D, Vanderauwera J, Wigerinck A, Drnec J (1993b) Omeprazole alone or in combination with clarithromycin for eradication of *H. pylori*: results of a randomized double-blind controlled study. Gastroenterology 104(4):A49

Burette A, Glupczynski Y, DePrez C, Crombez A (1993c) Lansoprazole plus roxithromycin and metronidazole for eradication of H pylori: results from a single-blind pilot study. Acta Gastroentrol Belg 56 [Suppl]:131

Burette A, Glupczynski Y, Deprez C, Ramdani B (1994) Two weeks omeprazole plus amoxicillin regimens for eradication of *H. pylori*. Am J Gastroenterol 89:A323

Burette A, Glupczynski Y, Deprez C, Ramdani B (1995) Omeprazole + amoxicillin + clarithromycin therapy for *H. pylori* infection. Gut 37 [Suppl 1]:A353

Burette A, Lamy V, Ramdani B, Capelli J, De Prez C, Glupczynski Y (1996) Lansoprazole (30 mg od vs bid) with amoxicillin and clarithromycin to cure *Helicobacter pylori* infection. Gut 39 [Suppl 2]4A:13

Burette A, Ramdani B, Deprez C, Glupczynski Y (1997a) Seven or twelve day triple therapies combining omeprazole with amoxicillin and clarithromycin to cure *H. pylori*. Gastroenterology 112:A2190

Burette A, Lamy V, Ligny G, Cabooter M, Ramdani B, Ectors M, Glupczynski Y, Laruelle N, Vandenhoven G, Noe M (1997b) Dual or triple therapy combining omeprazole with amoxicillin and/or clarithromycin for *H. pylori* infection. Gastroenterology 112:A2191

Börsch G, Labenz J, Gyenes E, Rühl GH (1991) Amoxicillin-omeprazole treatment for eradication of *Helicobacter pylori*. Eur J Gastroenterol Hepatol 3 [Suppl 1]:A38

Cammarota G, Fideli G, Montalto M, Tursi A, Renzi C, Papa A, Vecchio FM, Branca G, Certo M, Gasbarrini G (1994) Mucosa-associated lymphoid tissue in *Helicobacter pylori* infection: frequency and response to therapy. Am J Gastroenterol 89:A284

Cardelli A, Cordiano C, Giglio A, Lami F, Pilotto A, Pozzato P, Scarpulla G, Spadaccini A, Susi D, Olivieri A, Tosatto R, Roda E (1997) A new dual 7-day therapy is effective in eradicating *Helicobacter pylori* in duodenal ulcer patients. Gut 41 [Suppl 1]:A350

Caroli A, Kusstatscher S, Boni M, Grasso GA, Sperti C, Di Mario F, Puglisi A (1995a) Eradication of *Helicobacter pylori* infection: is there a double therapy still suitable? Gut 37 [Suppl 1]:A340

Caroli A, Kusstatscher S, Boni M, Grasso GA, Sperti C, Di Mario F, Puglisi A (1995b) High dose of amoxicillin improves the efficacy of double therapy for the eradication of *Helicobacter pylori* infection. UEGW A 1666

Carpintero P, Moreno JA, Perez Garcia JI, Hermida C, Gomez A, Garcia Valriberas R, Jimenez I, Pajares Garcia JM (1995) *Helicobacter pylori* eradication in dyspeptic patients with end stage renal failure. UEGW A 1684

Caselli M, Ruina M, Gallerani L, Fabbri P, Gaudenzi P, Alvisi V (1996) Azithromycin and increasing doses of omeprazole for the eradication of *Helicobacter pylori*. Gut 39 [Suppl 2]4A:01

Catalano F, Rizzo G, Ayoubi Khajekini MT, Branciforte G, Inserra G, Liberti A (1992) *Helicobacter pylori* positive dyspepsia: results of four days treatment. Ir J Med Sci 161 [Suppl 10]:T26

Catalano F, Terranova R, Branciforte G, Catanzaro R, Liberti A, Rutella E, Luca S (1994a) *Helicobacter pylori* eradication in elderly patients: comparison of two treatments. World congress LA A 105P

Catalano F, Catanzaro R, Liberti A, Branciforte G, Bentivegna C, Nuciforo G, Blasi A (1994b) *Helicobacter pylori* positive dyspepsia: results after six months suspension omeprazole/amoxicillin combined therapy. World congress LA A 107P

Catalano F, Catanzaro R, Liberti A, Baranciforte A, Brogna A, Bentivegna C, Blasi A (1995) Comparative efficacy of omeprazole in association with amoxicillin or clarithromycin in *Helicobacter pylori* positive functional dyspepsia. UEGW A 0164

Catalano F, Privitera U, Branciforte G, Catanzaro R, Bentivegna C, Brogna A, Blasi A (1996) Omeprazole vs two different doses of lansoprazole in triple therapy on *H. pylori* positive duodenal ulcer. Gut 39 [Suppl 2]4A:08

Catalano F, Catanzaro R, Brogna A, Brancoforte G, Bentivegna C, Liberti A (1997) Duodenal ulcer and funtional dyspepsia: different susceptibility of *Helicobacter pylori* to eradicating therapy. Gastroenterology 112:A2212

Caviglia R, Angelettia S, Luzi I, Marignani M, D'Ambra G, Pezzella C, Paoletti M, Annibale B, Delle Fave G (1995) Relationship between omeprazole pre-treatment and successful eradication rate on *H. pylori* (Hp) infection. Gastroenterology 108:A2132

Caviglia R, Paoletti M, Luzzi I, Angeletti S, Pica R, Marignani M, D'Ambra G, Iannoni C, Pezzella C, Annibale B, Della Fave G (1996) Omeprazole (omp) pretreatment, metronidazole (mtz) resistance do not affect significantly the eradication rate of *Helicobacter pylori* infection. Gastroenterology 112:A4511

Cayla R, Greaves RG, Mendelson MG, Lamouliatte HC, Gummet PA, Baron JH, Green RM, Roux D, Megraud F, Misiewicz JJ (1993) Omeprazole vs clarithromycin and omeprazole for eradication of *Helicobacter pylori* (*H. pylori*). UEGW A 101

Chen WH, Yang JC, Wang JT, Lin JT, Wang TH (1995) Comparison of three non-bismuth triple therapy for the eradication of *Helicobacter pylori*. UEGW A 1993

Chen MH, Wu WS, Cui Y, Li YY, Hu PJ (1996) Clinical study of one week clarithromycin combination therapy for the treatment of *H. pylori* infection. Helicobacter 1:271

Chen CY, Sheu MZ, Lee SC (1997) Intravenous dual therapy and oral new triple therapy in Helicobacter-related ulcer bleedings with major stigmat of recent hemorrhage. Gut 41 [Suppl 1]:A360

Chey WD, Fisher L, Elta GH, Barnett J, Nostrant T, Del Valle J, Hasler W, Scheiman JM (1997) One week, bid therapy for *H. pylori*: a randomized comparison of 2 strategies. Gastroenterology 112:A2162

Chiba N (1994) Low dose omeprazole (O) + clarithromycin (C) ± metronidazole (M) in the eradication of *H. pylori* (Hp): interim results. Am J Gastroenterol 89:A328

Chiba N (1996) Omeprazole and clarithromycin with and without metronidazoe for the eradication of *Helicobacter pylori*. Am J Gastroenterol 91:2139–2143

Ching CK, Chan YK, Ng WC (1997) The combination of omeprazole, amoxicillin and clarithromycin eradicates *Helicobacter pylori* in 95% of cases – 7-day equals 10-day therapy. Gastroenterology 112:A2189

Chow WH, Kwan WK, Leung CS, Wong KK (1996) Efficacy of low dose, short course of omeprazole + amoxicillin + metronidazole in the treatment of duodenal ulcer. Helicobacter 1:279

Cirillo M, De Falco R, Prota C, Landolfi C, Lobello R (1994) *Helicobacter pylori* eradication: omeprazole + amoxicillin versus ranitidine + amoxicillin versus triple therapy. A randomized-clinical trial. World congress LA A 80 P

Collins R, Keane C, O'Morain C (1991) Omeprazole and colloidal bismuth subcitrate ± adjuvant antibiotics in the treatment of *Helicobacter pylori* associated with duodenal ulcer disease. Gastroenterology 100:A48

Collins R, Beattie S, O'Morain C (1992) High dose omeprazole plus amoxycillin in the treatment of acute duodenal ulcer. Ir J Med Sci 161 [Suppl 10]:T33

Collins JSA, Johnston BT, Sloan JM, O'Morain C, Gilvary J, O'Connor HJ (1993a) Comparison of 3, 5, and 7 day triple therapy for *H. pylori* eradication. Acta Gastroentrol Belg 56 [Suppl]:A137

Collins R, Beattie S, Xia HX, O'Morain C (1993b) Short report: high-dose omeprazole and amoxicillin in the treatment of *Helicobacter pylori*-associated duodenal ulcer. Aliment Pharmacol Ther 7:313–315

Colombo E, Bortoli A, Meucci G, Teruzzi V, Imperiali G, Minoli G, Valduce H, Como, Garbagnate H, Rho H (1997) Lansoprazole vs omeprazole: one week triple therapy in peptic ulcer (preliminary results). Gastroenterology 112:A2195

Costa F, Amato G, Belcari C, Bellini M, Tumino E, Spataro M, Lambresa M, Manghetti M, Ciccorossi P, Maltinti G, Marchi S (1997) Treament of *Helicobacter pylori* infection with different doses of clarithromycin combined with amoxicillin and lansoprazole. Gastroenterology 112:A2166

Dal Bo N, Ferrana M, Salandin S, Dotto P, Del Bianco P, Vianello F, Plebani M, Rugge M, Grassi AS, Pasini M, Lecis PE, Vigneri S, Leandro G, Battaglia G, Di Mario F (1994a) Comparison of two different triple therapies with clarithromycin for *Helicobacter pylori* (Hp) eradication. Am J Gastroenterol 89:A333

Dal Bo N, Grasso GA, Pilotto A, Battaglia G, Ferrana M, Dotto P, Salandin S, Vianello F, Plebani M, Vigneri S, Rugge M, Del Bianco T, Di Mario F (1994b) Clarithromycin for the cure of *Helicobacter pylori* (H pylori) infection. Gut 35 [Suppl 5]:W64

Dammann H-G, Fölsch UR, Hahn EG, von Kleist DH, Klör H-U, Kirschner T, Kist M (1997) 7 vs 14 day treatment with pantoprazole, clarithromycin and metronidazole for cure of *H. pylori* infection in duodenal ulcer patients. Gut 41 [Suppl 1]:A349

Daskalopoulos G, Carrick J, Lian R, Lee A (1992) Optimising therapy for H pylori gastritis. Ir J Med Sci 161 [Suppl 10]:16

Daskalopoulos G, Lian JX, Carrick J, Lee A (1993) Metronidazole resistance significantly affects eradication of *Helicobacter pylori* infection. Gastroenterology 104(4):A133

Daskalopoulos G, Ho YY, Mehanna D, Chen K (1996) The role of quadruple therapy in the treatment of *Helicobacter pylori*. Gut 39 [Suppl 2]4A:19

de Boer WA, Driessen WMM (1994) Randomised study comparing one with two weeks of triple therapy for eradicating *Helicobacter pylori*. Gastroenterology 106:A410

de Boer WA, Driessen WMM (1995) Dual therapy of omeprazole plus amoxicillin versus quadruple therapy of omeprazole, bismuth, tetracycline and metronidazole for cure of *H. pylori* infection in ulcer patients. Gastroenterology 108:A2067

De Bona M, Bellamat A, Doglioni C, De Boni M (1994) Oral triple therapy for *Helicobacter pylori* eradication in dyspeptic patients: 12 months follow-up study. Gastroenterology 106:A355

de Korwin JD, Joubert M, Bazin N, Thiaucourt D, Protte E, Gissler C, Conroy MC, Duprez A, Merlin P, Forestier S (1993) Lansoprazole versus lansoprazole plus antibiotics in the treatment of *Helicobacter pylori* gastric infection. Gastroenterology 104(4):A67

De Koster E, Burette A, Nyst JF, Glupczynski Y, Deprez C, Deltendre M (1990) Hp treatment: the macrolide trail: one week erythromycin + CBS + omeprazole. Rev Esp Enferm Dig 78 [Suppl 1]:134–135

De Koster E, Nyst JF, Deprez C, Denis P, Buset M, De Reuck M, Deltendre M (1992a) *Helicobacter pylori* treatment: double vs. triple therapy: who needs bismuth? Gastroenterology 102:A58

De Koster E, Nyst JF, Deprez C, Jonas C, Denis P, Buset M, De Reuck M, Deltendre M (1992b) Hp treatment: disappointing results with amoxicillin plus omeprazole. Gastroenterology 102:A58

De Koster E, Deprez C (1993) Cimetidine + amoxicillin + metronidazole in *Helicobacter pylori* -associated relapsing duodenal ulcer: a preliminary report. Acta Gastroentrol Belg 56 [Suppl]:A133

De Koster E, Deprez C (1994) Cimetidine prophylaxis vs *Helicobacter pylori* eradication in patients with relapsing duodenal ulcer: report of on open multicenter study. World congress LA A 99P

De Medici A, Sacca N, Rodino S, Di Siena M, Giglio A (1994) Smoking does not have influence on the efficacy of omeprazole/amoxicillin combined therapy for eradication of *Helicobacter pylori*. UEGW OSLO III:A1439

De Medici A, Rodino S, Sacca N, De Siena M, Giglio A (1995) Comparison of two different therapeutic regimens in the eradication of *Helicobacter pylori*. UEGW A 1960

Delchier IC, Elamine I, Goldfain D, Chaussade S, Mancini L, Idström JP (1995) Comparison of omeprazole + amoxicillin versus omeprazole + amoxicillin + clarithromycin in the eradication of *Helicobacter pylori* (Hp) – results from a randomized study involving 120 patients. Gastroenterology 108:A2596

Deltendre M, Jonas C, Van Gossum M, De Koster E (1994) Omeprazole-amoxicillin and omeprazole-clarithromycin for eradication of *Helicobacter pylori*. Am J Gastroenterol 89:A337

Deltendre M, De Koster E, Van Gossum M, De Reuck M, Jonas C (1995a) Omeprazole based therapies for eradication of *Helicobacter pylori*. Gut 37 [Suppl 1]:A357

Deltendre M, De Koster E, Van Gossum M, De Reuck M, Jonas C (1995b) Omeprazole based therapies for eradication of *Helicobacter pylori*. UEGW A 0623

Di Mario F, Vigneri S, Termini R, Scialabba A, Savarino V, Mela GS (1993) One year relapse rate after h pylori eradication with omeprazole plus antimicrobials. Gastroenterology 104(4):A220

Di Mario F, Dal Bo N, Ferrana M, Salandin S, Dotto P, Del Bianco T, Vianello F, Vigneri F, Rugge M, Grassi SA, Battaglia G (1994a) Azithromycin in a triple therapy for eradicating *Helicobacter pylori*. Gut 35 [Suppl 2]:T249

Di Mario F, Ferrana M, Salandin S, Dotto P, Del Bianco T, Vianello F, Plebani M, Rugge M, Vigneri S, Battaglia G (1994b) Azithromycin: a new useful therapeutic strategy for the eradication of *Helicobacter pylori* infection. Modification of serum gastrin pepsinogens and anti-Hp antibodies (IgG). Gastroenterology 106:A989

Di Mario F, Dal Bo N, Grassi SA, Rugge M, Cassaro M, Donisi PM, Vianello F, Kusstatscher S, Salandin S, Grasso GA, Ferrana M, Battaglia G (1996) Azithromycin for the cure of *Helicobacter pylori* infection. Am J Gastroenterol 91:264–267

Dobrucali A, Tuncer M, Bal K, Uzunismail H, Yurdakul, Altin M, Oktay E (1995) One-day, high dose combined therapy of *Helicobacter pylori* infection. UEGW A 2061

Doppl WE, Waldherr M, Klor HU (1994) Low eradication rate of *Helicobacter pylori* after triple therapy. Am J Gastroenterol 89:A340

El-Omar E, Wirz A, McColl KEL (1995) Effect of *H. pylori* eradication on the severity of dyspeptic symptoms in DU patients – a one year follow-up study. Gut 37 [Suppl 1]:A342

Engstrand L, Genta RM, Scheynius A, Go MF, Graham DY (1994) Presence of intraepithelial *H. pylori* heat shock protein (HSP62) after successful treatment-a reflection of continuing chronic inflammation? Am J Gastroenterol 89:A154

Fakhreih S, Rahemi M, Dehbashi N, Saberi Firoozi M, Keshavarz AA, Alborzi I, Oboodi A, Massarrat S (1995) Eradication of *Helicobacter pylori* vs ranitidine maintenance therapy for prevention of duodenal ulcer rebleeding. UEGW A 2014

Ferrini G, Larcinese G, Semperlotti N (1994) Treatment with omeprazole and clarithromycin in duodenal ulcer associated with *Helicobacter pylori*. Am J Gastroenterol 89:A342

Ferrini G, D'Orazio A, Larcinese G, Pizzicanella G, Semperlotti N, Spadaccini A (1995a) Effect of roxatidine and amoxicillin plus tinidazole on the eradication of *Helicobacter pylori* in duodenal ulcer patients. UEGW A 2134

Ferrini G, De Fanis C, Della Sciucca A, Falcucci M, Grossi L, Lanetti G, Larcinese G, Lattanzio R, Lauri A, Marzio L, Mescia P, Moretta A, Pasto S, Sciampa G, Sedici A, Semperlotti N, Spadaccini A (1995b) Effect of omeprazole, clarithromycin and amoxicillin for a short time on *Helicobacter pylori* eradication. UEGW A 2133

Ferulano GP, Dilillo S, Sabino N, Scala F, De Paola P, Tucci D (1994) Omeprazole + amoxicillin vs omeprazole + amoxicillin + metronidazole in the eradication of *Helicobacter pylori*. Gastroenterology 106:A2925

Figueroa G, Acuna R, Troncoso M, Portell DP, Toledo MS, Albornoz V, Vigneaux J (1996) Low *H. pylori* reinfection rate after triple therapy in chilean duodenal ulcer patients. Am J Gastroenterol 91:1395–1399

Fiocca R, Villiani L, Luinetti O, Gianatti A, Boldorini R, Lazzaroni M, Bianchi Porro G, Trespi E, Perego M, Alvisi C, Cesana B, Solcia E (1992) *Helicobacter pylori* (Hp) eradication and sequential clearance of inflammation in duodenal ulcer patients treated with omeprazole and antibiotics. Ir J Med Sci 161 [Suppl 10]:T23

Fiocca R, Trespi E, Villani L, Broglia F, Luinetti O, Colla C, Solcia E (1995) High efficacy of a clarithromycin-amoxicillin-omeprazole association for *H. pylori* eradication and treatment of ulcer-like or reflux-like dyspeptic symptoms. Gut 37 [Suppl 1]:A336

Fixa B, Komarkova O, Krejsek J, Nozicka Z (1994) Effect of eradication of *Helicobacter pylori* on gastric mucosa and recurrence in duodenal ulcer disease. World congress LA A 104P

Forne M, Viver JM, Espinos JC, Coll J, Tressera S, Garau J (1995) Impact of colloidal bismuth subcitrate in the eradication rates of *Helicobacter pylori* infection-associated duodenal ulcer using a short treatment regimen with omeprazole and clarithromycin: a randomized study. Am J Gastroenterol 90:718–721

Fraser A, Moore L, Chua LE, Hollis B, Little SV (1996) An audit of low dose triple therapy for eradication of *Helicobacter pylori*. NZ Med J 290:11

Frevel M, Daake H, Janish H-D, Kellner H-U, Krezdorn H, Tanneberger D, Wack R, Cain CR (1997) Pantoprazole plus clarithromycin and metronidazole versus pantoprazole plus clarithromycin and amoxicillin for therapy of *H. pylori* infection. Gastroenterology 112:A2204

Fukuda Y, Mizuta T, Yamamoto I, Shimoyama T (1994) The novel anti-ulcer agent ecabet sodium (TA-2711) eradicates *Helicobacter pylori* inhabiting the gastric mucosa of the Japanese monkeys. UEGW OSLO III:A1448

Gasperoni S, Bronzetti R, Cardelli A (1994) A short effective therapy for HP infection. World congress LA A 85P

George LL, Borody TJ, Andrews P, Devine M, Moore-Jones D, Walton M, Brandl S (1990) Cure of duodenal ulcer after eradication of *Helicobacter pylori*. Med J Aust 153:145–149

Georgopoulus S, Spiliadis C, Stambolos P, Mentis A, Gianikaki L, Manika Z, Skandalis N (1995) Evaluation of the efficacy of clarithromycin in the eradication of *Helicobacter pylori* (Hp). Gut 37 [Suppl 1]:A339

Georgopoulos S, Mentis A, Karatapanis S (1996) Comparison of the efficacy of two short-term triple therapies based on clarithromycin in the eradication of *Helicobacter pylori* (Hp): A randomized study. Gut 39 [Suppl 2]4A:17

Georgopoulos SD, Ladas SD, Karatapanis S, Spiliadi Ch, Mentis AF, Tassios PS, Artikis V, Raptis SA (1997) Does follicular gastritis adversely affect *H. pylori* eradication rate? Gut 41 [Suppl 1]:A357

Gisbert JP, Boixeda D, Vila T, Martin-de-Argila C, Canton R, Redondo C, Arocena C (1994a) Modification of basal and stimulated pepsinogen levels after eradication of *Helicobacter pylori*. Am J Gastroenterol 89:A156

Gisbert JP, Boixeda D, Vila T, Martin-De-Argila T, de Rafael L, Alvarez Bareliola I, Arocena C (1994b) Modification of basal and stimulated gastrin levels after eradication of *Helicobacter pylori*. UEGW OSLO III:A1450

Gisbert JP, Boixeda D, Moreno L, Aller R, Urman J, Rincon MN, Higes MJ, Arpa MA, Martin de Argila C (1997) Which therapy should we use when a previous *Helicobacter pylori* eradicatoin therapy fails? Gut 41 [Suppl 1]:A341

Glupczynski Y, Burette A, DePrez C, Ramdani B (1993) Omeprazole plus roxythromycin and metronidazole for eradication of *Helicobacter pylori*: results of a single-blind pilot study. Acta Gastroenterol Belg 56 [Suppl]:135

Goddard AF, Logan RPH, Lawes S, Hawkey CJ, Spiller RC (1996) Metronidazole or tinidazole in combination with omeprazole and clarithromycin for the eradication of *H. pylori*: a randomized and double-blind comparison. Gastroenterology 112:A1239

Goh KL, Parasakthi N, Peh SC, Wong NW, Tan KK, Lo YL, Chin SC (1993) Efficacy of combination therapy of omeprazole with antibiotics in the eradication of *Helicobacter pylori*. Gastroenterology 104:A89

Govosdis B, Triantafillidis JK, Tsami-Pandi A, Cheracakis P, Barbatzas C (1994a) Effect of the administration of omeprazole plus amoxicillin on the rate of *Helicobacter pylori* eradication from dental plaque and saliva of patients with active duodenal ulcer. UEGW OSLO III:A1513

Govosdis B, Triantafillidis JK, Tsami-Pandi A, Cheracakis P, Barbatzas C (1994b) Comparison of the effect of the administration of omeprazole plus amoxicillin vs lansoprazole plus amoxicillin on the *Helicobacter pylori* eradication from dental plaque and saliva of patients with active duodenal ulcer. World congress LA A 66P

Graham DY, Graham KS, Malaty HM, El-Zimiaty H, Genta RM, Cole RA, Yousfi MM, Al-Assi MT, Neil G (1995) Variability with omeprazole-amoxicillin combinations for treatment of *Helicobacter pylori* infection. Gastroenterology 108:A2099

Greaves RG, Cayla R, Mendelson MG, Lamouliatte H, Gummet PA, Baron JH, Megraud F, Logan RH, Misiewicz JJ (1994) Omeprazole versus clarithromycin and omeprazole for eradication of *H. pylori* infection. Gastroenterology 106:A1238

Greenberg PD, Cello JP (1996) Prospective double-blind treatment of *Helicobacter pylori* in patients with non-ulcer dyspepsia. Gastroenterology 112:A1240

Gudjonsson H, Bardhan KD, Hoie O, Kristensen ES, Scheutz E, Kliebe-Frisch C, Duggan AE (1997) High *H. pylori* eradication rate with one week triple regimen containing ranitidine bismuth citrate (RBC). Gut 41 [Suppl 1]:A363

Gupta AM, Korsten MA, Gentry RT, Lieber CS (1994) Eradication of *Helicobacter pylori* increases antral gastric alcohol dehydrogenase (ADH) activity. World congress LA A 699P

Gurbuz AK, Giardiello FM, Dagalp K, Karaeren N, Alper A, Pasricha P (1994) Clarithromycin and omeprazole for *Helicobacter pylori* gastritis: an unsatisfactory regimen. Gastroenterology 106:A3627

Habu Y, Mizuno S, Kiyota K, Yoshida S, Inokuchi H, Kimoto K, Kawai K (1996) Triple therapy of omeprazole + amoxicillin + clarithromycin if effective for the cure of *Helicobacter pylori* infection in gastric and duodenal ulcer patients. -results of a randomized study involving 120 patients in Japan. Gastroenterology 112:A1238

Hackelsberger A, Miehlke S, Lehn N, Stolte M, Malfertheiner P, Bayerdörffer E (1996) *Helicobacter pylori* eradication vs. short term acid suppression: long term consequences for gastric body mucosa. Gastroenterology 112:A1218

Hentschel E, Brandstätter G, Dragosics B, Hirschl AM, Nemec H, Schütze K, Taufer M, Wurzer H (1993) Effect of ranitidine and amoxicillin plus metronidazole on the eradication of *Helicobacter pylori* and the recurrence of duodenal ulcer. N Engl J Med 328:308–312

Hermida C, Moreno JA, Carpintero P, Mateos JM, Gagravalos R, Pajares JM (1996) Triple therapy (omeprazole + amoxicillin + clarithromycin) for *Helicobacter pylori* eradication in patients with chronic gastritis. Twelve days better than six. Gut 39 [Suppl 2]4A:11

Hermida C, Fernadez-Munoz J, Perez-Poveda JJ, Abad F, Pajares JM (1997) Triple therapy omeprazole (O) + amoxicillin (A) + clarithromycin (C) for *Helicobacter pylori* (Hp) infection. 6 vs 12 days. Results and cost analysis. Gut 41 [Suppl 1]:A344

Hirschl AM, Hentschel E, Berger J, Nemec H, Rotter ML (1991) Treatment of *Helicobacter pylori* infections with amoxicillin plus metronidazole: bacteriological, serological and histological results. Eur J Gastroenterol Hepatol 3:1–3

Ho AS, Lee SC, Hsu CT (1996) What's the clinically favored triple therapy? Gut 39 [Suppl 2]4A:09

Hogan DL, Rapier RC, Dreilinger A, Chose MA, Bausch PM, Einstein WM, Nyberg LM, Isenberg JI (1996) Duodenal bicarbonate secretion: eradication of *Helicobacter pylori* and duodenal structure and functions in humans. Gastroenterology 110:705–716

Hosking SW, Ling TKW, Yung MY, Cheng A, Chung SCS, Leung JWC, Li AKC (1992) Randomized controlled trial of short term treatment to eradicate *Helicobacter pylori* in patients with duodenal ulcer. BMJ 305:502–504

Hosking SW, Ling TKW, Chung SCS, Cheng AFB, Sung JJY, LI AKC (1994) Duodenal ulcer healing by eradication of *Helicobacter pylori* without anti-acid treatment: randomised controlled trial. Lancet 343:508–510

Hu PJ, Li YY, Chui Y, Hazell SL, Mitchell HM, Lee A (1994) The effect of modified triple therapy on the healing of duodenal ulcer and eradication of *Helicobacter pylori* infection. World congress LA A 84P

Hu FL, Wang ECK, Wang JM, Jia BQ (1995) Role of *Helicobacter pylori* eradication in duodenal ulcer healing and relapse. UEGW A 2280

Huber FE (1993) Vierwöchige Kombinationstherapie erfolgreich. Krankenhaus Artz 66:118–119

Hudson N, Brydon WG, Eastwood MA, Ferguson A, Palmer KR (1995) Successful *Helicobacter pylori* eradication incorporating a one-week antibiotic regimen. Aliment Pharmacol Ther 9:47–50

Huelin-Benitez J, Jimenez Perez M, Sanchez Galdon S, Duran Campos A, Cardenas Martinez A, Espana Contreras P, de la Cruz J, Lozano JM, Maldonado G (1997) Short-course treatment to eradicate *H. pylori* in 246 patients with peptic ulcer disease. Gut 41 [Suppl 1]:A388

Hunt R, Schwartz H, Fitch D, Fedorak R, Al Kawas F, Vakil N, H pylori study group (1995) Dual therapy of clarithromycin (Cl) and omeprazole (Om) for the treatment of patients with duodenal ulcers (DU) associated with *H. pylori* (Hp) infection. Gut 37 [Suppl 1]:A17

Jan CM, Wu DC, Su YC, Perng DS, Wang WM, Chen LT, Chen CY (1994) The hemodynamic changes of gastroduodenal regional blood flow after Hp eradication in DU scar patients. World congress LA A 709P

Jaspersen D, Koerner T, Schorr W, Hammar CH (1994) *Helicobacter pylori*-eradication prevents relapse bleeding in duodenal ulcer hemorrhage. UEGW OSLO III:A1459

Jaup BH (1991) Omeprazole – eller Vismutbaserad Trippel-korttidsterapi mot *Helicobacter pylori*. En pilotstudie. Hygia 101:160

Jaup B, Norrby A (1994) Low dose short term triple therapy for eradication of *Helicobacter pylori*. Am J Gastroenterol 89:A451

Jaup B, Norrby A (1995a) Low dose, short term triple therapy for cure of *Helicobacter pylori* infection and healing of peptic ulcers. Am J Gastroenterol 90:943–945

Jaup BH, Norrby A (1995b) Comparison of two low dose one-week triple therapy regimens with and without metronidazole for the cure of *H. pylori* infection. GUT 37 [Suppl 1]:A170

Johnston BJ, Reed PJ (1994) Patient comment on successful *Helicobacter pylori* eradication treatment. Am J Gastroenterol 89:A357

Kadayifci A, Simsek H, Tatar G (1997) Low cost regimen for *H. pylori* eradication with clarithromycin combinations. Gastroenterology 112:A2205

Kalach N, Benhamou PH, Raymond J, Bergeret M, Barbet P, Briet F, Flourié B, Senouci L, Gendrel D, Dupont C (1995) A controlled study of the efficacy of lansoprazole in combination with two different dual antibiotic associations during *Helicobacter pylori* (H pylori) gastric infection in children. Gastroenterology 108:A1231

Kalantzis N, Gabriel P, Giannopoulos ATH, Scandalis N, Spiliadis CH, Mavratzotis D, Xiromeritou B, Karamanolis DG, Varvagiannis G, Stefanidis D (1994) Comparative study on the efficacy of omeprazole in combination with clarithromycin or clarithromyin + ornidazole in healing duodenal ulcer and eradicating *Helicobacter pylori*. World congress LA A 65P

Kamberoglou D, Giorgiou S, Doulgeroglou V, Tzias V, Lagoudakis M (1995) High eradication rate of *Helicobacter pylori* (Hp) after one week triple therapy regimen. UEGW A 0519

Katelaris PH, Patchett SE, Zhang ZW, Domizio P, Farthing MJG (1995) A randomized prospective comparison of clarithromycin versus amoxicillin in combination with omeprazole for eradication of *Helicobacter pylori*. Aliment Pharmacol Ther 9:205–208

Katicic M, Presecki V, Marusie M, Prskalo M, Ticak M, Sabarie B, Colic-Cvrlje V, Dominis M, Kalenie S, Dzebro S, Papa B (1996) Eradication of *H. pylori* infection with five different drug regimens. Gut 39 [Suppl 2]4A:23

Katicic M, Presecki V, Marusic M, Prskalo M, Ticak M, Sabaric B, Dominis M, Kalenic S, Dzebro S, Colic-Cvrlje V, Papa B, Naumovski-Mihalic S, Plecko V (1997) Eradication of *H. pylori* infection with two triple-therapy regimens of 7, 10 and 14 days duration. Gut 41 [Suppl 1]:A367

Kihira K, Kimura K, Satoh K, Takimoto T, Saifuku K, Taniguchi Y, Koijma T, Tokumaru K, Yamamoto H (1996a) Effect of 1-week triple therapy for *Helicobacter pylori* infection with lansoprazole or ranitidine and clarithromycin and metronidazole. Gastroenterology 112:A2581

Kihira K, Satoh K, Ido K, Yodhida Y, Kimura K (1996b) Ranitidine will be alternative to lansoprazole in short-term low-dose triple therapy for *Helicobacter pylori* infection. Helicobacter 1:276

Kimura K, Kenichi I, Saifuko K, Taniguchi Y, Satoh K, Takimoto T, Kihira K, Yoshida Y (1994) One-hour topical therapy for the eradication of *H. pylori*. Am J Gastroenterol 90:205–214

Kist M, Strobel S, Fölsch UR, Kirchner T, Hahn EG, von Kleist DH, Klör H-U, Dammann H-G (1997) Prospective assessment of the impact of primary antibiotical resistances on cure rates of *Helicobacter pylori* infections. Gut 41 [Suppl 1]:A328

Kodama R, Fuijoka T, Fujiyama K, Kawasaki H, Kubota T, Nasu M (1994) Combination therapy with clarithromycin and sofalcone for eradication of *Helicobacter pylori*. Eur J Gastro Hepatol [Suppl] 1:125–128

Koelz HR, Beglinger C, Inauen W, Blum AL (1995) Double-blind comparison of three different amoxicillin (amo) plus omeprazole (ome) regimens for eradication of *Helicobacter pylori* (Hp) in patients with peptic ulcer. Gastroenterology 108:A2594

Kordecki H, Kosic R, Milkiewicz P, Kubisa D (1996) Does eradication of *Helicobacter pylori* decrease the risk of mucosal lesions in patients taking NSAID? Gut 39 [Suppl 2]3A:29

Krause R, Müller G, Ullmann U (1993) Effect of a short-term therapy with omeprazole and amoxicillin on H pylori eradication: ulcer healing and relapse in patients with peptic ulcer. Acta Gastroentrol Belg 56 [Suppl]:A137

Krause R, Pruitt R, Lukasik N, Thomas J, Fennerty B (1997) 10 vs 14 day triple therapy with lansoprazole (Prevacid), amoxicillin, and clarithromycin in the eradication of *Helicobacter pylori* (Hp). Gut 41 [Suppl 1]:A373

Kung NS, Sung JJY, Ng PW, Yuen WF, Chung E, Lim BH, Kwok SPY, Ma HC (1996) Two-day versus one-week anti-Helicobacter therapy in controlled bleeding ulcers: a prospective randomized trial. Gut 39 [Suppl 2]4A:06

Labenz J, Gyenes E, Rühl GH, Börsch G (1992a) Efficiency of oral triple therapy (BSS/metronidazole/tetracycline) to eradicate Hp in DU disease. Ir J Med Sci 161 [Suppl 10]:T11

Labenz J, Gyenes E, Rühl GH, Börsch G (1992b) Pretreatment with omeprazole endangers the efficacy of amoxicillin/omeprazole treatment to eradicate Hp. Ir J Med Sci 161 [Suppl 10]:15

Labenz J, Gyenes E, Rühl GH, Börsch G (1992c) Kurzzeittherapie mit hochdosiertem Omeprazol und Amoxicillin Zur Helicobacter-pylori-Eradikation. Med Klin 87:118–119

Labenz J, Gyenes E, Rühl GH, Börsch G (1992d) Two weeks treatment with amoxicillin/omeprazole for eradication of *Helicobacter pylori*. Z Gastroenterol 30:776–778

Labenz J, Gyenes E, Rühl GH, Bauer FE, Börsch G (1993a) Amoxicillin plus omeprazole versus triple therapy for eradikation of *Helicobacter pylori* in duodenal ulcer disease: a prospective, randomized and controlled study. Gut 34:1167–1170

Labenz J, Gyenes E, Rühl GH, Börsch G (1993b) Omeprazole plus amoxicillin: efficacy of various treatment regimens to eradicate *Helicobacter pylori*. Am J Gastroenterol 88:491–495

Labenz J, Rühl GH, Bertrams J, Börsch G (1993c) Amoxicillin plus omeprazole for eradication of *Helicobacter pylori* in duodenal ulcer disease. UEGW A 96

Labenz J, Rühl GH, Bertrams J, Börsch G (1993d) Amoxicillin plus omeprazole for eradication of *Helicobacter pylori* in gastric ulcer disease. UEGW A 99

Labenz J, Stolte M, Domian C, Bertrams J, Aygen S, Börsch G (1993e) Omeprazole plus amoxicillin or clarithromycin for eradication of Hp in DU disease. Acta Gastroentrol Belg 56 [Suppl]:A139

Labenz J, Rühl GH, Bertrams J, Börsch G (1994a) Medium-or high-dose omeprazole plus amoxicillin eradicates *Helicobacter pylori* in gastric ulcer disease. Did Dis Sci 39:1483–1487

Labenz J, Stolte M, Jorias J, Sollböhmer M, Bertrams J, Börsch G (1994b) Role of acid inhibition in omeprazole-enhanced amoxicillin treatment of *Helicobacter pylori* infection in peptic ulcer disease. UEGW OSLO III:A1462

Labenz J, Stolte M, Rühl GH, Bertrams J, Börsch G (1994c) Low-dose short-term omeprazole enhanced antibiotic double therapy (clarithromycin plus metronidazole) of *Helicobacter pylori* infection. UEGW OSLO III:A1164

Labenz J, Stolte M, Rühl GH, Becker T, Tillenburg B, Sollböhmer M, Börsch G (1995a) One-week low-dose triple therapy for the eradication of *Helicobacter pylori*. Eur J Gastroenterol Hepatol 7:9–11

Labenz J, Adamek RJ, Idström JP, Peitz U, Tillenburg B, Börsch G (1995b) Duodenal ulcer healing and *Helicobacter pylori* eradication by one-week low-dose triple therapy with omeprazole, clarithromycin and metronidazole. UEGW A 0129

Labenz J, Adamek RJ, Stolte M, Opferkuch W, Becker T, Tillenburg T, Börsch G (1995c) Efficacy and safety of two simple on-week triple therapy schedules for *Helicobacter pylori*. Gastroenterology 108:A2072

Labenz J, JP, Peitz U, Tillenburg B, Becker T, Stolte M (1995d) Efficacy and tolerability of one-week low-dose triple therapy consisting of pantoprazole, clarithromycin and metronidazole for cure of *Helicobacter pylori* infection. UEGW A 0292

Lahaie RG, Lemoyne M, Poitras P, Gagnon M, Martin F, Boivin M, Plourde V (1995) A randomized trial of the efficacy of three regimens for the eradication of *Helicobacter pylori*. Gastroenterology 108:A2095

Laine L, Stein C, Neil G (1995) Limited efficacy of omeprazole-based dual and triple therapy for *Helicobacter pylori*: a randomized trial employing "optimal dosing." Am J Gastroenterol 90:1407–1410

Laine L, Estrada R, Trujilo M, Fukanaga K, Neil G (1996) Randomized comparison of 7, 10 and 14 days of omeprazole, amoxicillin and clarithromycin for treatment of *Helicobacter pylori*. Gastroenterology 112:A4510

Laine L, Estrada R, Trujillo M, Emami S (1997) Randomized comparison of ranitidine bismuth citrate (RBC)-based triple therapies for *H. pylori*. Gut 41 [Suppl 1]:A382

Lambert JR, Taupin D, Yeomans N, Goy J, Nicholson L, Gregorevic B, Lin SK, Midolo P, Korman M (1994) Dose dependent effect of omeprazole with amoxicillin in *Helicobacter pylori* eradication. A randomized controlled trial. World congress LA

Lamouliatte H, Megraud F, DeMascarel A, Barberis C, Bernard PH, Cayla R, Quinton A (1989) Does omeprazole improve amoxycillin therapy directed towards *Campylobacter pylori*-associated chronic gastritis? Klin Wochenschr 67 [Suppl XVIII]:37

Lamouliatte H, de Mascarel A, Megraud F, Barberis C, Bernard PH, Cayla R, Quinton A (1990) Omeprazole improves amoxicillin therapy directed towards *Helicobacter pylori* associated gastritis. Gastroenterology 98:A75

Lamouliatte H, Bernard PH, Boulard A, Cayla R, de Mascarel A, Megraud F (1991) *Helicobacter pylori* eradication prevents duodenal ulcer relapse. Gastroenterology 100:A104

Lamouliatte H, Bernardh PH, Cayla R, Megr·ud F, De Mascarel A, Quinton A (1992) Controlled study of omeprazole-amoxicillin-tinidazole vs ranitidine-amoxicillin-tinidazole in *Helicobacter pylori* associated duodenal ulcers (DU). Final and long-term results. Gastroenterology 102:A106

Lamouliatte H, Cayla R, Megr·ud F, Zerbib F, Stablo M, Bouchard S, Quinton A (1993a) Randomized controlled trial with omeprazole and antibiotics in a combined treatment for *Helicobacter pylori* eradication. Preliminary results. Acta Gastroentrol Belg 56 [Suppl]:A139

Lamouliatte H, Dorval ED, Picon L, Cayla R, Loulergue J, de Muret A, Sallerin V, Megraud F (1993b) Fourteen days triple therapy using lansoprazole amoxicillin and tinidazole achieves a high eradication rate in H pylori positive patients. Acta Gastroentrol Belg 56 [Suppl]:139

Lamouliatte HC, Cayla R, Megraud F, Zerbib F, Stablo M, Bouchard S, Quinton A (1993c) Amoxicillin-clarithromycin-omeprazole: the best therapy for *Helicobacter pylori* infection? Acta Gastroentrol Belg 56 [Suppl]:A140

Lamouliatte H, Cayla R, Zerbib F, Megraud F (1994a) Dual therapy (DT) versus triple therapy (TT) for *Helicobacter pylori* (*H. pylori*) eradication: preliminary results of a randomized controlled trial. Gastroenterology 106:A3335

Lamouliatte H, Cayla R, Zerbib F, Megraud F (1994b) Randomized controlled trial for *Helicobacter pylori* eradication: dual therapy (DT) versus triple therapy (TT). UEGW OSLO III:A79

Lamouliatte H, Cayla R, Forestier S, De Mascarel A, Zerbib F, Talbi P, Megraud F (1995a) Dual therapy versus triple therapy: high dose of lansoprazole plus amoxicillin in combination or not with clarithromycin for *Helicobacter pylori* infection. Gut 37 [Suppl 1]:A365

Lamouliatte H, Cayla R, Forestier S, de Mascarel A, Zerbib F, Talbi F, Megraud F, Joubert-Collin M (1995b) Dual therapy versus triple therapy: high dose lansoprazole plus amoxicillin in combination or not with clarithromycin for *Helicobacter pylori* infection. UEGW A 1295

Lamouliatte H, Cayla R, Zerbib F, Megraud F, de Mascarel A (1995c) Seven days triple therapies with lansoprazole and low dose of clarithromycin plus amoxicillin or tinidazole for *Helicobacter pylori* eradication: preliminary results of a randomized study. UEGW A 1298

Lamouliatte H, Ruszniewski P, Flejou JF, Megraud F, Clyti N, Slama A (1996a) Effect of 3 doses of ranitidine (300, 600, 1200 mg/day) combined with two antibiotics in the eradication of *Helicobacter pylori*. Gastroenterology 112:A2587

Lamouliatte H, Cayla R, Talbi P, Zerbib F, Megraud F, de Mascarel A (1996b) Randomised study comparing two seven days triple therapies with lansoprazole and low dose od clarithromycin plus amoxicillin or tinidazole for *Helicobacter pylori* eradication. Gastroenterology 112:A2589

Lamouliatte H, Cayla R, Zerbib F, Megraud F, de Mascarel A (1996c) Triple therapy with PPI-amox-icillin-clarithromycin for *H. pylori* eradication: the optimal regimens in 1966. Gastroenterology 112:A2586

Lamouliatte H, Florent CH, Vicari F, Megraud F, Forestier F (1996d) Effect of lansoprazole and amoxicillin plus metronidazole on the eradication of *Helicobacter pylori*. Gastroenterology 112:A2588

Lamouliatte H, Talbi P, Cayla R, Zerbib F, Megraud F (1996e) Randomized study comparing two seven days triple therapies with lansoprazole and low dose of clarithromycin plus amoxicillin or tinidazole for *H. pylori* eradication. Gut 39 [Suppl 2]:4A:20

Lamouliatte H, The Aquitanine-Gastro Association, de Mascarel A, Megraud F, Samoyeau R (1997) Double-blind study comparing once daily versus twice daily dosage of PPI with amoxicillin-clari-thromycin for *H. pylori* cure. Gut 41 [Suppl 1]:A340

Lamy V, Ramdani B, Cappelli J, Glupczynski Y, De Prez C, Burette A (1996) Lansoprazole (30 mg OD vs BID) with amoxicillin and clarithromycin to cure *H. pylori* infection. Helicobacter 1:270

Lazzaroni M, Marconi G, Bargiggia S, Minguzzi M, Bianchi Posso G (1995) Efficacy of omeprazole combined with antibiotics for *Helicobacter pylori* eradication and duodenal ulcer recurrence. Eur J Gastroenterol Hepatol 7:117–119

Lee CK, Wyeth J, Sercombe JC, Pounder RE, Pasi J, Lee CA (1995) *H. pylori* detection and eradication in haemophilic patients. Gut 37 [Suppl 1]:A177

Lerang F, Moum B, Ragnhildstveit E, Efskind PS, Hauge T, Tolås P, Henriksen M (1994a) Alternative triple therapy for *Helicobacter pylori* related peptic ulcer disease. Am J Gastroenterol 89:A371

Lerang F, Moum B, Ragnhildstveit E, Efskind PS, Hauge, Tolås P, Henriksen M, Nicolaysen H (1994b) Alternative triple therapy for *Helicobacter pylori* related ulcer disease. World congress LA A 89P

Lerang F, Moum B, Ragnhildstveit E, Haug JB (1995a) *Helicobacter pylori* (Hp) infection and met-ronidazole (mtz) resistance. Gut 37 [Suppl 1]:A343

Lerang F, Moum B, Ragnhildstveit E, Hauge T, Aubert E, Henriksen M, Sandvei PK, Tolkarings P, Söberg T, Efskind PS (1995b) Simple low cost triple therapy with bismuth for *Helicobacter pylori* (Hp) positive peptic ulcer disease (PUD). UEGW A 0551

Lerang F, Moum B, Haug JB, Berge T (1996) Highly effective triple therapy with omeprazole amoxicillin and clarithromycin in previous *H. pylori* treatment failures. Gut 39 [Suppl 2]4A:25

Lerang F, Moum B, Haug JB, Tolås P, Berge T (1997) Highly effective second-line anti-*H. pylori* therapy: omeprazole, amoxicillin and clarithromycin in patients previously have failed metronidazole-based therapy. Gastroenterology 112:A2214

Liberti A, Catalano F, Terranova R, Brogna A, Branciforte G, Catanzaro R, Bentivegna C, Luca S (1995) Hp positive functional dyspepsia in elderly patients: comparison of two treatments. Gastro-enterology 108:A2118

Lidtk FE, Siebert U, Tegeler R, Meineke I, Radzn HJ, Sattler B, Lepsien G (1994) Long-term results of various treatment regimens on *Helicobacter pylori* (Hp)-positive ulcer patients. Am J Gastroenterol 89:A378

Lind T, Veldhuysen van Zanten SJO, Unge P, Spiller RC, Bayerdörffer E, O'Morain C, Wrangstadh M, Idström JP (1995) The MACH 1 study: optimal one-week treatment for *Helicobacter pylori* defined? Gut 37 [Suppl 1]:A15

Lobo AJ, McNulty CAM, Uff JS, Dent J, Eyre-Brook IA, Wilkonson SP (1994) Preservation of gastric antral mucus is associated with failure of eradication of *Helicobacter pylori* by bismuth, metron-idazole and tetracycline. Aliment Pharmacol Ther 8:181–185

Logan RPH, Gummet PA, Misiewicz JJ, Karim QM, Walker MM, Baron JH (1991) One week eradi-cation regimen for *Helicobacter pylori*. Lancet 338:1249–1252

Logan RPH, Gummett PA, Hegarty BT, Walker MM, Baron JH, Misiewicz JJ (1992a) Clarithromycin and omeprazole for *Helicobacter pylori*. Lancet 340:239

Logan RPH, Rubio MA, Gummet PA, Hegarty B, Walker MM, Baron JH, Misiewicz JJ (1992b) Om-eprazole and amoxicillin suspension for *Helicobacter pylori*. Ir J Med Sci 161 [Suppl 10]:16

Logan RPH, Schaufelberger H, Misiewicz JJ, Gummet PA, Karim QN, Walker M, Baron JH (1993a) The dose and frequency of omeprazole are important in treating *H. pylori* with dual therapy. Gastroenterology 104:A186

Logan RPH, Schaufelberger HD, Gummet PA, Baron JH, Misiewicz JJ (1993b) The effect of patient compliance on Helicobacter. UEGW A 98

Logan RPH, Gummet PA, Misiewicz JJ, Karim QN, Walker MM, Baron JH (1994a) One week's anti-*Helicobacter pylori* treatment for duodenal ulcer. Gut 35:15–18

Logan RPH, Barchan KD, Celestin LR, Theodossi A, Palmer K, Reed PI (1994b) Clarithromycin (Cl) and omeprazole (Om) in the prevention of duodenal ulcer (DU) recurrence and eradication of *Helicobacter pylori* (Hp). Am J Gastroenterol 89:A372

Logan RPH, Gummett HD, Schaufelberger HD, Greaves RRFH, Mendelson GM, Walker MM, Thomas PH, Baron JH, Misiewicz JJ (1994c) Eradication of *Helicobacter pylori* with clarithromycin and omeprazole. Gut 35:323–326

Logan RPH, Bardhan KD, Celestin LR, Theodossi A, Palmer KR, Reed PI, Baron JH, Misiewicz JJ (1995a) Eradication of *Helicobacter pylori* and prevention of recurrence of duodenal ulcer: a randomized, double-blind, multicenter trial of omeprazole with or without clarithromycin. Aliment Pharmacol Ther 9:417–423

Logan RPH, Goddard AF, Tonge KA, Gummet PA, Hawkey CJ, Misoewicz JJ, Baron JH (1995b) Eradication of *Helicobacter pylori* using clarithromycin, omeprazole and amoxicillin for one week. Gut 37 [Suppl 1]:A350

Londong W, Gorgas R, Pommerlen W, Marsch-Ziegler U, Semler P, Rost K-L, Idström JP (1995) Effect of different omeprazole doses combined with amoxicillin on intragastric pH, amoxicillin bioavailability and *Helicobacter pylori* eradication in duodenal ulcer patients. Gastroenterology 108:A2597

Loo VG, Sherman P, Matlow AG (1992) *Helicobacter pylori* infection in a pediatric population: in vitro susceptibilities to omeprazole and eight antimicrobial agents. Antimicrob Agents Chemother 36:1133–1135

Luna P, del Castillo G, Farias R, Zerbo O, Romanelli O, Dezi R, Valero J, Kogan Z, Ianella M, Boerr L, Corti R (1997) Efficacy and tolerability of a seven-day triple scheme with pantoprazole, amoxicillin and clarithromycin for eradication of Helicoacter pylori. Gastroenterology 112:A2211

Lynch DAF, Sobala GM, Gallacher B, Dixon MF, Axon ATR (1992) Effectiveness of a five times daily triple therapy regime for eradicating *Helicobacter pylori*. Ir J Med Sci 161 [Suppl 10]:T16

Maconi G, Bordi C, Cesana B, Pilato FP, Damilano I, Franceschi M (1996) High vs Standard dose omeprazole plus amoxicillin for treatment of *H. pylori* positive duodenal ulcer. A multicentre, nationwide randomized trial. Gut 39 [Suppl 2]4A:26

Macri G, Garcea MR, Passaleva MT, Romano M, Galli A, Surrenti E, Salvadori G, Surrenti C (1995) Does eradication of *Helicobacter pylori* reduce the recurrence of duodenal ulcer bleeding? UEGW A 1709

Maier M, Schilling D, Dorlars D, Wegener K, Köhler B, Benz C, Riemann JF (1994) Eradication of *Helicobacter pylori* compared to ranitidine maintenance therapy after peptic ulcer bleeding – a prospective randomized trial. World congress LA A 93 P

Malfertheiner P, Bayerdörffer E, Diete U, Gil J, Lind T, Misiuna P, O'Morain C, Sipponen P, Spiller RC, Stasiewicz J, Treichel H-C, Ujszászy L, Unge P, Veldhuyzen van Zanten SJO, Zeijlon L (1997) The GU-MACH study: eradication of Helicobacter pyori, ulcer healing and relapse rate in gastric ulcer patients. Omeprazole and clarithromycin in combination with either amoxicillin or metronidazole. Gut 41 [Suppl 1]:A356

Manes G, Dominguez-Munos JE, Uomo G, Gigliotti T (1996) Maintenance therapy with ranitidine enhances reinfection with *H. pylori* after successful eradication. Gut 39 [Suppl 2]3A:01

Mantzaris GJ, Petraki Kal, Christoforidis P, Amberiadis P, Florakis N, Triantafyllou G (1997) Comparison of two 10-day regimens, omeprazole + standard triple therapy and omeprazole-amoxicillin-clarithromycin for eradication of *Helicobacter pylori* (Hp) infection and healing of duodenal ulcer. Gastroenterology 112:A2221

Marchi S, Costa F, Di Matteo G, Dobrilla G, Dodero M, Fratton A, Gandolfi L, Iaquinto G, Loriga P, Marzio L, Pacini D, Saggioro A, Savarino G, Spinelli P, Zamboni G, Tosatto R, Oliveri A (1997) Ranitidine bismuth citrate in co-prescription with clarithromycin 1g/day or 1.5 g/day are equally effective in the eradication of *H. pylori* and healing of duodenal ulcers. Gastroenterology 112:A2224

Martinez-Gomez MJ, Sanz JC, Sanchez Perez V, Gimeno M, Alarcon T, Lopez-Brea M (1994) Treatment and follow-up of spanish children with gastritis by *H. pylori* during a 3 year period. Am J Gastroenterol 89:A376

Massarrat S, Saberi-Firoozi M, Fattahi S, Zare M, Javan A, Etaati H (1995) Efficacy of triple therapy of amoxicillin + omeprazole or amoxicillin + tinidazole + omeprazole for eradication of *Helicobacter pylori* and prevention of DU relapse. UEGW A 2022

Mattle WP (1994) Omeprazole plus clarithromycin in eradicating *Helicobacter pylori* (Hp): (a seven or fourteen day course of treatment with two omeprazole regimes). World congress LA A 64 P

Megraud F, Lehn N, Lind T, Bayerdorffer E, O'Morain C, Spiller RC, Unge P, Veldhuyzen van Zanten S, Wrangstadh M, Burman C-F (1997a) *Laboratoire de Bacteriologie, Hopital Pellegrin, Bordeaux, France. The MACH 2 study. *Helicobacter pylori* resistance to antimicrobial agents and its influence on clinical outcome. Gastroenterology 112:A1622

Megraud F, Pichavant R, Palegry D, French PC, Roberts PC, Williamsson R (1997b) Ranitidine bismuth citrate (RBC), co-prescribed with clarithromycin is more effective in the eradication of *Helicobacter pylori* than omeprazole with clarithromycin. Gut 41 [Suppl 1]:A337

Meining A, Höchter W, Weingart J, Simon T, Krämer W, Klann H, Bolle KH, Sommer A, Lehn N, Stolte M, Bayerdörffer E (1996) Omeprazole-clarithromycin-metronidazole versus omeprazole-amoxicillin for cure of *Helicobacter pylori* infection in duodenal ulcer patients. Gastroenterology 112:A1236

Meloni M, Cicu A, Carboni GP, Pischedda F, Diana O, Bandiera F, Senna A (1995) Short-term, low-dose triple therapy in gastritis *Helicobacter pylori* correlated. UEGW A 1741

Mendelson M, Greaves R, Logan R, Hegarty B, Baron J, Misiewicz JJ (1992) Eradication of *Helicobacter pylori* with clarithromycin and omeprazole. Gut 33 [Suppl 2]:S27

Messa C, Di Leo A, Greco B, Caradonna L, Amati L, Linsalata M, Giorgio I, Jirillo E (1996) Successful eradicating treatment of *Helicobacter pylori* in patients with chronic gastritis: gastrin levels of cytokines, epidermal growth factor and polyamines before and after therapy. Immunopharmacol Immunotoxicol 18:1–3

Midolo PD, Lambert JR, Turnidge J (1994) Metronidazole resistance – a predictor of failure to eradicate *Helicobacter pylori* by triple therapy. Am J Gastroenterol 89:A390

Midolo PJ, Lambert JR, Turnidge J (1996) Metronidazole resistance: a predictor of failure of *Helicobacter pylori* eradication by triple therapy. J Gastroenterol Hepatol 11:290–292

Millar MR, Pike J (1992) Bactericidal activity of antimicrobial agents against slowly growing *Helicobacter pylori*. Antimicrob Agents Chemother 36:185–187

Misiewicz JJ, Harris AW, Bardhan KD, Levi S, Langworthy H (1996) Over 95% of the patients remain *H. pylori* negative 6 months after one week low-dose eradication therapy. Gut 39 [Suppl 2]4A:14

Miwa H, Ohkura R, Murai T, Yamada T, Watanabe H, Iwazaki R, Ogihara T, Watanabe S, Sato N (1997) Effectiveness of two weeks OAC therapy for *H. pylori* infection in Japan. Gastroenterology 112:A2188

Miyaji H, Ito S, Azuma T, Ito Y, Suto H, Yamasaki Y, Sato F, Ohtaki Y, Hirai M, Kuriyama M, Kohli Y, Keida Y (1997) The prevalence of the drug resistance in *Helicobacter pylori* and the effects of the resistance on the eradication therapy in Japan. Gastroenterology 112:A2183

Moayyedi P, Axon ATR (1994a) Efficacy of a new one week triple therapy regime in eradicating *Helicobacter pylori*. Gut 35 [Suppl 2]:T248

Moayyedi P, Tompkins DS, Axon ATR (1994b) Determination of the optimum dose of omeprazole in a new triple therapy regimen for eradicating *Helicobacter pylori*. Gut 35 [Suppl 5]:W63

Moayyedei P, Thompkins DS, Axon ATR (1995) Efficacy of ten days of clarithromycin, amoxicillin and omeprazole in eradicating *Helicobacter pylori* infection. Gut 37 [Suppl 1]:A176

Moayyedi P, Tompkins DS, Ragunathan PL, Axon ATR (1996) Relevance of metronidazole resistance in predicting failure of omeprazole, clarithromycin and tinidazole to eradicate *Helicobacter pylori*. Gut 39 [Suppl 2]1A:07

Moayyedi P, Langworthy H, Tompkins DS, Mapstone N, Chalmers DM, Axon ATR (1997) The optimum 5 day therapy against *Helicobacter pylori*. Gastroenterology 112:A2196

Mones J, Ricard E, Sainz S (1996) *Helicobacter pylori* eradication. omeprazole, amoxicillin and clarithromycin: 1 week vs 2 weeks. Gastroenterology 112:A2583

Morgando A, Perotto C, Todros L, Sanseverino P, De Marco L, Pugliese G, Ferrari A, Marchiaro G, Ponzetto A (1995) *Helicobacter pylori* eradication for duodenal ulcer: no reinfection and rare recurrence at two years. UEGW A 2034

Mosca S, Rocco VP, De Caprio M, Gigliotti T (1995a) Influence of smoking ion the efficacy of omeprazole + amoxicillin therapy for eradication of *Helicobacter pylori*. UEGW A 1930

Mosca S, Rocco VP, De Caprio M, Gigliotti T (1995b) Comparison of two double therapies (nizatidine plus amoxicillin v/s omeprazole plus amoxicillin) in patients with *Helicobacter pylori* positive duodenal ulcer. UEGW A 1932

Moshkowitz M, Konikoff FM, Peled Y, Santo M, Hallak A, Bujanover Y, Tiomny E, Gilat T (1995) High *Helicobacter pylori* numbers are associated with low eradication rate after triple therapy. Gut 36:845–847

Möllhaupt B, Flöckiger T, Fröhli P, Engelhart G, Hörlimann R (1996) One week low dose triple therapies with lansoprazole or omeprazole are equally effective for *H. pylori* eradication and ulcer healing. Gastroenterology 112:A1241

Nair P, O'Shea C, Wicks ACW (1995) *Helicobacter pylori* eradication in the long term management of peptic ulcer disease in general practice. UEGW A 1372

Nakata H, Imoto K, Kasamatsu T, Tamaki Y, Tamaki H (1996) Effect of lansoprazole and clarithromycin plus amoxicillin on the eradication of *Helicobacter pylori*. Helicobacter 1:276

Nebiki H, Arakawa T, Yamada H, Ohkawa K, Harihara S, Ito H (1994) Absence of effect of eradication of *Helicobacter pylori* on gastric ulcer relapse unlikely to duodenal ulcer. Am J Gastroenterol 89:A394

Neri M, Susi D, Di Iorio P, Seccia G, Laterza F, Cuccurullo F (1994a) High-dose omeprazole with clarithromycin for one week: an effective dual therapy regimen for H pylori infection. Gastroenterology 106:A429

Neri M, Susi D, Laterza F, Di Iorio P, Seccia G, Mezzetti A, Cuccurullo F (1994b) Omeprazole, bismuth and clarithromycin in the sequential treatment of *Helicobacter pylori* infection. Aliment Pharmacol Ther 8:469–471

Neri M, Susi D, Laterza D, Carbone F, Cuccurullo F (1995) Omeprazole and clarithromycin vs omeprazole and amoxicillin: a comparison of one-week and two-week treatments. Gut 37 [Suppl 1]:A364

Noach LA, Bosma NB, Tytgat GNJ (1993) CBS and clarithromycin: alternative therapy for *Helicobacter pylori* infection in patients with metronidazole resistant strains? UEGW A 102

O'Connor HJ, Loane J, Cunnae K (1996) One-week triple therapy for *Helicobacter pylori* incorporating high-dose clarithromycin – a prospective study. Gastroenterology 112:A2585

O'Riordan T, Mathai E, Tobin E, McKenna D, Keane C, Sweeney E, O'Morain CO (1990) Adjuvant antibiotic therapy in duodenal ulcers treated with colloidal bismuth subcitrate. Gut 31:999–1002

Otero W, Sierra F, Gutierrez O, Quinteroa F (1995) Omeprazole plus amoxicillin in *H. pylori* eradication and duodenal ulcer healing. Reinfection and ulcer recurrence in an area of high prevalence of infection. Gastroenterology 108:A2074

Ozmen MM, Johnson CD (1995) Is short term triple therapy with lansoprazole, clarithromycin, and metronidazole a definitive answer for *Helicobacter pylori* eradication? Am j Gastroent 90:1542–1543

Pajares JM, Blanco M Perez-Miranda M, Jimenez-Alonso I, Garcia Gravalos R (1994) Comparison of two triple therapies: anti-H2 or CBS plus two antibiotics to eradicate Hp and to prevent recurrence of DU. UEGW OSLO III:A1488

Parasakthi N, Goh KL, Peh SC, Wong NW, Nazarina AR, Chuah SY, Lo YL, Ong KK (1995) Clarithromycin in the treatment and eradication of *Helicobacter pylori* in duodenal ulcer patients. Gut 37 [Suppl 1]:A385

Patchett S, Beattie S, Keane C, O'Morain C (1991) Eradicating *Helicobacter pylori* and symptoms of non-ulcer dyspepsia. BMJ 303:1238–1240

Patchett S, Beattie S, Keane C, O'Morain C (1992) Short report: short-term triple therapy for H pylori-associated duodenal ulcer disease. Aliment Pharmacol Ther 6:113–117

Patchett SE, Katelaris PH, Zhang ZW, Domizio P, Lowe DG, Farthing MJG (1994) A randomised prospective comparison of omeprazole and clarithromycin versus omeprazole and amoxicillin for the eradication of *Helicobacter pylori*. Gastroenterology 106:A2007

Pazzi P, Carli G, Dalla Libera M, Scagliarini R, Gamberini S, Merighi A, Gullini S (1995) Early assessment of *Helicobacter pylori* eradication by brush-cytology. UEGW A 1725

Pedrazzoli J Jr, Magalh'es AFN, Ferraz JGP, Trevisan M, De Nucci G (1994) Triple therapy with sucralfat is not effective in eradicating *Helicobacter pylori* and does not reduce duodenal ulcer relapse rates. Am J Gastroenterol 89:1501–1504

Peitz U, Nusch A, Tillenburg B, Becker T, Stolte M, Börsch G, Labenz J (1996a) Highly effective well tolerated one-week triple therapy with omeprazole, clarithromycin and amoxicillin for *Helicobacter pylori* (Hp) infection. Gastroenterology 112:A3928

Peitz U, Nusch A, Tillenburg B, Stolte M, Börsch G, Labenz J (1996b) High cure rate of *H. pylori* (Hp) infection by one-week therapy with omeprazole (ome) metronidazole (met) and clarithromycin (cla) despite a negative impact by met resistance. Gut 39 [Suppl 2]1A:03

Peitz U, Tillenburg B, Becker T, Stolte M, Börsch G, Labenz J (1996c) Highly effective well tolerated one-week triple therapy with omeprazole, clarithromycin and amoxicillin for *Helicobacter pylori* (Hp) infection. Gastroenterology 112:A3927

Peitz U, Nusch A, Sulliga M, Becker T, Stolte M, Börsch G, Malfertheiner P, Labenz J (1997) Second line treatment of *Helicobacter pylori* (HP) infection. Gut 41 [Suppl 1]:A385

Perotto C, Morgando A, Sanseverino P, Ferrari A, Saracco G, Todros L, Barletti C, Rosina F, DeAngelis C, Smedile A, Marchiaro G, Ponzetto A (1995) 97% cure for *Helicobacter pylori* infection in duodenal ulcer patients. UEGW A 2037

Peterson WL, Sontag SJ, Ciociola AA, Syker DL, McSorley DL, Webb DD and the *H. pylori* ulcer group (1995) Ranitidine bismuth citrate plus clarithromycin is effective in the eradication of *Helicobacter pylori* and prevention of duodenal ulcer relapse. Gut 37 [Suppl 1]:A19

Peura D, Lin Z, Balaban D, Shifflett J, Parolisi S (1996) The effect of two dosage regimens of omeprazole plus bid clarithromycin on *H. pylori* eradication and short-term dyspeptic symptom relief. Gastroenterology 112:A1242

Pieramico O, Zanetti MV, Innerhofer M (1996) Omeprazole-based dual and triple therapy for the eradication of *H. pylori* infection in peptic ulcer disease: a randomized trial. Gastroenterology 112:A4507

Pilotto A, Di Mario F, Franceshi M, Grassi SA, Battaglia G, Dal Bo N, Bozzola L, Ferrana M, Scagnelli M, Salandin S, Azzini CF (1994a) Triple therapy (omeprazole + azithromycin + metronidazole) versus double therapy (omeprazole + azithromycin) for eradication of *Helicobacter pylori* in the elderly. UEGW OSLO III:A1493

Pilotto A, Franceschi M, Battaglia G, Grassi SA, Bozzola L, Dal Bo N, Ferrana M, Scagnelli M, Salandin S, Di Mario F (1994b) Eradication of *Helicobacter pylori* in the elderly: triple versus double therapies. Am J Gastroenterol 89:A403

Pilotto A, Franceschi M, Bozzola L, Battaglia G, Scagnelli M, Fabrello R, Dal Bo N, Vianello F, Ferrarese S, Di Mario F (1994c) Double therapy (omeprazole plus azithromycin or clarithromycin) for eradication of *Helicobacter pylori* in the elderly. Am J Gastroenterol 89:A402

Pilotto A, Franceshi M, Di Mario F, Battaglia G, Bozzola L, Scagnelli M, Fabrello R, Dal Bo N, Ferranese S, Azzini CF (1994d) Azithromycin + omeprazole versus clarithromycin + omeprazole for eradication of *Helicobacter pylori* in the elderly. UEGW OSLO III:A1494

Pilotto A, Franceschi M, Bozzola L, Fortunato A, Dal Bo N, Scagnelli M, Fabrello R, Soffiato G, Meli V, Oleani G, Di Mario F (1995) The cure for *Helicobacter pylori* (Hp) infection with double of triple omeprazole-based therapies in the elderly: effects on eradication rate, chronic gastritis and serum anti-Hp antibodies and pepsinogens. Gastroenterology 108:A3643

Pilotto A, Franceschi M, Bozzola L, Di Mario F, Buda A, Valerio G (1997) Lansoprazole, clarithromycin and/or amoxicillin and metronidazole for one-week to cure *Helicobacter pylori* infection in elderly. Gastroenterology 112:A2207

Pommerlen W, Schultze V, Lembacke B, Wrangstadh M, London G, the Berlain omeprazole amoxicillin study group (1995) Dose-response of twice daily dosing of omeprazole combined with amoxicillin on *Helicobacter pylori* eradication in duodenal ulcer patients. Gastroenterology 108:A2598

Popovic N, Glisic M, Popovic P, Milosavljevic T, Todorovic K, Matejic O (1996) Comparison of two double therapies (ranitidine plus amoxicillin v/s omeprazole plus amoxicillin) in patients with *Helicobacter pylori* positive duodenal ulcer. Gut 39 [Suppl 2]4A:07

Popovic N, Bulajic M, Glisic M, Popovic P, Milosaljevic T, Popovic N, Matejic O (1997) Comparison of two triple therapies (ranitidine plus amoxicillin plus tinidazole v/s omeprazole plus amoxicillin plus tinidazole) in patients with *Helicobacter pylori* positive duodenal ulcer. Gut 41 [Suppl 1]:A377

Powell KU, Bell GD, Bowden A, Harrison G, Trowell JE, Gant P, Jones PH (1994) *Helicobacter pylori* eradication therapy: a comparison between either omeprazole or ranitidine in combination with amoxicillin plus metronidazole. Gut 35 [Suppl 5]:W61

Pryce DI, Harris AW, Gabe SM, Karim QM, Beveridge I, Langworthy H, Walker MM, Misiewicz JJ, Baron JH (1996) One week of lansoprazole, clarithromycin and metronidazole eradicates *Helicobacter pylori*. Gastroenterology 112:A2584

Przytulski K, Niezychowski W, Regula J, Butruk E (1996) Efficacy of clarithromycin, tinidazole and omeprazole in duodenal ulcer disease with *Helicobacter pylori* infection in Poland: A pilot study. Helicobacter 1:278

Qureshi H, Ahmed W, Syed S, Zia Lodi T, Zuberi SJ (1995) *Helicobacter pylori* clearance and eradication with triple therapy in duodenal ulcer patients. J Pak Med Assoc 45:1–3

Rauws EAJ, Noach LA, Heebels AE, Brink ME, Tytgat GNJ (1990a) Short-term regimens to eradicate *Helicobacter pylori*. World Congress in Gastroenterology Sydney FP 566

Rauws EAJ, Tytgat GNJ (1990b) Cure of duodenal ulcer associated with eradication of *Helicobacter pylori*. Lancet 335:1233–1235

Reilly TG, Poxon V, Walt RP (1995) The eradication of *Helicobacter pylori* in practice: an audit of three years clinical experience with peptic ulcer patients. Gut 37 [Suppl 1]:A345

Reinauer S, Goerz G, Ruzicka T, Susanto F, Humfeld S, Reinauer H (1994) *Helicobacter pylori* in patients with systemic sclerosis: detection with 13Curea breath test and eradication. Acta Derm Venerol 74:361–363

Rejchrt S, Bures J, Tichy M, Kresjsek J, Kolesar J, Pidrman V (1994) Serum acute phase reactants and interleukin-6 in duodenal ulcer treated by omeprazole and amoxicillin. UEGW OSLO III:A1496

Rizzo G, Catalano F, Ayoubi Khajekini MT, Brancoforte G, Liberti A (1993) Duodenal ulcer *Helicobacter pylori* positive: first results of the association with omeprazole and amoxicillin. UEGW A 100

Rokkas T, Mavrogeorgis A, Liatsos C, Rallis E, Kalegiropoulos N (1993a) Evaluation of the combination of omeprazole and amoxycillin in eradicating *H. pylori* and preventing relapses in duodenal ulcer patients. UEGW A 99

Rokkas T, Mavrogeorgis A, Rallis E, Giannikos N (1993b) *H. pylori* eradication reduces the possibility of rebleeding in peptic ulcer disease. UEGW A 3

Rokkas T, Karameris A, Anagnostopoulos J, Mavrogeorgis A, Liatsos C, Giannikos N (1994) *Helicobacter pylori* eradication rates and long term clinical course in duodenal ulcer patients treated either with triple therapy or amoxicillin/omeprazole. World congress LA A 117P

Rossi P, Stornelli G, Resta S, Neve D, Rosci L, Puoti C (1995) Evaluation of the effectiveness of a low-dose. UEGW A 0342

Rossi P, Pauluzi OA, Tavanti A, Caracciolo F, Gurnari M, Nardi F, Pauluzi P (1996) Bismuth vs omeprazole in a triple therapy for eradication of *Helicobacter pylori* in duodenal ulcer patients. Gastroenterology 112:A1230

Rubinstein G, Dunkin K, Howard AJ (1994) The susceptibility of *Helicobacter pylori* to 12 antimicrobial agents omeprazole and bismuth salts. J Antimicrob Chemother 34:409–413

Saberi-Firoozi M, Massarrat S, Zare S, Fattahi M, Javan A, Etaati H, Dehbashi N (1995) Effect of triple therapy or amoxicillin plus omeprazole or amoxicillin plus tinidazole plus omeprazole on duodenal ulcer healing, eradication of *Helicobacter pylori* and prevention of ulcer relapse over a 1-year follow-up period. Am J Gastroenterol 90:1419–1423

Sacca N, De Medici A, Rodino S, De Siena M, Giglio A (1996) Duodenal ulcer *Helicobacter pylori* Hp) positive: therapy with ranitidine (R) + clarithromycine (C) + metronidazole (M) versus omeprazole (O) + clarithromycine + metronidazole. Gut 39 [Suppl 2]4 A:18

Safe AF, Warren B, Corfield A, McNulty CA, Watson B, Mountford RA, Read A (1993) Role of serology in monitoring treatment for *Helicobacter pylori* infection in elderly patients. Age Ageing 22:256–259

Saggjoro A, GISU (1997) A one-week triple therapy vs a two-week dual therapy for eradication and healing of *H. pylori* (Hp) positive duodenal ulcers (DU): results from a randomized. double-blind clinical trial. Gastroenterology 112:A2208

Sainz MJ, Sola-Vera J, Ricart E, Sancho FJ, Balanzo J (1997) *Helicobacter pylori* eradication with omeprazole, amoxicillin and clarithromycin: one week vs two weeks and reinfection rate at one year. Gastroenterology 112:A2206

Saladin S, Battaglia G, Dal Bo N, Lecis PE, Pilotto A, Ferrana M, Vianello F, Kusstatsscher S, Di Mario F (1995) Clarithromycin for the cure of *Helicobacter pylori* infection: one or two weeks of treatment? Gastroenterology 108:A2112

Santander C, Perez-Miranda M, Gomez Cedenilla A, Carpintero P, Grivalos RG, Pajares JM (1994) *Helicobacter pylori* eradication vs maintenance therapy for the prevention of recurrent bleeding from duodenal ulcer. Gut 35 [Suppl 5]:W67

Santander C, Gravalos RG, Cedenilla AG, Pajares JM (1995) Maintenance treatment vs *Helicobacter pylori* eradication therapy in preventing rebleeding of the peptic ulcer disease. Gastroenterology 108:A2064

Savarino V, Mansi C, Mele MR, Bisso G, Mela GS, Saggioro A, Caroli M, Vigneri S, Termini R, Olivieri A, Tosatto R, Celle G (1997a) Eradication of *Helicobacter pylori* using one-week therapy combining ranitidine bismuth citrate with two antibiotics. Gastroenterology 112:A2223

Savarino V, Zentilin P, Bisso G, Pivari M, Mele MR, Mela GS, Mansi C, Vigneri S, Termini R, Celle G (1997b) On-week triple therapy combining omeprazole or ranitidine with two antibiotics for eradication of *Helicobacter pylori* infection. Gastroenterology 112:A2215

Scheiman JM, Chey WD, Behler EM, Crause I, Elta GH (1996) One-week therapy for *Helicobacter pylori*. A randomized trial of two treatment regimens. J Clin Gastroenterol 23:170–173

Schulz TB, Kjellevold Y, Rynstrand E, Rolke H (1994) Triple therapy in a central hospital. UEGW OSLO III:A1503

Schütze K, Hentschel E (1995) Duodenal ulcer healing after 7-day treatment: a pilot study with lansoprazole, amoxicillin and clarithromycin. Z Gastroenterol 33:651–653

Sebesta C, Weiss W, Schmid A, Gschwantier M, Scherz M, Ruckser R, Kier P, Hintenberger W (1996) Seven-day low-dose triple therapy with lansoprazole, clarithromycin and metronidazole as a first line therapy in patients with *H. pylori*-positive peptic disorders. Helicobacter 1:279

Seppälä K, Färkkilä M, Nuutinen H, Hakala K, Väänänen H (1992) Triple therapy of *Helicobacter pylori* infection in peptic ulcer. Scand J Gastroenterol 27:973–976

Sheu BS, Lin CY, Lin XZ, Shiesh SC, Yang HB, Chen CY (1996a) Long-term outcome of triple therapy in *Helicobacter pylori*-related nonulcer dyspepsia: a prospective controlled assessment. Am J Gastroenterol 91:441–447

Sheu B-S, Yang H-B, Su I-J, Lin X-Z (1996b) A three-day course of intravenouse omeprazole plus antibiotics for *H. pylori*-positive bleeding duodenal ulcer. Gut 39 [Suppl 2]4A:05

Signorelli S, Svanoni F, Negrini F, Girola M, Bonassi U (1994) Dyspeptic syndrome and eradication of *Helicobacter pylori* (Hp). World congress LA A 686P

Sobala GM, Lynch DAF, Gallacher B, Dixon MF, Axon ATR (1992) Eradication of *H. pylori* prevents duodenal ulcer recurrence. Ir J Med Sci 161 [Suppl 10]:T7

Sobhani I, Chastang CL, deKorwin JD, Lamouliatte H, Mégraud F, Guerre J, Elouare-Blanc L (1995) Antibiotic versus maintenance therapy in the prevention of duodenal ulcer recurrence. Gastroenterol Clin Biol 19:252–258

Soliman ASG, Trudgill NJ, Hardy PG, Riley SA (1996) *Helicobacter pylori* eradication in selected patients on long term acid suppression in general practice. Gastroenterology 112:A1211

Spadaccini A, De Fanis C, Sciampa G, Pantaleone U, Di Virgilio M, Magnarini C, Pizzicanella G (1995a) Double vs triple therapy in the eradication of *Helicobacter pylori*: our results and reflections. UEGW A 1736

Spadaccini A, De Fanis C, Sciampa G, Pantaleone U, Di Virgilio M, Magnarini C (1995b) Ranitidine vs omeprazole: short-term triple therapy in patients with *Helicobacter pylori* positive duodenal ulcer. Gut 37 [Suppl 1]:A168

Spadaccini A, Masciulli V, De Fanis C, Sciampa G, Pantaleone U, Di Virgilio M, Magnarini C, Pizzicanella G (1995c) Ranitidine vs omeprazole: short-term triple therapy in patients with *Helicobacter pylori* positive duodenal ulcer. UEGW A 1734

Spadaccini A, De Fanis C, Sciampa G, Pantaleone U, Di Virgilio M, Pizzicannella G (1997) Lansoprazole or ranitidine bismuth citrate triple therapies for *Helicobacter pylori* eradication: Results of an open randomized study. Gut 41 [Suppl 1]:A389

Spinzi GC, Imperiali G, Teruzzi V, Songia M, Minoli G, Baratelli G, Posca M, Scarpis M, Snider L (1993) Prevention of duodenal ulcer relapse with amoxicillin and omeprazole. UEGW A 62

Spinzi GC, Bortoli A, Colombo E, Fertitta A, Lesinigo E, Minoli G (1996) Dual therapy of omeprazole plus amoxicillin versus omeprazole plus clarithromycin for cure of *Helicobacter pylori* (Hp) in ulcer patients. Gastroenterology 112:A1232

Stupnicki TH, Taufer M, Denk H, Ratschek M, Spath P, Graf K (1994a) Efficacy of triple therapy (sucralfat/amoxicillin/metronidazole) in eradication *Helicobacter pylori* and duodenal (DU) healing – follow-up to one year. Am J Gastroenterol 89:A414

Stupnicki TH, Taufer M, Denk H, Ratschek M, Spath P, Graf K (1994b) Duodenal ulcer (DU) treated (sucralfat/amoxicillin/metronidazole) with *Helicobacter pylori* (Hp) eradication. Preliminary follow up to one year. World congress LA A 119P

Stupnicki T, Taufer M, Denk H, Ratschek M, Spath P, Graf K (1995) Eradication of *Helicobacter pylori* (Hp) and duodenal ulcer (DU) healing after combined treatment with sucralfat (amoxicillin (AM) and metronidazole (MTZ) – follow up to one year. UEGW A 0088

Stölzle L, Klann H, Topf G, Seib HJ (1997) Ten days treatment with pantoprazole, amoxicillin and metronidazole for cure of *Helicobacter pylori* infection. Gastroenterology 112:A2210

Sung JY, Ling TKW, Suen R, Chung SCS (1994) Can sucralfate replace bismuth in triple therapy for the treatment of *Helicobacter pylori* (Hp) associated duodenal ulcers (DU). World congress LA A 87P

Sung JJY, Chung SCS, Ling TKW, Yung MY, Leung VKS, Ng NKW, Li MKK, Cheng AFB, Li AKC (1995a) Antibacterial treatment of gastric ulcer associated with *Helicobacter pylori*. N Engl J Med 332:139–142

Sung JY, Leung VKS, Chung SCS, Ling TKW, Suen R, Augustine RN, Cheng FB, Li AKC (1995b) Triple therapy with sucralfat, tetracycline, and metronidazole for *Helicobacter pylori*-associated du-

298   P. Unge

odenal ulcers. Can sucralfate replace bismuth in triple therapy for the treatment of *Helicobacter pylori* (Hp) associated duodenal ulcers (DU). Am J Gastroent 90:1424–1427

Sung JY, Ling TKW, Suen R, Leung VKS, Ng EKW, Chung SCS (1995c) Amoxicillin plus omeprazole versus triple therapy for the eradication of *H. pylori* and healing of duodenal ulcers. Gut 37 [Suppl 1]:A21

Tachibana M, Kuwayama H (1997) Comparative study on efficacy and side-effects of sucralfate and lansoprazole in eradicating *Helicobacter pylori* when combined with metronidazole-amoxicillin dual therapy. Gastroenterology 112:A2222

Takats A, Gero G, Penyige J, Ovari Z, Mark GY, Boga B, Molnar GY, Szentmihalyi A (1993) Comparative investigations with therapies containing various antibiotics on eradication of *Helicobacter pylori*. UEGW A 97

Takats A, Racz I, Boga B, Gero G (1994) Efficacy of a "one-day-triple-therapy" with potentialisation of omeprazole for eradication of *Helicobacter pylori*. Am J Gastroenterol 89:A455

Takimoto T, Satoh K, Taniguchi Y, Kihira K, Saifuku K, Kumakura Y, Yoshida Y, Kimura K (1996) Effect of lansoprazole and clarithromycin plus metronidazole on the eradication of *Helicobacter pylori*. The Second Meeting of the Japanese Research for *Helicobacter pylori* Related Gastroduodenal Diseases, 16–17 April 1996, A67

Tan WC, Hogan J, Lombard M, Krasner N (1995a) Eradication of *Helicobacter pylori* with three different drug regimens. UEGW A 0441

Tan ACITL, den Hartog G, Meijer JWR, Thies JE, de Vries RAA, Mulder CJJ (1995b) No additional value of bismuthsubcitrate to combination omeprazole/amoxicillin therapy in the eradication of *Helicobacter pylori*. UEGW A 1490

Tham TCK, Collins JSA, McCormick C, Sloan JM, Bamford K, Watson RGP (1995) Ramdomised controlled trial of ranitidine and omeprazole and their combination with antibiotics in the eradication of *Helicobacter pylori*. Gastroenterology 108:A2110

Treiber G, Klotz U (1994) *Helicobacter pylori* (Hp) eradication rates do not depend on higher omeprazole levels. Am J Gastroenterol 89:A416

Treiber G, Ammon S, Schneider E (1997) AMOC – a short new quadruple therapy vs standard triple therapy for *Helicobacter pylori* eradication. Gut 41 [Suppl 1]:A352

Truesdale RA, Chamberlain CE, Martin DF, Maydonovitch CL, Peura DA (1990) Long-term follow-up and antibody response to treatment of patients with *Helicobacter pylori*. Gastroenterology 98:A140

Tucci A, Corinaldesi R, Stanghellini V, Varoli O, Paparo GF, Gasperoni S, Biasco G, Di Febo G, Santaguida G, Barbara L (1991) One-day therapy for *Helicobacter pylori* eradication. Gastroenterology 100:A177

Tucci A, Corinaldesi R, Stanghellini V, Varoli O, Paparo GF, Gasperoni S, Biasco G, Di Febo G, Santaguida G, Barbara L (1993) One-day therapy for treatment of *Helicobacter pylori* infection. Dig Dis Sci 38:1670–1673

Tucci A, Poli L, Varioli O, Paparo GF, De Giorgio R, Stanghellini V, Corinaldesi R (1994) Evaluation of two therapeutic regimens for the treatment of *Helicobacter pylori* infection. Ital J Gastroenterol 26:107–110

Tursi A, Cammarota G, Montalto M, Papa A, Fideli G, Gasbarrini G (1996a) The use of azithromycin in short-term low-dose triple therapies for *Helicobacter pylori* infection. Am J Gastroentrol 91:817–818

Tursi A, Cammarota G, Papa A, Montalto M, Fideli G, Gasbarrini G (1996b) Short-term low-dose triple therapy with lansoprazole plus amoxicillin and clarithromycin for *Helicobacter pylori* eradication. Am J Gastroenterol 91:668–670

Tyszkiewicz T, Gerlee M, Wadström T (1994) Lansoprazole/amoxicillin versus omeprazole/amoxicillin in *H. pylori* eradication. Am J Gastroenterol 89:A459

Unge P, Gad A, Gnarpe H, Olsson J (1989) Does omeprazole improve antimicrobial therapy directed towards gastric *Campylobacter pylori* in patients with antral gastritis? Scand J Gastroenterol 24 [Suppl 167]:49–54

Unge P, Gad A, Eriksson K, Bergman B, Carling L, Ekström P, Glise H, Gnarpe H, Junghard O, Lindholmer C, Sandzén B, Strandberg L, Stubberöd A, Weywadt L (1993) Amoxicillin added to omeprazole prevents relapse in the treatment of duodenal ulcer patients. Eur J Gastroenterol Hepatol 5:325–331

Unge P, Gad A, Back S, Carling L, Hallerbäck B, Svenheden A, Weywadt L, Zeijlon L (1994) Local treatment for H pylori eradication in duodenal ulcer patients comparing modified and immediate release amoxicillin tablets. Gastroenterology 106:A1269

Unge P, Jönsson B, Stålhammar N-O (1995) The cost effectiveness of *Helicobacter pylori* eradication versus maintenance and episodic treatment in duodenal ulcer patients in Sweden. Pharmacoeconomics 8:410–427

Utzon P, Aabakken L, Sandstad O, Guldvog I, Skar V (1994) Eradication of *Helicobacter pylori* with 10 or 14 days of bismuth triple regimes. UEGW OSLO III:A1516

Va S, Neves B, Duarte C, Quina M (1995) A comparison of dual and triple therapy for *Helicobacter pylori* eradication in duodenal ulcer. UEGW A 0512

Valle J, Seppälä K, Sipponen P, Kosunen T (1991) Disappearance of gastritis after eradication of *Helicobacter pylori*. Scand J Gastroenterol 26:1057–1065

van der Hulst RWM, Weel JFL, van der Ende A, ten Kate FJ, Dankert J, Tytgat GNJ (1996) Therapeutic options after failed *Helicobacter pylori* eradication therapy. Am J Gastroenterol 91:2333–2337

Van Ganse E, Burette A, Glupczynski Y, Deprez C (1993) Lansoprazole plus roxithromycin and metronidazole for eradication of *H. pylori*: results of a pilot study. Barcelona EDDW A 102

van Oijen AHAM, Dekkers CPM, Festen HPM, de Koning RW, Jansen JBMJ (1997) Lansoprazole + amoxicillin + metronidazole versus lansoprazole + amoxicillin + placebo for cure of *H. pylori* infection in patients with non-ulcer dyspepsia. Gastroenterology 112:A2197

Veenendaal RA, Götz JM, Meijer JL, Biemond I, Bernards AT, Offerhaus GJA, Lamers CBHW (1996a) Comparison of omeprazole and clarithromycin versus omeprazole, clarithromycin and metronidazole in the treatment oc *Helicobacter pylori*. Gastroenterology 112:A1233

Veenendaal RA, Götz JM, Meijer JL, Biemond I, Bernards AT, Offerhaus GJA, Lamers CBHW (1996b) Comparison of omeprazole and clarithromycin versus omeprazole, clarithromycin and metronidazole in the treatment of *Helicobacter pylori*. Gut 39 [Suppl 2]4A:03

Veldhuyzen van Zanten S, Hunt R, Cockeram A, Schep G, Malatjalian D, Matisko A, Jewell D (1994) Adding omeprazole 20 mg once a day to metronidazole/amoxicillin treatment of Hp-gastritis: a randomized double-blind trial. The importance of metronidazole resistance. Am J Gastroenterol 89:A417

Veldhuyzen van Zanten SJO, Bradette M, Farley A, BAyerdörffer E, Lind T, O'Morain C, Sipponen P, Spiller R, Unge P, Sinclair P, Wrangstadh M, Zeijlon L (1997) The Du-mach study: Eradication of *Helicobacter pylori*, ulcer healing and relapse in duodenal ulcer patients. Omeprazole and clarithromycin in combination with either amoxicillin or metronidazole. Gut 41 [Suppl 1]:A381

Vetvik K, Schrumpf E, Mowinkel P, Aase S, Andersen KJ (1994) Effects of omeprazole and eradication of *Helicobacter pylori* on gastric and duodenal mucosal enzyme activities and DNA in duodenal ulcer patients. Scand J Gastroenterol 29:995–1000

Vigneri S, Termini R, Savarino V, Di Mario F, Mela GS, Pisciotta G, Mansi C, Badalamenti S (1996) Two years relapse rate after *H. pylori* eradication with omeprazole plus antimicrobials in duodenal ulcer. Gastroenterology 112:A1243

Wagner S, Varrentrapp M, Haruma K, Lange P, Mller M, Schorn T, Soudah B, Bär W, Gebel M (1991) The role of omeprazole (40 mg) in the treatment of gastric *Helicobacter pylori* infection. Z Gastroenterol 29:595–598

Wagner S, Bleck J, Gebel M, Bär W, Manns M (1992) What treatment is best for gastric *Helicobacter pylori* infection. Ir J Med Sci 161 [Suppl 10]:16

Webb DD (1996a) Treatment of *Helicobacter pylori*: key success factors. *Helicobacter pylori* and gastroduodenal disorders IBC third annual: H2B-306

Webb DD (1996b) Treatment of *Helicobacter pylori*: key success factors. *Helicobacter pylori* and gastroduodenal disorders IBC third annual. H2B-305

Webb DD (1996c) Treatment of *Helicobacter pylori*: key success factors. *Helicobacter pylori* and gastroduodenal disorders IBC third annual. H2B-T09

Webb DD (1996d) Treatment of *Helicobacter pylori*: key success factors. *Helicobacter pylori* and gastroduodenal disorders IBC third annual. H2B-T11

Witzel L, Leder K (1997) Cure of *Helicobacter pylori* in duodenal ulcer disease with triple therapy consisting of pantoprazole, clarithromycin and metronidazole. Gastroenterology 112:A2209

Wu CS, Yang CC, Yeh YH, Wu YZ, Huang YF, Kuo CL, Huang MH (1996) One week therapy for eradicating *H. pylori* and healing peptic ulcer without maintenance H2-blocker usage-A new dimension for ulcer treatment. Helicobacter 274

Wurzer H, Rodrigo L, Archambault A, Rokkas T, Skandalis N, Fedorak R, Bazzoli F, Hentschel H, Mora P, Stamler D, Megraud F (1996) Short-course therapy with amoxicillin-clarithromycin triples for 10 days (ACT-10) eradicates *H. pylori* and heals duodenal ulcer. Gut 39 [Suppl 2]4A:33

Wyeth JW, Pounder RE, DeKoster E, Misiewicz JJ, O'Morain CA, Rauws EAJ, Duggan AE (1994) GR122311X (ranitidine bismuth citrate) with antibiotics for the eradication of *Helicobacter pylori*. Gastroenterology 106:A1366

Wyeth JW, Pounder RE, DeKoster E, Misiewicz JJ, O'Morain CA, Rauws EAJ, Duggan AE (1994) GR122311X (ranitidine bismuth citrate) with antibiotics for the eradication of *Helicobacter pylori*. Gastroenterology 106:A 1366

Xia HX, Daw MA, Beattie S, Keane CT, O'Morain CA (1992a) The influence of metronidazole resistance on triple therapy for *Helicobacter pylori* associated duodenal ulcer. Gastroenterology 102:A947

Xia HX, Daw MA, Sant S, Beattie S, Keane CT, O'Morain CA (1992b) Metronidazole resistance in *Helicobacter pylori* and antimicrobial trials. Ir J Med Sci 161 [Suppl 10]:T30

Yang JC, Yang CK, Shun CT, Wang JT, Lee SC, Wang TH (1996) Intragastric distribution of *Helicobacter pylori* after treatment with regimens containing omeprazole. Gut 39 [Suppl 2]4A:34

Yousfi MM, El-Zimaity HMT, Al-Assi MT, Cole RA, Genta RM, Graham DY (1995) Metronidazole, omeprazole and clarithromycin (MOC): an effective combination therapy for *Helicobacter pylori* infection. Gastroenterology 108:A2115

Yousfi MM, El-Zimaity HMT, Cole RA, Genta RM, Graham DY (1996) One week triple therapy with omeprazole, amoxicillin and clarithromycin for treatment of *Helicobacter pylori* infection. Gastroenterology 112:A2580

Zala G, Wirth HP, Flury R, Bauer S (1993a) Omeprazole/amoxicillin: eradikation or *H. pylori* before or after ulcer therapy? UEGW A 100

Zala G, Wirth HP, Wüst J, Flury R, Giesendanner S (1993b) Metronidazole resistant H pylori: omeprazole/amoxicillin worth while to try? UEGW A 100

Zala G, Wirth HP, Giezendanner S, Fiury R, Wüst J (1994) Omeprazole/amoxicillin: impaired eradication of H pylori by smoking but not by omeprazole pre-treatment. Gastroenterology 106:A708

Zala G, Schwery St, Flury R, Meyenberger C, Fried M, Wirth HP (1995) The negative influence of smoking on *Helicobacter pylori* eradication depends on the therapy regimen. Gastroenterology 108:A2060

Zhou DY, Yang HT, Zuo JS, Xu KT, Wang LL (1991) Treatment of *Helicobacter pylori* infection with omeprazole combined with antibiotics. Microb Ecol Health Dis 4(spec issue):S185

Helicobacter pylori and the Future: An Afterword

N.S. MANN and T.U. WESTBLOM

Science is the great antidote to the poison of enthusiasm and superstition.

Adam Smith (1723–1790)

1 Introduction

As seen throughout the chapters of this volume, the field of *Helicobacter* research has come a long way. The association of gastritis and peptic ulceration with the spiral-shaped bacterium *Helicobacter pylori* was first noted only 15 years ago (MARSHALL and WARREN 1984) even though there had been single reports on human gastric spiral organisms in the past (KRIENITZ 1906; FREEDBERG and BARRON 1940). *H. pylori* was successfully cultured in 1982, and 2 years later the name *Campylobacter pyloridis* was proposed (MARSHALL et al. 1984). However, for grammatical reasons, the name was changed to *Campylobacter pylori* (MARSHALL and GOODWIN 1987). By 1988 sufficient morphological evidence based on electron microscopic studies had accumulated to justify a new genus: *Helicobacter* (GOODWIN et al. 1989).

The epidemiology of *H. pylori* and its role in the causation of gastritis, duodenal ulcer, gastric ulcer, gastric lymphoma, gastric carcinoma, and nonulcer dyspepsia have been extensively studied and reported (GRAHAM 1989; GRAHAM et al. 1991b; BLASER 1990; Moss and CALAM 1992; PARSONNET et al. 1991, 1994;

Department of Medicine, Texas A&M University, College of Medicine, Central Texas Veterans Health Care System, 1901 S. First Street, Temple, TX 76504, USA

LOFFELD et al. 1990). Invasive and noninvasive tests in the diagnosis of *H. pylori* have been developed (BRESLIN and O'MORAIN 1997; WESTBLOM 1993). The mechanisms whereby *H. pylori* causes peptic ulcer have been evaluated, and the role of gastrin and gastric acid in the pathogenesis of *H. pylori*-induced peptic ulcer has been studied (EL-OMAR et al. 1995; COURILLON-MALLET et al. 1995). The eradication of *H. pylori* by various combinations of antibiotics and their efficacy in the management of peptic ulcer have been reported (WOLFSEN and TALLEY 1993; JASPERSEN et al. 1995). Finally, the role of *H. pylori* in the pathogenesis of non-gastrointestinal diseases, for example, coronary artery disease (MENDALL et al. 1994; LIP et al. 1996) has been published. In this afterword, we summarize these various aspects and try to project the future, including the possible development of a vaccine against *H. pylori*.

2 Epidemiology and Transmission

H. pylori is a common chronic bacterial infection with worldwide distribution. The rate of infection is higher in lower socioeconomic groups and in Third World countries. Poor sanitary conditions and crowded living quarters are important in the acquisition of *H. pylori* infection (DOOLEY et al. 1989; DWYER et al. 1988; GRAHAM et al. 1991a,b). Fecal-oral spread may be important in the transmission of infection. It can be spread from contact with gastric secretions at the time of endoscopy (LANGENBERG et al. 1990). Municipal water supply can also be a source of infection (KLEIN et al. 1991).

In the future, with the wider use of seroepidemiological and molecular tests, differences in various population groups will be further characterized and elucidated. It is possible that some insects are involved in the mechanical transmission of *H. pylori* by the fecal-oral route as flies have already been shown to be capable of harboring *H. pylori* (GRUBEL et al. 1997).

3 Gastritis, Peptic Ulcer, Gastric Cancer, and Gastric Lymphoma

H. pylori is associated with chronic gastritis, which subsequently increases the risk of prepyloric and duodenal ulcer. Since *H. pylori* can attach itself only to the gastric mucosa (and *not* the duodenal mucosa), it seems that metaplastic gastric tissue in the duodenal bulb is a prerequisite for the development of duodenal ulcer. Gastric metaplasia in the duodenal bulb is an acquired microscopic lesion which occurs in response to hyperchlorhydria; it is also associated with active or healed duodenal ulcer (WYATT et al. 1990; CARRICK et al. 1989; HARA et al. 1988). It is estimated that about 20% of persons infected with *H. pylori* will develop peptic ulcers.

Chronic gastritis may progress to atrophy and intestinal metaplasia – which may progress to adenocarcinoma. The risk of gastric cancer is increased five times as a result of *H. pylori* infection. Gastric lymphoma is also associated with *H. pylori*. Some cases of gastric lymphoma have regressed after eradication of *H. pylori*; however, in other, often more severe cases eradication of *H. pylori* had no effect on the lymphoma.

Production of ammonia by *H. pylori* may be important in the pathogenesis of gastritis. It is possible that earlier age at infection with *H. pylori*, genetic predisposition, blood group O, and differences in the strains of *H. pylori* explain why some persons develop clinicopathological syndromes after *H. pylori* infection. Some strains of *H. pylori* produce a specific protein (CagA) which is a 120-kDa protein. CagA-producing strains of *H. pylori* are more commonly associated with peptic ulcer and gastric cancer. *H. pylori* may also interact with gastrointestinal hormones (see below) to produce peptic ulcer disease.

In the future, various strains of *H. pylori* will be studied in detail; the role of locally produced ammonia will be further elucidated and the interaction of environmental factors with *H. pylori* infection in the pathogenesis of gastritis, dyspepsia, peptic ulcer, gastric adenocarcinoma, and gastric lymphoma will be explored in detail.

4 *H. pylori* and Hormones, Pathogenesis of Duodenal Ulcer

The mechanism whereby *H. pylori* causes duodenal and gastric ulcers is not completely understood. *H. pylori* and the "gastrin link" to duodenal ulcer was first suggested in 1989 (LEVI et al. 1989). *H. pylori* infection increases serum gastrin which increases gastric acid (CALAM 1994). In the rat, *H. pylori* causes hypergastrinemia through the production of luminal ammonia, which causes G-cell hyperfunction (LICHTENBERGER et al. 1995). *H. pylori* infection increases gastric acid secretion during fasting, during stimulation with meal, and during infusion with gastrin-releasing peptide (EL-OMAR et al. 1995).

Eradication of *H. pylori* lowers gastrin-mediated acid secretion (EL-OMAR et al. 1993; MOSS and CALAM 1993). In the antrum of *H. pylori*-infected patients there is significant decrease in D-cells, which are responsible for producing somatostatin. Somatostatin normally inhibits gastrin release. It is possible that changes in gastrin physiology are due to changes in somatostatin levels (MCHENRY et al. 1993).

H. pylori also decreases acid secretion transiently after initial infection. Chronic *H. pylori* infection causes gastric atrophy, which decreases acid secretion and may be associated with gastric cancer. Gastric mucosa infected with *H. pylori* produces cytokines such as interleukins, tumor-necrosis factor α, interferon-γ, and platelet-activating factor. These cytokines may release gastrin from antral G-cells. Tumor necrosis factor α may inhibit release of somatostatin from D-cells, leading in turn to increased expression of gastrin. It has been shown that *H. pylori* produces *N*-α-methylhistamine, which is a potent H3 receptor agonist. H3 receptors are involved in production of gastric acid. Idiopathic gastric acid hypersecretion

(COLLEN and JENSEN 1994) has been recently described. These patients had basal acid output greater than 10.0 MEq/h. However, their *H. pylori* status was not evaluated. It is possible that underlying *H. pylori* infection in some of these cases is responsible for gastric hypersecretion. In the future, the role of *H. pylori* in the production and regulation of some gastrointestinal hormones will be further elucidated, and the pathogenesis of *H. pylori*-induced peptic ulcer will be explained. It will be interesting to study the interplay of *H. pylori*, gastrin, gastric acid secretion, and H3 receptors.

The mucus-bicarbonate layer which covers the luminal surface of the duodenal mucosa has a protective effect. Patients with duodenal ulcer have decreased basal and stimulated duodenal mucosal bicarbonate production (DUNN 1993). Eradication of *H. pylori* results in normal bicarbonate production in the duodenum (HOGAN et al. 1996). In the future, it will be interesting to evaluate the effect of various strains of *H. pylori* on the duodenal bicarbonate. It is likely that "ulcerogenic" strains of *H. pylori* would more adversely affect the duodenal mucus-bicarbonate layer.

5 Diagnosis, Treatment, Vaccines

The various tests used to diagnose *H. pylori* are described by Westblom and Bhatt in this volume. The urea breath test is more reliable than the antibody tests which can be performed on either serum or saliva. However, urea breath tests usually involve use of radioactive material, for example, [14C]urea. [13C]urea is a non-radioactive isotope, but the test is expensive and not easily available. The antibody tests obviously cannot be used to confirm eradication of *H. pylori* since antibody levels do not decline quickly enough after antibiotic treatment. If endoscopy is performed, rapid urease tests such as CLO test and PyloriTek are reliable. Since CLO test and PyloriTek involve the use of infected tissue, the material should be carefully disposed of. The practice of putting slides of positive CLO and PyloriTek on the charts for purposes of documentation must be strongly discouraged, as a Polaroid photograph can be taken and substituted in the patient record (MANN et al. 1991). Culturing the antral tissue is not generally required; however, in the future when resistant strains of *H. pylori* may become more prevalent, culture will be needed to select the most appropriate antibiotic. In untreated patients, the noninvasive UBT and IgG serology are reliable in predicting *H. pylori* status (CUTLER et al. 1995; THIJS et al. 1996). Routine testing for *H. pylori* can be very expensive (GREENBERG et al. 1996), and a case can be made for empirically treating all ulcer patients with antibiotics. However, recent investigations show that a significant number of ulcer patients are not associated with *H. pylori* or nonsteroidal anti-inflammatory drugs (LANAS et al. 1995). In the future it is anticipated that new noninvasive and cost-effective diagnostic methods will be developed and refined.

Comparing ulcer patients with and without *H. pylori* infection may further elucidate the pathogenic mechanisms involved.

Antibiotic treatment of *H. pylori* is discussed in the chapter by Unge. Various
combinations of H2 blockers, proton-pump inhibitors, bismuth, and antibiotics are
able to eradicate *H. pylori* in 75%–90% of cases. The duration of antibiotic
treatment, cost effectiveness, and side effects are extensively discussed. As in the
treatment of any infectious disease, resistant strains of *H. pylori* are emerging which
may require the discovery of new and more effective antibiotics and/or development of alternative methods of treatment and prevention, i.e., vaccines. As mentioned above, the emergence of such resistant strains may increase the need for
culturing of antral tissue for proper selection of effective antibiotics.

An ounce of prevention is better than a pound of treatment. In a widespread
disease such as *H. pylori* there is no question about the need for an effective vaccine.
Early childhood infection with *H. pylori* may be responsible for later development
of gastric carcinoma or lymphoma. It is obvious that vaccination of children
against *H. pylori* may prevent the occurrence of gastric malignancy later in life.
Vaccination is generally designed to have a preventive and not a therapeutic role.
However, in experimental animals such as ferrets and mice, vaccination against
Helicobacter species has also been found to be effective in eradicating existing
infection (CUENCA et al. 1996; CORTHESY-THEULAZ et al. 1995). In the future it is
possible that an oral vaccine against *H. pylori* will be developed which prevents and
eradicates human *H. pylori* infection.

6 *H. pylori* and Nongastrointestinal Diseases

Recently there has been a tendency to implicate *H. pylori* in the pathogenesis of
many nongastrointestinal diseases. It has been suggested that there is a significant
correlation between *H. pylori* and coronary artery disease (PATEL et al. 1995).
However, more recent studies have questioned such an association (DELANEY et al.
1996). A link has been suggested between *H. pylori* infection and chronic inflammatory skin conditions such as rosacea (REBORA et al. 1994). However, this
association is not generally accepted. Growth retardation in children infected with
H. pylori has been reported (PATEL et al. 1994). *H. pylori* has also been implicated in
the pathogenesis of migraine and beneficial effect of *H. pylori* eradication on migraine has been reported (GASBARRINI et al. 1998). Ammonia production by
H. pylori has been suggested as a precipitating factor in hepatic encephalopathy in
cirrhotic patients.

H. pylori is a common and widespread infection, especially among lower socioeconomic classes and in institutionalized patients. Care should be taken before
an etiological role is assigned to *H. pylori* in nongastrointestinal diseases. At this
time *H. pylori* infection appears to be confined to the gastric mucosa, and only one
case of *H. pylori* bacteremia has been reported. As such, *H. pylori* is unlikely to

cause systemic disseminated disease. However, it is not unlikely that in the future some immunosuppressed patients, for example, HIV patients and patients on chemotherapy, may develop *H. pylori* bacteremia resulting in multiorgan involvement, and like Whipple's disease may come to be recognized as a systemic disease.

Although the majority of peptic ulcers seem to be caused by *H. pylori*, a significant minority (up to 40% in some populations) seem not to be associated with *H. pylori* or nonsteroidal anti-inflammatory drugs. These ulcers may represent "old-fashioned" peptic ulcers which may require the use of more traditional treatments focusing on acid control. If not all peptic ulcers are associated with *H. pylori*, empirical treatment of all peptic ulcer patients with antibiotics may not be cost effective. Consequently there will be a need for better noninvasive, inexpensive diagnostic tests in the future.

The role of *H. pylori* in the pathogenesis of peptic ulcer disease, gastric malignancy, chronic gastritis, dyspepsia, and possibly systemic diseases is still evolving. As evidenced throughout the chapters of this volume, we can expect many interesting developments in this arena in the 21st century.

References

Blaser MJ (1990) Helicobacter pylori and the pathogenesis of gastroduodenal inflammation. J Infect Dis 161:626–633

Breslin NP, O'Morain CA (1997) Noninvasive diagnosis of Helicobacter pylori infection: a review. Helicobacter 2:111–117

Calam J (1994) Helicobacter pylori. Eur J Clin Invest 24:501–510

Carrick J, Lee A, Hazell S, Ralston M, Daskalopoulos G (1989) Campylobacter pylori, duodenal ulcer, and gastric metaplasia: possible role of functional heterotopic tissue in ulcerogenesis. Gut 30:790–797

Collen MJ, Jensen RT (1994) Idiopathic gastric acid hypersecretion. Comparison with Zollinger-Ellison syndrome. Dig Dis Sci 39:1434–1440

Corthesy-Theulaz I, Porta N, Glauser M, Saraga E, Vaney AC, Haas R, Kraehenbuhl JP, Blum AL, Michetti P (1995) Oral immunization with Helicobacter pylori urease B subunit as a treatment against Helicobacter infection in mice. Gastroenterology 109:115–121

Courillon-Mallet A, Launay JM, Roucayrol AM, Callebert J, Emond JP, Tabuteau F, Cattan D (1995) Helicobacter pylori infection: physiopathologic implication of N α-methyl histamine. Gastroenterology 108:959–966

Cuenca R, Blanchard TG, Czinn SJ, Nedrud JG, Monath TP, Lee CK, Redline RW (1996) Therapeutic immunization against Helicobacter mustelae in naturally infected ferrets. Gastroenterology 110:1770–1775

Cutler AF, Havstad S, Ma CK, Blaser MJ, Perez-Perez GI, Schubert TT (1995) Accuracy of invasive and noninvasive tests to diagnose Helicobacter pylori infection. Gastroenterology 109:136–141

Delaney BC, Hobbs FD, Holder R (1996) Association of Helicobacter pylori infection with coronary heart disease. Eradication of the infection on grounds of cardiovascular risk is not supported by current evidence. BMJ 312:251–252

Dooley CP, Cohen H, Fitzgibbons PL, Bauer M, Appleman MD, Perez-Perez GI, Blaser MJ (1989) Prevalence of Helicobacter pylori infection and histologic gastritis in asymptomatic persons. N Engl J Med 321:1562–1566

Dunn BE (1993) Pathogenic mechanisms of Helicobacter pylori. Gastroenterol Clin North Am 22:43–57

Dwyer B, Kaldor J, Tee W, Marakowski E, Raios K (1988) Antibody response to Campylobacter pylori in diverse ethnic groups. Scand J Infect Dis 20:349–350 el-Omar E, Penman I, Dorrian CA, Ardill JE, McColl KE (1993) Eradicating Helicobacter pylori infection lowers gastrin mediated acid secretion by two thirds in patients with duodenal ulcer. Gut 34:1060–1065

el-Omar EM, Penman ID, Ardill JE, Chittajallu RS, Howie C, McColl KE (1995) Helicobacter pylori infection and abnormalities of acid secretion in patients with duodenal ulcer disease. Gastroenterology 109:681–691

Freedberg AS, Barron LE (1940) The presence of spirochetes in human gastric mucosa. Am J Dig Dis 7:443–445

Gasbarrini A, De Luca A, Fiore G, Gambrielli M, Franceschi F, Ojetti V, Torres ES, Gasbarrini G, Pola P, Giacovazzo M (1998) Beneficial effects of Helicobacter pylori eradication on migraine. Hepatogastroenterology 45:765–770

Goodwin CS, Armstrong JA, Chilvers T, Peters M, Collins MD, Sly L, McConnell W, Harper WES (1989) Transfer of Campylobacter pylori and Campylobacter mustelae to Helicobacter gen. nov. as Helicobacter pylori comb. nov. and Helicobacter mustelae comb. nov., respectively. Int J Syst Bacteriol 39:397–405

Graham DY (1989) Campylobacter pylori and peptic ulcer disease. Gastroenterology 96:615–625

Graham DY, Adam E, Reddy GT, Agarwal JP, Agarwal R, Evans DJ Jr, Malaty HM, Evans DG (1991a) Seroepidemiology of Helicobacter pylori infection in India. Comparison of developing and developed countries. Dig Dis Sci 36:1084–1088

Graham DY, Malaty HM, Evans DG, Evans DJ Jr, Klein PD, Adam E (1991b) Epidemiology of Helicobacter pylori in an asymptomatic population in the United States. Effect of age, race, and socioeconomic status. Gastroenterology 100:1495–1501

Greenberg PD, Koch J, Cello JP (1996) Clinical utility and cost effectiveness of Helicobacter pylori testing for patients with duodenal and gastric ulcers. Am J Gastroenterol 91:228–232

Grubel P, Hoffman JS, Chong FK, Burstein NA, Mepani C, Cave DR (1997) Vector potential of houseflies (Musca domestica) for Helicobacter pylori. J Clin Microbiol 35:1300–1303

Hara M, Harasawa S, Tani N, Miwa T, Tsutsumi Y (1988) Gastric metaplasia in duodenal ulcer. Histochemical considerations of its pathophysiological significance. Acta Pathol Jpn 38:1011–1018

Hogan DL, Rapier RC, Dreilinger A, Koss MA, Basuk PM, Weinstein WM, Nyberg LM, Isenberg JI (1996) Duodenal bicarbonate secretion: eradication of Helicobacter pylori and duodenal structure and function in humans. Gastroenterology 110:705–716

Jaspersen D, Koerner T, Schorr W, Brennenstuhl M, Raschka C, Hammar CH (1995) Helicobacter pylori eradication reduces the rate of rebleeding in ulcer hemorrhage. Gastrointest Endosc 41:5–7

Klein PD, Graham DY, Gaillour A, Opekun AR, Smith EO (1991) Water source as risk factor for Helicobacter pylori infection in Peruvian children. Gastrointestinal Physiology Working Group. Lancet 337:1503–1506

Krienitz W (1906) Ueber das Auftreten von Spirochäten verschiedener Form im Mageninhalt bei Carcinoma ventriculi. Dtsch Med Wochenschr 28:872

Lanas AI, Remacha B, Esteva F, Sainz R (1995) Risk factors associated with refractory peptic ulcers. Gastroenterology 109:1124–1133

Langenberg W, Rauws EA, Oudbier JH, Tytgat GN (1990) Patient-to-patient transmission of Campylobacter pylori infection by fiberoptic gastroduodenoscopy and biopsy. J Infect Dis 161:507–511

Levi S, Beardshall K, Haddad G, Playford R, Ghosh P, Calam J (1989) Campylobacter pylori and duodenal ulcers: the gastrin link. Lancet 1:1167–1168

Lichtenberger LM, Dial EJ, Romero JJ, Lechago J, Jarboe LA, Wolfe MM (1995) Role of luminal ammonia in the development of gastropathy and hypergastrinemia in the rat. Gastroenterology 108:320–329

Lip GH, Wise R, Beevers G (1996) Association of Helicobacter pylori infection with coronary heart disease. Study shows association between H pylori infection and hypertension. BMJ 312:250–251

Loffeld RJ, Stobberingh E, Flendrig JA, Arends JW (1990) Presence of Helicobacter pylori in patients with non-ulcer dyspepsia revealing normal antral histological characteristics. Digestion 47:29–34

Mann NS, Mann SK, Hyder SA (1991) In vitro endoscopic Polaroid photography for CLO test of Helicobacter pylori. J Clin Gastroenterol 13:599–601

Marshall BJ, Goodwin CS (1987) Revised Nomenclature of Campylobacter pyloridis. Int J Syst Bacteriol 37:68

Marshall BJ, Warren JR (1984) Unidentified curved bacilli in the stomach of patients with gastritis and peptic ulceration. Lancet 1:1311–1315

Marshall BJ, Royce H, Annear DI, Goodwin CS, Pearman JW, Warren JR, Armstrong JA (1984) Original Isolation of Campylobacter pyloridis from human gastric mucosa. Microbios Lett 25:83–88

McHenry L Jr, Vuyyuru L, Schubert ML (1993) Helicobacter pylori and duodenal ulcer disease: the somatostatin link? Gastroenterology 104:1573–1575

Mendall MA, Goggin PM, Molineaux N, Levy J, Toosy T, Strachan D, Camm AJ, Northfield TC (1994) Relation of Helicobacter pylori infection and coronary heart disease. Br Heart J 71:437–439

Moss S, Calam J (1992) Helicobacter pylori and peptic ulcers: the present position. Gut 33:289–292

Moss SF, Calam J (1993) Acid secretion and sensitivity to gastrin in patients with duodenal ulcer: effect of eradication of Helicobacter pylori. Gut 34:888–892

Parsonnet J, Friedman GD, Vandersteen DP, Chang Y, Vogelman JH, Orentreich N, Sibley RK (1991) Helicobacter pylori infection and the risk of gastric carcinoma. N Engl J Med 325:1127–1131

Parsonnet J, Hansen S, Rodriguez L, Gelb AB, Warnke RA, Jellum E, Orentreich N, Vogelman JH, Friedman GD (1994) Helicobacter pylori infection and gastric lymphoma. N Engl J Med 330:1267–1271

Patel P, Mendall MA, Khulusi S, Northfield TC, Strachan DP (1994) Helicobacter pylori infection in childhood: risk factors and effect on growth. BMJ 309:1119–1123

Patel P, Mendall MA, Carrington D, Strachan DP, Leatham E, Molineaux N, Levy J, Blakeston C, Seymour CA, Camm AJ et al (1995) Association of Helicobacter pylori and Chlamydia pneumoniae infections with coronary heart disease and cardiovascular risk factors. BMJ 311:711–714

Rebora A, Drago F, Picciotto A (1994) Helicobacter pylori in patients with rosacea. Am J Gastroenterol 89:1603–1604

Thijs JC, van Zwet AA, Thijs WJ, Oey HB, Karrenbeld A, Stellaard F, Luijt DS, Meyer BC, Kleibeuker JH (1996) Diagnostic tests for Helicobacter pylori: a prospective evaluation of their accuracy, without selecting a single test as the gold standard. Am J Gastroenterol 91:2125–2129

Westblom TU (1993) The comparative value of different diagnostic tests for Helicobacter pylori. In: Goodwin CS, Worsley BW (eds) Helicobacter pylori: biology and clinical practice. CRC, Boca Raton, pp 329–342

Wolfsen HC, Talley NJ (1993) The diagnosis and treatment of duodenal and gastric ulcer. In: Goodwin CS, Worsley BW (eds) Helicobacter pylori: biology and clinical practice. CRC, Boca Raton, pp 365–395

Wyatt JI, Rathbone BJ, Sobala GM, Shallcross T, Heatley RV, Axon AT, Dixon MF (1990) Gastric epithelium in the duodenum: its association with Helicobacter pylori and inflammation. J Clin Pathol 43:981–986

Subject Index

Printing: Saladruck, Berlin
Binding: Buchbinderei Lüderitz & Bauer, Berlin

Current Topics in Microbiology and Immunology

Volumes published since 1989 (and still available)

Vol. 218: **Berns, Kenneth I.; Giraud, Catherine (Eds.):** Adeno-Associated Virus (AAV) Vectors in Gene Therapy. 1996. 38 figs. IX,173 pp. ISBN 3-540-61076-6

Vol. 219: **Gross, Uwe (Ed.):** Toxoplasma gondii. 1996. 31 figs. XI, 274 pp. ISBN 3-540-61300-5

Vol. 220: **Rauscher, Frank J. III; Vogt, Peter K. (Eds.):** Chromosomal Translocations and Oncogenic Transcription Factors. 1997. 28 figs. XI, 166 pp. ISBN 3-540-61402-8

Vol. 221: **Kastan, Michael B. (Ed.):** Genetic Instability and Tumorigenesis. 1997. 12 figs.VII, 180 pp. ISBN 3-540-61518-0

Vol. 222: **Olding, Lars B. (Ed.):** Reproductive Immunology. 1997. 17 figs. XII, 219 pp. ISBN 3-540-61888-0

Vol. 223: **Tracy, S.; Chapman, N. M.; Mahy, B. W. J. (Eds.):** The Coxsackie B Viruses. 1997. 37 figs. VIII, 336 pp. ISBN 3-540-62390-6

Vol. 224: **Potter, Michael; Melchers, Fritz (Eds.):** C-Myc in B-Cell Neoplasia. 1997. 94 figs. XII, 291 pp. ISBN 3-540-62892-4

Vol. 225: **Vogt, Peter K.; Mahan, Michael J. (Eds.):** Bacterial Infection: Close Encounters at the Host Pathogen Interface. 1998. 15 figs. IX, 169 pp. ISBN 3-540-63260-3

Vol. 226: **Koprowski, Hilary; Weiner, David B. (Eds.):** DNA Vaccination/Genetic Vaccination. 1998. 31 figs. XVIII, 198 pp. ISBN 3-540-63392-8

Vol. 227: **Vogt, Peter K.; Reed, Steven I. (Eds.):** Cyclin Dependent Kinase (CDK) Inhibitors. 1998. 15 figs. XII, 169 pp. ISBN 3-540-63429-0

Vol. 228: **Pawson, Anthony I. (Ed.):** Protein Modules in Signal Transduction. 1998. 42 figs. IX, 368 pp. ISBN 3-540-63396-0

Vol. 229: **Kelsoe, Garnett; Flajnik, Martin (Eds.):** Somatic Diversification of Immune Responses. 1998. 38 figs. IX, 221 pp. ISBN 3-540-63608-0

Vol. 230: **Kärre, Klas; Colonna, Marco (Eds.):** Specificity, Function, and Development of NK Cells. 1998. 22 figs. IX, 248 pp. ISBN 3-540-63941-1

Vol. 231: **Holzmann, Bernhard; Wagner, Hermann (Eds.):** Leukocyte Integrins in the Immune System and Malignant Disease. 1998. 40 figs. XIII, 189 pp. ISBN 3-540-63609-9

Vol. 232: **Whitton, J. Lindsay (Ed.):** Antigen Presentation. 1998. 11 figs. IX, 244 pp. ISBN 3-540-63813-X

Vol. 233/I: **Tyler, Kenneth L.; Oldstone, Michael B. A. (Eds.):** Reoviruses I. 1998. 29 figs. XVIII, 223 pp. ISBN 3-540-63946-2

Vol. 233/II: **Tyler, Kenneth L.; Oldstone, Michael B. A. (Eds.):** Reoviruses II. 1998. 45 figs. XVI, 187 pp. ISBN 3-540-63947-0

Vol. 234: **Frankel, Arthur E. (Ed.):** Clinical Applications of Immunotoxins. 1999. 16 figs. IX, 122 pp. ISBN 3-540-64097-5

Vol. 235: **Klenk, Hans-Dieter (Ed.):** Marburg and Ebola Viruses. 1999. 34 figs. XI, 225 pp. ISBN 3-540-64729-5

Vol. 236: **Kraehenbuhl, Jean-Pierre; Neutra, Marian R. (Eds.):** Defense of Mucosal Surfaces: Pathogenesis, Immunity and Vaccines. 1999. 30 figs. IX, 296 pp. ISBN 3-540-64730-9

Vol. 237: **Claesson-Welsh, Lena (Ed.):** Vascular Growth Factors and Angiogenesis. 1999. 36 figs. X, 189 pp. ISBN 3-540-64731-7

Vol. 238: **Coffman, Robert L.; Romagnani, Sergio (Eds.):** Redirection of Th1 and Th2 Responses. 1999. 6 figs. IX, 148 pp. ISBN 3-540-65048-2

Vol. 239: **Vogt, Peter K.; Jackson, Andrew O. (Eds.):** Satellites and Defective Viral RNAs. 1999. 39 figs. XVI, 179 pp. ISBN 3-540-65049-0